This book is to be returned on or before
the last date stamped below.

TOXICOLOGICAL ASPECTS OF FOOD

TOXICOLOGICAL ASPECTS OF FOOD

Edited by

KLARA MILLER

The British Industrial Biological Research Association,
Carshalton, Surrey, UK

ELSEVIER APPLIED SCIENCE
LONDON and NEW YORK

ELSEVIER APPLIED SCIENCE PUBLISHERS LTD
Crown House, Linton Road, Barking, Essex IG11 8JU, England

Sole Distributor in the USA and Canada
ELSEVIER SCIENCE PUBLISHING CO., INC.
52 Vanderbilt Avenue, New York, NY 10017, USA

WITH 62 ILLUSTRATIONS AND 65 TABLES

British Library Cataloguing in Publication Data

Toxicological aspects of food.
1. Food poisoning
I. Miller, Klara
615.9′54   RA1258

Library of Congress Cataloging-in-Publication Data

Toxicological aspects of food.

Includes index.
1. Food poisoning.   2. Food contamination.   I. Miller,
Klara.
RA1258.T695   1987   615.9′54   87-5404

ISBN 1-85166-080-1

615·954
TOX

The selection and presentation of material and the opinions expressed are the sole responsibility of the author(s) concerned

Phototypesetting by Keyset Composition, Colchester, Essex
Printed in Great Britain at the University Press, Cambridge

FOREWORD

There are enormous geographical inequalities in the amount and variety of foodstuffs available to the consumer and, while famine or threat of famine afflicts many third-world countries, the developed countries enjoy an abundance of relatively cheap food in almost bewildering variety. The success of the more affluent countries in meeting the increasing food demands of their populace has been achieved in a number of ways including: (a) amplification of agricultural food production, (b) control of losses during storage, (c) control of losses during distribution and in the home, i.e. increased shelf-life, and (d) more efficient use of available resources. In all these areas, new chemicals and new technologies have played an indispensable role.

Amplification of food production is exemplified by the increase in yield of maize in the USA from $2 \cdot 3$ tons/ha to $5 \cdot 5$ tons/ha in the period 1945–1970. These increased yields have only been achievable by the use of agrochemicals: fertilizers, pesticides and herbicides. It has been a major achievement of the agricultural industry to make two or three ears of corn grow where one grew previously, but an achievement heavily reliant on the associated agrochemical industry. Nor is increased efficiency necessarily confined to production of plant foods; by use of anabolic agents and veterinary drugs, production of animal products also may be enhanced.

In many third-world countries, an already parlous situation is made worse by the substantial proportion of food lost between production and consumption due to vermin or microbial spoilage. Even foods which may still appear edible to the consumer may be contaminated by mycotoxins elaborated by field or storage fungi, with consequent hazards to health. Once again, in more fortunate areas, such losses and contamination have been minimised by the use of chemicals (fungicides, fumigants) or new technologies such as irradiation in controlling germination in stored foodstuffs. Extension of shelf-life by means of, *inter alia*, preservatives and anti-oxidants has facilitated the feeding of vast urban populations with minimal losses while reducing the health hazards from pathogenic micro-organisms or chemical spoilage products.

New technologies have also emerged to meet the increasing demands for food, leading to more efficient use of food raw materials, e.g. in re-formed meat products, and the development of novel foods to meet general nutritional needs or specific dietary goals. Using such new technologies and additives, it is also now possible to exploit novel sources of nutrients and convert these into palatable foods, further opening up possibilities for increasing food supplies from hitherto unconventional sources.

While nostalgia might have us wish that we could return to earlier methods of agriculture and food preparation, this is clearly an impracticable proposition; it would be quite impossible to meet current and future demands for food using only 'organically grown' raw materials (whatever that means) distributed in completely unprocessed form. However, once adequate supplies of food are assured and at a price that the consumers can afford, the broader issues of food safety also need to be addressed. Indeed, food safety assurance has assumed an increasing importance in the field of food science and technology, and would always be a consideration whenever new processes or new chemicals are introduced into the food chain. Both at national and international level, regulatory agencies have been established with the express purpose of ensuring that the safety of food supplies is not compromised and, where necessary, legislative procedures have been adopted to control potential hazards. Implicit in this regulatory activity is a need objectively and scientifically to establish the nature and quantitative dose-dependence of the potential toxic hazard; from this need has grown, over the past thirty years or so, the developing and increasingly mature science of food toxicology. The requirements of this scientific discipline and the problems encountered in the safety evaluation process are dealt with in the first section of this book, which also helps to put into perspective the relative hazards from sources other than food additives and contaminants.

The current debate on food safety has had an important emotional dimension which has, to some extent, clouded the real issues. The emphasis has been most heavily placed on man-made chemicals used in agriculture and food processing to the neglect of other, and in some cases more serious, hazards. In this climate, risk–benefit assessments have not always been seen in context. Whilst the concept of 'zero hazard' from chemicals used in food production and processing is attractive, it is both unrealistic and irrational. There can be no doubt that food-borne microbial infections and intoxications constitute a hazard to the consumer of far greater magnitude than the properly controlled use of the chemicals, fungicides and preservatives used to combat them. It is ironic that higher levels of potently toxic and carcinogenic mycotoxins have been found in so-called 'health foods' produced without the benefits of anti-microbials than in comparable conventional food products. In this situation, even an imprecise assessment of residual hazard would clearly indicate that, although the net hazard might not be zero, it is significantly reduced by the use of fungicides in production and storage. Similarly, the benefits accruing from the use of anti-oxidants in controlling food spoilage and associated loss of nutrients, or accumulation of toxic oxidation products, may be seen as outweighing any net risk associated with their use.

The very toxicological techniques, both experimental and epidemiological, which have been applied to assessment of the safety-in-use of food additives and man-made contaminants have also helped to identify and quantify hazards arising from the presence of natural toxicants which are, and always have been, present in traditional food sources. A very great number of quite highly toxic components have been identified even in staple foods, particularly of plant origin, and are known to have caused death and morbidity in some circumstances. Examples such as favism, lathyrism, tropical ataxic neuropathy or even deaths from eating 'greened' potato serve to remind us that foods which may be valuable and innocuous in most circumstances are not totally without risk. However, any attempt to exclude such foods from the diet in pursuit of zero-risk would lead to a much more serious problem of food shortage and malnutrition. While such issues are not directly addressed in this book, they do impinge on the safety evaluation of foods from novel, non-traditional sources. There is no doubt that, if the potato were not a well-established food and was being evaluated as a novel food source, it would not pass the stringent safety requirements which are currently applied; the levels of glycoalkaloids such as solanine would be considered unacceptably high. It follows, as is pointed out in the section on novel foods later, that new foods/processes currently being evaluated will be safer than some of those which they replace. It also follows that, if the standards applied are too rigorous, potentially valuable and safe food sources may be lost. On a more positive note, knowledge of naturally occurring toxicants in plant foods has enabled the plant breeder to be alerted to the dangers and to develop low-toxicant varieties such as the low-glucosinolate, low-erucic acid strains of rape. In this instance, novelty has been linked to safety and irrational neophobia would have led to a higher risk or the abandonment of a very valuable food crop. Critics of scientific progress in the field of food and agriculture would be well advised to learn from these examples; mankind has *not* learned from historical experience to select a safe diet which carries no risk, and new technologies can give increased margins of safety.

Suspicion of processed foods has led to a suspicion of the processes themselves and a firm belief in some quarters that 'good' food equates with domestically prepared food. This belief does not stand close examination in the light of the discovery of a number of potent mutagens and carcinogens in foods subjected to high temperatures in such traditional cooking procedures as roasting, grilling and frying. There is at least circumstantial evidence to suggest that polycyclic aromatic hydrocarbons and other pyrolysis products like the amino imidazoarenes may be implicated in the aetiology of human cancer and any proposed novel food process which carried such risks would be considered a non-starter. A valuable result of research in this area is the identification of the types of food materials and cooking procedures which carry the greatest potential for the formation of mutagens, and sound advice can now be given on how to reduce the hazard. Unfortunately, old habits die hard and the domestic cook is not subject to the same regulatory constraints as the commercial food processor!

While the foregoing might be taken as somewhat reassuring, and there can be no doubt that advances in food toxicology have played and continue to play a part in assuring the safety of the food supply, there are still a number of problems which require fundamental research towards a solution. One such problem, albeit a multi-faceted one, is that of food intolerance, whether of an immunological nature or resulting from other mechanisms. It has to be admitted that, at present, there is no suitable predictive model for the food toxicologist to apply prospectively, and most knowledge in this area has been derived from retrospective case studies, not always well founded. It is little comfort to the sufferer to point out that the consequences are only rarely of a life-threatening nature and that the incidence of intolerance to natural dietary components is probably greatly in excess of that to food additives. While one regulatory approach is to ensure that, by adequate labelling, the presence of the components or additives responsible can be identified and exposure avoided, improvements on this position are clearly needed.

Another problem facing the regulatory toxicologist is the undue weight placed on some toxicological end-points, such as cancer, at the expense of a more balanced overall evaluation. This has in large measure been dictated by a response to political pressure and ill-considered legislation in some countries. A reappraisal is needed in order to put other toxic manifestations into a proper context, particularly those which relate to major causes of human morbidity such as cardio- and cerebro-vascular disease, while recognising the comparative irrelevance of some lesions seen in common laboratory animal species which seem to have no counterpart in man. Better experimental models and a clearer understanding of the mechanisms of pathogenesis are needed in order to discharge the duty of ensuring that the safety evaluation process is soundly based.

This book addresses all the problems referred to above and which face the regulatory toxicologist when considering the potential hazards posed by food contaminants, natural and man-made, and when evaluating the safety of new foods, food additives or technological processes. Distinguished experts in the various specialist fields have provided their insight into the nature of the problems and how they might be attacked. There is clearly no room for complacency as the industrialised world becomes more and more complex, but the success of the scientific approach to identifying and controlling potential hazards in the food supply may be judged by the availability of adequate amounts of generally safe, wholesome and nutritious food.

R. WALKER
Professor of Food Science
Department of Biochemistry
University of Surrey
Guildford, UK

CONTENTS

xi

Section III. Cooking, Preservation and Storage

Section IV. Food and Food Components

LIST OF CONTRIBUTORS

A. E. BENDER
2 Willow Vale, Fetcham, Leatherhead, Surrey KT22 9TE, UK.

D. M. CONNING
The British Nutrition Foundation, 15 Belgrave Square, London SW1X 8PS, UK.

P. S. ELIAS
Federal Research Centre for Nutrition, Postfach 3640, D-7500 Karlsruhe 1, Federal Republic of Germany.

SHOJI FUKUSHIMA
First Department of Pathology, Nagoya City University Medical School, 1 Kawasumi, Mizuho-cho, Mizuho-ku, Nagoya 467, Japan.

MASAO HIROSE
First Department of Pathology, Nagoya City University Medical School, 1 Kawasumi, Mizuho-cho, Mizuho-ku, Nagoya 467, Japan.

NOBUYUKI ITO
First Department of Pathology, Nagoya City University Medical School, 1 Kawasumi, Mizuho-cho, Mizuho-ku, Nagoya 467, Japan.

JOHN CHR. LARSEN
Institute of Toxicology, National Food Agency, Mørkhøj Bygade 19, DK-2860 Søborg, Denmark.

A. MALASPINA
The Coca-Cola Company, PO Drawer 1734, Atlanta, Georgia 30301, USA.

KLARA MILLER
*Immunotoxicology Department, The British Industrial Biological
Research Association, Woodmansterne Road, Carshalton, Surrey SM5
4DS, UK.*

E. POULSEN
*Institute of Toxicology, National Food Agency, Mørkhøj Bygade 19,
DK-2860 Søborg, Denmark.*

ENRICA QUATTRUCCI
*Istituto Nazionale della Nutrizione, Via Ardeatina 546, 00179 Roma,
Italy.*

FRANCIS J. C. ROE
19 Marryat Road, Wimbledon Common, London SW19 5BB, UK.

CAROL A. SHIVELY
*Hershey Foods Corporation, Technical Center, PO Box 805, Hershey,
Pennsylvania 17033-0805, USA.*

STANLEY M. TARKA JR
*Hershey Foods Corporation, Technical Center, PO Box 805, Hershey,
Pennsylvania 17033-0805, USA.*

YOSHIO UENO
*Department of Toxicology and Microbial Chemistry, Faculty of
Pharmaceutical Sciences, Science University of Tokyo, 12 Ichigaya
Funagawara-Machi, Shinjuku-ku, Tokyo 162, Japan.*

G. VETTORAZZI
World Health Organisation, 1211 Geneva 27, Switzerland.

MARY E. ZABIK
*Department of Food Science and Human Nutrition, Michigan State
University, East Lansing, Michigan 48824-1224, USA.*

Chapter 1

THE IMPORTANCE OF TOXICOLOGY IN FOOD SCIENCE

G. Vettorazzi

World Health Organization, Geneva, Switzerland

INTRODUCTION

The enormous popularity of toxicology among the life sciences in the years following the United Nations Conference on the Human Environment in 1972 (UNEP, 1978) has resulted in a general feeling that all the problems caused to man and his biosphere by natural and man-made pollution will be healed or mended by the outright application of the principles and advances of toxicology. Today, however, toxicology as a discipline appears to be undergoing a moment of reflection and, recently, it has been pointed out that most difficulties in the field are not technical but political, psychological and sociological (Chenoweth, 1985).

Toxicology, from a trivial discipline buried in medical school curricula, suddenly emerged in the 1970s as a leading developmental specialty at the very forefront of science. Then, because of its inherent multidisciplinary character, it split inevitably into an array of associations with many cognate sciences. Thus, in addition to some of the well-established fields such as clinical (Conso, 1984; Temple, 1984), forensic (Cravey and Baselt, 1981; Maes, 1984; Oliver, 1980; Pohl, 1984), and environmental toxicology (Duffus, 1980; Guthrie and Perry, 1980; Somani and Cavender, 1981), a

1

variety of branches have been developed for which clear lines of demarcation were often difficult to draw.

Today many areas of specialization are open to the basically trained toxicologist. Here is a list that by no means should be interpreted as being exhaustive: analytical (Everson and Oehme, 1981), aquatic (Pearson *et al.*, 1980), chemical (Galli *et al.*, 1978), ecological toxicology (Hammons, 1981; Truhaut, 1977), environmental genotoxicology (Sawicki, 1982), evaluative (Kassel, 1984), experimental (Bertelli, 1979; WHO/EURO, 1984), food regulatory and regulatory (Vettorazzi, 1978, 1980, 1981), genetic (Thilly and Liber, 1980), industrial toxicology (Lauwerys, 1982; Lewis, 1984), neurotoxicology (Blum and Manzo, 1985), nutritional (Hathcock, 1982; Truhaut and Ferrando, 1978), ophthalmic toxicology (Ballantyne *et al.*, 1977), phytotoxicology (Kingsbury, 1980), preventive (Preziosi *et al.*, 1984), relay toxicology (Ferrando *et al.*, 1978), reproductive toxicology (Dixon, 1983), toxicovigilance (Roche, 1979) and tropical toxicology (Schvartsman, 1976; Smith and Bababunmi, 1980). An attentive reader of the current literature might also come up against certain folklore, such as barefoot toxicology (Abbou, 1979), courtroom toxicology (Houts *et al.*, 1981) or shuttle toxicology (Miller, 1984).

Important associations of toxicology are undoubtedly food science and nutrition; in this regard, if the science of toxicology has developed fast during the last decades, food science and technology as well as nutrition have equally advanced at a very rapid pace. These advances brought about the appearance of a large number and variety of foodstuffs on the market shelves. Highly organized curricula have made food science a multi-disciplinary academic specialty which incorporates the sciences of chemistry, biochemistry, nutrition, bacteriology, engineering, etc. and which concerns itself with production, processing, composition, nutrition, acceptability and safety of food. There is today sufficient documentation to show that food is an extremely complex chemical mixture (even without considering the presence of extraneous materials), and the impact of these chemicals on the metabolic and homeostatic mechanisms of the human body is still in many respects the object of speculation, in spite of the great advances of physiological and medical sciences. It will thus be difficult to ignore the contributions of the food scientist when food safety evaluations are carried out (Vettorazzi, 1975). Food science interfaces with toxicology in many aspects which are all geared towards a common goal: the safety and acceptability of food. This chapter will describe briefly some of these aspects which are today of significance for the advances of toxicology as a food science. They will be described only in their essential elements with the objective of identifying important operational interactions in the activities and responsibilities of the food scientist and food toxicologist.

MICROBIAL AND PARASITIC ENTITIES

The presence in food of bacteria, rickettsia, viruses, molds and parasitic protozoa/metazoa may cause human illness, characterized as food 'poisoning' or food 'intoxication' if the responsible agent grew in or on food and produced a toxin, or it may cause a food 'infection' if a parasite is ingested with the food and chooses the human organism as its host. Most food-borne illnesses of this type are well known and have been thoroughly characterized and extensively reviewed (Marth, 1981; Mundt, 1982; Rechcigl, 1983a; Riemann and Bryan, 1979). Efforts in this field are today mainly directed towards the establishment of control measures which would eliminate or reduce the incidence of these diseases. It is the responsibility of the food toxicologist to ensure that adequate technical and scientific support is developed and provided to those in charge of this control. Today this is mainly carried out by actively promoting investigations on new methods of detection and quantification of microbial contaminants which will be more effective, in terms of accuracy, time and cost, and by optimizing processing conditions such as dehydration and ultra-high temperature sterilization to ensure destruction or inhibition of microbial growth, including microbial toxic metabolites and enzymes. The outcomes of these trends are of great value in evaluating the role of microbiological criteria for foods and food ingredients (NRC/NAS, 1985). In addition to the development of methodology and dynamic optimization of conditions, there are two other aspects of growing importance today which underline the interface of toxicology and food science: one is the host/gut flora interaction and the other is the safety assessment of enzyme preparations of microbial origin used in food technology in mobilized and immobilized forms.

The gut microflora may influence the outcome of toxicity in a number of ways, reflecting their importance in relation to the nutritional status of the host animal, to the metabolism of xenobiotics prior to absorption, and to the biliary conjugation products. This was recognized by the Joint FAO/WHO Expert Committee on Food Additives (JECFA) on several occasions when it drew attention to the need for studies on metabolism involving the intestinal microflora in toxicological evaluation of food additives and contaminants (WHO/FAO, 1971, 1975). Diet and gut flora interactions in toxicology today form a topic of broad interest (Hentges, 1983; Rowland and Walker, 1983; Mallett, 1984; WHO, 1987a).

The increasing use of enzymes in food technology has made it imperative that consideration be given to the toxicological evaluation of enzymes as a class of food additives. More and more enzymes derived from microbial sources are used today. These enzyme preparations are generally not single enzymes but often have enzymatic activities besides that of the main principle and also contain non-enzymatic proteins, metabolites, and other residues from the source material. In addition, residues of substances used in their manufacture and adjuncts such as buffers, inorganic salts, diluents, or stabilizers are often present. Consequently, for toxicological evaluation the expression of the amount of the enzyme preparation used in terms of activity is less relevant than a statement in terms of weight. In addition to concern regarding the possible hazard arising from the presence of toxins associated with enzyme preparations from micro-organisms, particularly with reference to mycotoxins (Moreau, 1979; Kurata and Ueno, 1984) and the possible allergic reactions following inhalation or dermal application, there is also the possibility of mutations accruing in the organism which could affect the food enzyme adversely through the emergence of new, potentially toxic products. Furthermore, the increasing use of immobilizing enzymes calls for the evaluation of the immobilizing substrates as well as the immobilizing techniques (WHO/FAO, 1971, 1974, 1978). Guidelines for the evaluation of these substances as well as principles helping to establish specifications for identity and purity were formulated (WHO, 1982, 1986); the food scientist and the food toxicologist ought to be cognizant of these advances.

TOXICANTS FROM NATURAL SOURCES

Many apparently wholesome and healthful foods contain naturally occurring substances which have undesirable effects on humans and animals. The ingestion of these foods can bring about toxic outcomes which may become evident in the form of aspecific acute reactions, such as in the case of inborn intolerances in hypersensitive individuals, or they can manifest their presence through well-characterized clinical syndromes, as in instances of mushroom poisoning, skeletal deformities, aortic ruptures and neoplastic phenomena.

Furthermore, early in the history of scientific investigation of ailments it was noticed that certain foods contained small amounts of materials whose effects, although not toxic, were nevertheless interfering with the nutritional quality. These factors, today of primary concern to the nutritional toxicologist, became known as co-nutrients, and include substances such as antienzymes, antivitamins and estrogens.

The interest in naturally occurring toxic factors in food is as old as medicine, and man has learned through the years the laborious task of refraining from edibles which, by experience, caused obvious objectionable consequences to his well-being. Today this problem becomes even more arduous with the discovery that the amounts of the harmful substance consumed daily may be very minute, and no observable physiological effect can be obtained from a single intake. Consequently, careful studies are now directly aimed towards the evaluation of long-term impact on animals, and extrapolation of results obtained in laboratory animals to those anticipated in man has become the normal procedure. In this manner, several toxic factors already have been characterized (NAS, 1973; Liener, 1980; Rodricks and Pohland, 1981; Rechcigl, 1983b). Many more, however, are still awaiting basic biochemical and pharmacological investigations as well as extensive epidemiological studies. The task of ascertaining more clearly and systematically the role of food-borne toxicants in human pathology is of relatively recent date.

There are signs of renewed interest in contaminants from natural sources, especially because of the importance of the recurrent problems they cause in developing areas of the world. The International Programme on Chemical Safety (IPCS) is presently preparing an extensive review on pyrrolizidine alkaloids and their role as causative agents of veno-occlusive diseases (Tandon et al., 1977, 1978; WHO, 1987b). The food scientist and the food toxicologist in the developing world are continuously challenged by the appearance of new fields of investigation from toxicants found in common foods of natural origin. It should, however, be recognized that the problem generally affects localized areas and, with the exception of a very few (e.g. mycotoxins), contaminants from natural sources are not commonly found in foods circulating in international trade at levels which may cause public health concern.

An interesting field of expansion is today represented by the presence of 'pressor' amines in a number of common foods either naturally or as a result of processing. As an example, baby foods containing banana may contain up to 25 ppm of 5-hydroxytryptamine (serotonin). Thus a baby of 7 kg consuming 200 g of such a food would ingest 0·7 mg/kg body weight, and about 70% of this amount would be absorbed from the intestine (Vettorazzi, 1972, 1974). Amines related to the common aromatic amino acids tyrosine, histidine, and tryptophan include many of the most physiologically active compounds in the animal body. Histamine, tryptamine, tyramine, and norepinephrine are known examples. These amines are formed in the animal and plant tissues when the corresponding amino acids are decarboxylated by endogenous enzymes during life, or by bacterial action after death. These substances are referred to collectively as pressor amines because they act as potent vasoconstrictors and hence elevate the blood pressure. Normally these compounds are rapidly deaminated after ingestion through the action of the enzyme monoamine oxidase. A study by Price and Smith (1971) demonstrated that about 5% of the tyramine content of cheese may be absorbed from the buccal cavity, thus bypassing intestinal and hepatic monoamine oxidase. It would be of interest to determine whether other physiologically active amines present in food, with weakly basic pK_a values like that of tyramine, behave in an analogous manner, and in what amounts they can be found in the undissociated state at the pH of saliva.

Patients on antidepressant drugs that are monoamine oxidase inhibitors are advised to avoid consuming food rich in pressor amines. It is, however, known that pesticides used in agriculture seem to present a mode of action which involves inhibition of the monoamine oxidase system (Aziz and Knowles, 1973; Beeman and Matsumura, 1973). The use of such pesticides on crops naturally rich in physiologically active amines or their precursors may well pose new and hitherto unidentified health problems (Vettorazzi, 1974). Further investigation in this area would foster a close interaction between the food scientist (identification and quantification of pressor amines in common foods with special regard to overprocessed ones) and the food toxicologist (correlating levels of amines in foods with residues of agricultural compounds inhibiting the monoamine oxidase system, estimating intakes with the reported cases involving alimentary migraine and hypertensive conditions in the general population).

CONTAMINANTS FROM VARIOUS SOURCES

The term 'contaminant' and particularly 'food contaminant' means different things to different people. No satisfactory scientific definition of the term has ever been provided. The existing definitions are legal interpretations varying from place to place, from country to country. It could not be expected otherwise since definitions imply the possibility of making classifications and vice versa, and at the present time from the biological and toxicological viewpoints this is not possible. To quote just one example, trace elements occur in all foods as natural or inherent components of plant and animal tissues and fluids. They may also be present as a result of accidental or deliberate addition. A number of them have been unequivocally established as essential elements in mammalian nutrition. Several can be beneficial under some conditions. Some of them, such as arsenic, lead, cadmium and mercury, are frequently classified as toxins because their toxicity to man and animal is relatively high and their biological activity is largely confined to toxic reactions. However, all trace elements can be toxic if consumed in sufficiently large quantities or for protracted periods of time. There is also evidence that the toxicity or the beneficial effect of a particular element can be greatly influenced by the extent to which elements or compounds present in the diet affect absorption, excretion or body metabolism. Furthermore, there is ample evidence of interactions of vitamins with essential minerals, vitamins amongst themselves, vitamins with toxic minerals, and interactions of essential minerals with toxic metals. Such interactions may have a direct bearing on the significance of establishing 'safe' levels of intake and 'safe' limits in food for many contaminants and they may influence the range between nutritionally required amounts and toxic levels (Vettorazzi, 1982). If a scientific definition of food contaminants is not possible at the present time, the concept of contamination is clear in everybody's mind. Popularly, a food contaminant is a substance which could be found in food but which should not be present at all or at least it should not be present at the level found. According to the Office of Technology Assessment of the US Congress, environmental contaminants fall into three categories: synthetic or natural organic chemicals, metals or their organic and inorganic derivatives, and natural or synthetic radioactive substances (OTA, 1979). The US Food and Drug Administration defines environmental contaminants as added, poisonous, or deleterious substances that cannot be avoided by good manufacturing practices, and that may make food injurious to health.

Environmental contaminants can enter food directly or indirectly as a result of such human activities as agriculture, mining, industrial operations or energy production. The increasing sensitivity of analytical methods and the establishment in many countries of control requirements have brought about the need to introduce some quantification in toxicology for both levels of intake and levels in food for food contaminants (Vettorazzi, 1983a). The technical advances of the analytical sciences have also permitted the detection of many hitherto unsuspected chemicals in minute amounts in food. It should, however, be realized that the presence of a trace amount of an extraneous substance in food should not be taken as posing in itself a hazard to man.

Current recommendations with regard to 'safe' levels of intake for food additives and pesticide residues have been based on concepts such as that of Acceptable Daily Intake (ADI). This concept was developed by the Joint FAO/WHO Expert Committee on Food Additives (JECFA), an internationally sponsored expert committee whose original function was that of providing safety evaluations of food additives. However, when the mandate of JECFA was extended to include, in its toxicological assessment, food contaminants as well as food additives, the ADI concept was not found to be suitable as a toxicological end-point for assessment (Vettorazzi and Kouthon, 1981), and the above committee developed the concept of Provisional Tolerable Weekly Intake (PTWI), which should be applied to cumulative toxic elements (WHO/FAO, 1972). This concept has proven to be useful and its application to the toxicological assessment of cadmium, mercury and lead carried out in 1972 still holds true today. No advances were made from 1972 until 1982 in the methodology of assessment applied to toxic metals in food, except for the development of an administrative definition of irreducible limits (WHO, 1978). An irreducible level of a food contaminant was defined as that concentration of a substance which cannot be eliminated from a food without involving the discarding of that food altogether, severely compromising the ultimate availability of major food supplies. In 1982, however, a major breakthrough in the methodology of assessment of food contaminants took place (WHO, 1982). The concept of an ADI expressed from zero to an upper limit was not found appropriate for contaminants or substances which are both essential nutrients and unavoidable constituents of food; thus for copper and zinc, which are both essential to human nutrition but cause toxicity at higher levels of intake, the committee established provisional maximum tolerable daily intakes (PMTDI) (expressed in two figures, one indicating the level of essentiality and the other the level of safety). For tin, a metal contaminant with no cumulative properties, a provisional maximum daily intake (expressed in one figure) was established. As noted previously, provisional tolerable weekly intakes (PTWI) (expressed in one figure) had been established for metal contaminants with cumulative properties (e.g. cadmium, mercury and lead). Finally, since phosphorus (as phosphate) is an essential nutrient as well as an unavoidable constituent of food, a maximum daily intake (expressed in one figure) was established for this substance. This applies to diets that are nutritionally adequate in

TABLE 1
End-points of Assessment
(WHO/FAO, 1972; WHO, 1978, 1982, 1983, 1984, 1986)

Food Additives	
Acceptable Daily Intake (ADI)	0–*x*
Contaminants	
(a) with cumulative properties:	
Provisional Tolerable Weekly Intake (PTWI)	*x'*
(b) with no cumulative properties:	
(i) essential and toxic:	
Provisional Maximum Tolerable Daily Intake (PMTDI)	*x''*
(ii) not essential but toxic:	
Provisional Maximum Tolerable Daily Intake (PMTDI)	*x–y*
(iii) essential and unavoidable:	
Maximum Tolerable Daily Intake (MTDI)	*x'''*

TABLE 2
Evaluations
(WHO/FAO, 1972; WHO, 1978, 1982, 1983, 1984, 1986)

Constituent	mg/person	mg/kg body weight
Arsenic (PMTDI)		0·002
Cadmium (PTWI)	0·5	0·008 3
Copper (PMTDI)		0·05–0·5[a]
Iron (PMTDI)		0·8[b]
Lead (PTWI)	3·0	0·05[c]
Mercury, total (PTWI)	0·3	0·005
Mercury, methyl (PTWI)	0·2	0·003 3[d]
Phosphorus (MTDI)		70·0
Tin, inorganic (PMTDI)		2·0
Zinc (PMTDI)		0·3–1·0[a]

[a] The first figure expresses the daily dietary requirements; the second figure expresses the toxicologically safe level.
[b] This figure applies to iron from all sources except for iron oxides and hydrated oxides used as colouring agents and iron supplements taken during pregnancy and lactation or for specific clinical requirements.
[c] Not applicable to infants and children.
[d] This figure applies to diets that are nutritionally adequate in respect of calcium.

respect of calcium; if the calcium intake were high, the intake of phosphate could be proportionately higher, and the reverse relationship would also apply (Tables 1 and 2).

In setting limits for contaminants, as well as in determining the extent of the introduction of such substances into food supplies, the practitioner in food science and the practitioner in food toxicology interact continuously. The end result should be a balanced merging of the two key specialties for the benefit of food safety.

RESIDUAL CHEMICALS UTILIZED IN FOOD PRODUCTION AND PROCESSING

Many substances utilized in food processing and food production may be found in trace amounts in the final food products. Amongst these xenobiotics are residues of pesticides used in agriculture and in preserving fruits and raw agricultural produce as well as processing aids. A wide range of pesticide chemicals is needed for the control of pests and diseases on many types of edible plants throughout the world. Frequently the use of a pesticide for a specific purpose does not lead to a residue. However, if a residue is present in food products measures should be taken to ensure that it will not harm the consumer. Processing aids are substances or materials, not including apparatus or utensils and not consumed as food ingredients by themselves, which are intentionally used in the processing of raw materials, foods or other ingredients to serve a certain technological purpose during treatment or processing and which may result in the unintentional but unavoidable presence of residues or derivatives in the final product. The list of processing aids is long and varied and it includes anti-foaming agents, catalysts, clarifying/filtration aids, colour stabilizers, contact freezing and cooling agents, desiccating/anti-caking agents, detergents, enzyme preparations, enzyme immobilizing agents and supports, extraction solvents, flocculating agents, flour treatment agents, ion exchange resins, membranes and molecular sieves, lubricants, propellants and packaging gases, washing and peeling agents and the like. This impressive list, encompassing hundreds of substances, gives a perspective of the complexities involved in the establishment of safety measures necessary to ensure the consumer's protection. The toxicological implications of such a variety of residual chemicals on the health of the consumer and the undeniable usefulness of these substances in food production and processing, impose upon the agriculturist, the food technologist, the practitioner of food science and toxicology, as well as the regulator, the difficult task of keeping in equilibrium consumer preferences and his welfare—a never ending exercise full of surprises and hopes surrounded by a permanent halo of uncertainties!

SUBSTANCES INTENTIONALLY ADDED TO FOOD

Perhaps no area other than the toxicological evaluation of food additives can better illustrate the close relationship between food science and toxicology (regulatory aspects are discussed in detail in Chapter 2). The role and the importance of food scientists in the safety assessment of chemicals intentionally added to food have been often highlighted by the Joint FAO/WHO Expert Committee on Food Additives. In 1960, the committee expressed the opinion that it was the responsibility of toxicologists, oncologists and food scientists to evaluate the carcinogenic risk of food additives (WHO/FAO, 1961). In 1964, the same committee reiterated the point that evaluation of acceptability of a food additive is the function of toxicologists, oncologists and food scientists (WHO/FAO, 1965). In 1975, the same committee was faced with the task of evaluating compounds which either contained unique impurities or which gave rise to transformation products, and it recognized the need to consult with food technologists and other specialists in the matter at an early stage of the toxicological testing of food additives (WHO/FAO, 1975).

Food additives are non-nutritive substances added intentionally to food, generally in small quantities, to improve its appearance, flavour, texture or storage properties. Many of them are xenobiotics, others are either body constituents or may be transformed by metabolism into one or more substances which are normally utilized by the body. Food scientists and technologists had developed and utilized many of these substances; the list of additives in existence today is no less impressive than the one which classifies processing aids. The use of additives in food preservation and processing is as old as recorded civilization: man has used vinegar and spices to improve the qualities of certain foods; salt and smoke have been used for preservation of meat and fish; the process of fermentation has been used to prepare bread, beer and cheese. The modern concern about the use of additives in food is mainly directed to the impact that continuous ingestion of additives may have on the health of the consumer; this public concern has resulted in a situation whereby many countries have found it necessary to regulate their use. However, historically, the regulatory process was not aimed at protecting the consumer's health but to discourage fraudulent practice; often food was adulterated by the addition of certain substances to endow its appearance with qualities it did not possess, hence the intervention of public bodies to prevent such practices.

As science progressed and public perception became more refined about the health/food relationship, the regulatory process also became more active. The present food regulatory situation is quite complex and it lies at the crossroads of many components: avoidance of fraud, food production and processing, economy, trade, public health, the law, and others. However, as has been rightly noted (Hutt, 1985), the pressing regulatory problems of today are scientific, not legal, in nature. Laws can reflect science and in the absence of scientific knowledge can make arbitrary rules, but no law can predetermine science. Scientific progress must therefore be at the forefront of every regulatory development relating to food.

An objective and reliable toxicological evaluation of food additives is crucial for the modern regulatory process. If the toxicological recommendations are based on the careful study of all technological and biological data available at the time of the evaluation, and the administrative decisions regarding the use and limitation of use of a particular additive are based on the toxicological recommendations, it follows that the availability of a sufficient and adequate scientific data base is pivotal to the whole regulatory process (Vettorazzi, 1983b).

It is at this point that the food scientist and the practitioner of toxicology play a decisive role, and by no means should they retreat to their laboratories at the first sign of regulatory controversy. The task of the food scientist and food technologist is not, however, over after assisting in the evaluation exercise; they will also have to ensure that all the recommendations and decisions ensuing from the overall process are put into effect in the daily operations related to the procurement of raw material, food formulation, processing, packaging and delivery of the final product to the consumer.

REFERENCES

Abbou, R. (1979). Barefoot toxicologists and industrial ecotoxicology. In: *Actualités Toxicologiques*, L. Roche (Ed.), Masson, Paris.

Aziz, S. A. and Knowles, C. O. (1973). Inhibition of monoamine oxidase by the pesticide chlordimeform and related compounds. *Nature*, **242**, 417–8.

Ballantyne, B., Gazzard, M. F. and Swanston, D. W. (1977). Applanation tonometry in ophthalmic toxicology. In: *Current Approaches in Toxicology*, Ballantyne, B. (Ed.), John Wright and Sons, Bristol.

Beeman, R. W. and Matsumura, F. (1973). Chlordimeform: a pesticide acting upon amine regulatory mechanisms. *Nature*, **242**, 273–4.

Bertelli, A. (1979). Nuovi Aspetti di Tossicologia Sperimentale e Clinica, C. G. Ed. Medico-Scientifiche, Torino, Italy.

Blum, K. and Manzo, L. (Eds) (1985). *Neurotoxicology*, Marcel Dekker, Basel/New York.

Chenoweth, M. B. (1985). Perspectives in toxicology. *Ann. Rev. Pharmacol. Toxicol.*, **25**, 33–40.

Conso, F. (1984). Clinical toxicology. In: *Workshop on Manpower Development and Training*. WHO/EURO Interim Document 18; IPCS Joint Seminar 9; CEC/EUR 9619. WHO Regional Office for Europe, Copenhagen, Denmark.

Cravey, R. H. and Baselt, R. C. (Eds) (1981). *Introduction to Forensic Toxicology*, Biomedical Publications, Davis, California.

Dixon, R. L. (1983). Laboratory aspects of reproductive toxicology. In: *Scope 20: Methods for Assessing the Effects of Chemicals on Reproductive Functions*, V. B. Vouk and P. J. Sheehan (Eds), John Wiley and Sons, Chichester.

Duffus, J. H. (1980). *Environmental Toxicology*, Arnold, London.

Everson, R. J. and Oehme, F. W. (1981). *Analytical Toxicology Manual*, American College of Veterinary Toxicologists, Kansas State University, Manhattan, Kansas.

Ferrando, R., Truhaut, R., Raynaud, J.-P. and Spanoghe, J.-P. (1978). Toxicity by relay. III. Safety for human consumer of the use of Carbadox, a feed additive for swine, as estimated by a seven year relay toxicity on dogs. *Toxicology*, **II**, 167–83.

Galli, C. L., Paoletti, R. and Vettorazzi, G. (Eds) (1978). *Chemical Toxicology of Food*, Elsevier/North-Holland Biomedical Press, Amsterdam, Holland.

Guthrie, F. E. and Perry, J. J. (Eds) (1980). *Introduction to Environmental Toxicology*, Elsevier/North-Holland Biomedical Press, Amsterdam.

Hammons, A. S. (Ed.) (1981). *Methods for Ecological Toxicology: A Critical Review of Laboratory Multispecies Tests*, Ann Arbor Science Publishers, Ann Arbor, Michigan.

Hathcock, J. N. (Ed.) (1982). *Nutritional Toxicology*, Academic Press, New York.

Hentges, D. J. (Ed.) (1983). *Human Intestinal Microflora in Health and Disease*, Academic Press, New York.

Houts, M., Baselt, R. C. and Cravey, R. H. (1981). *Courtroom Toxicology*, Matthew Bender, New York.

Hutt, P. B. (1985). Food technology and food law: an uneasy partnership. *Food Technol.*, **39**(8), 14–18.

Kassel, S. (1984). Assessment of need and demand for evaluative toxicology. In: *Workshop on Manpower Development and Training*. WHO/EURO Interim Document 18; IPCS Joint Seminar 9; CEC/EUR 9619, WHO Regional Office for Europe, Copenhagen, Denmark.

Kingsbury, J. M. (1980). Phytotoxicology. In: *Casarett and Doull's Toxicology*, J. Doull, C. D. Klaassen and M. O. Amdur (Eds), Macmillan Publishing Co., New York.

Kurata, H. and Ueno, Y. (1984). *Toxigenic Fungi: Their Toxins and Health Hazards*, Kodansha, Tokyo/Elsevier, Amsterdam.

Lauwerys, R. R. (1982). *Toxicologie Industrielle et Intoxications Professionelles*, Masson, Paris.

Lewis, K. (1984). A career in toxicology. In: *Workshop on Manpower Development*

G. VETTORAZZI

and Training. WHO/EURO Interim Document 18; IPCS Joint Seminar 9; CEC/ EUR 9619, WHO Regional Office for Europe, Copenhagen, Denmark.

Liener, I. E. (Ed.) (1980). *Toxic Constituents of Plant Foodstuffs*, Academic Press, New York.

Maes, R. A. A. (Ed.) (1984). *Proc. Ann. European Meeting, Int. Assoc. Forensic Toxicologists*, Elsevier, Amsterdam.

Mallett, A. (1984). Diet and gut flora in toxicology. *BIBRA Bull.*, **23**(9), 398–400.

Marth, E. H. (1981). Foodborne hazards of microbial origin. In: *Food Safety*, H. R. Roberts (Ed.), John Wiley and Sons, New York.

Miller, A. (1984). Shuttle toxicology. *Food Chem. Toxicol.*, **22**, 1025–6.

Moreau, C. (1979). *Moulds, Toxins and Food*, John Wiley and Sons, Chichester/ New York.

Mundt, J. O. (1982). Hazards of food borne bacterial infections and intoxications. In: *Nutritional Toxicology*, Vol. 1, J. N. Hathcock (Ed.), Academic Press, New York.

NAS (1973). *Toxicants Occurring Naturally in Foods*, National Academy of Sciences, Washington, DC.

NRC/NAS (1985). *An Evaluation of the Role of Microbiological Criteria for Foods and Food Ingredients*. Sub-committee on Microbiological Criteria; Committee on Food Protection; Food and Nutrition Board, National Research Council; National Academy of Sciences. National Academy Press, Washington, DC.

Oliver, J. S. (1980). *Forensic Toxicology*. Proc. European Meeting Int. Assoc. Forensic Toxicologists, Croom Helm, London.

OTA (1979). *Environmental Contaminants in Food*, Office of Technology Assessment, Congress of the United States, Washington, DC.

Pearson, J. G., Foster, R. B. and Bishop, W. E. (Eds) (1980). *Aquatic Toxicology and Hazard Assessment*, Proc. Fifth Ann. Symp. Aquatic Toxicology, ASTM, Philadelphia.

Pohl, K. D. (1984). *Forensische Toxikologie: eine Einführung in die Laboratoriumspraxis der Giftanalyse*, Kriminalistik Verlag, Heidelberg.

Preziosi, P., Sampaolo, A., and Silano, V. (1984). Changing need for toxicologists in Italy resulting from European Community legislation. In: *Workshop on Manpower Development and Training*. WHO/EURO Interim Document 18; IPCS Joint Seminar 9; CEC/EUR 9619, WHO Regional Office for Europe, Copenhagen, Denmark.

Price, D. and Smith, S. E. (1971). Cheese reaction and tyramine, *Lancet*, **i**, 130.

Rechcigl, M., Jr (Ed.). (1983a). *CRC Handbook of Foodborne Diseases of Biological Origin*, CRC Press, Boca Raton, Florida.

Rechcigl, M., Jr (Ed.) (1983b). *Handbook of Naturally Occurring Food Toxicants*, CRC Press, Boca Raton, Florida.

Riemann, H. and Bryan, F. L. (1979). *Food-borne Infections and Intoxications*, 2nd edn, Academic Press, New York.

Roche, L. (Ed.) (1979). Toxicovigilance. In: *Proc. Meeting of WHO/World Federation of Associations of Clinical Toxicology Centers and Poison Control Centers*, Geneva, Switzerland, June 1978, Masson, Paris.

Rodricks, J. V. and Pohland, A. E. (1981). Food hazards of natural origin. In: *Food Safety*, H. R. Roberts (Ed.), Wiley-Interscience Publication.

Rowland, I. R. and Walker, R. (1983). The gastrointestinal tract in food toxicology. In: *Toxic Hazards in Food*, D. M. Conning and A. B. G. Landsdown (Eds), Croom Helm, London/Canberra.

Sawicki, E. (Ed.) (1982). *Handbook of Environmental Genotoxicology*, CRC Press, Boca Raton, Florida.

Schvartsman, S. (Ed.) (1976). *Proc. First Congr. Tropical Toxicology*, Manaus, Brazil, April 11–14 (in Portuguese).

Smith, R. L. and Bababunmi, E. A. (Eds) (1980). *Toxicology in the Tropics* (International Symposium), Taylor and Francis, London.

Somani, S. M. and Cavender, F. L. (Eds) (1981). *Environmental Toxicology: Principles and Policies*, Thomas, Springfield, Illinois.

Tandon, H. D., Tandon, B. N., Tandon, R. and Nayak, N. C. (1977). A pathological study of the liver in an epidemic outbreak of veno-occlusive disease. *Ind. J. Med. Res.*, **65**, 679–84.

Tandon, H. D., Tandon, B. N. and Mattocks, A. R. (1978). An epidemic of reno-occlusive disease of the liver in Afghanistan. *Am. J. Gastroenterol.*, **72**, 607–13.

Temple, A. R. (Ed.) (1984). *Symposium on Medical Toxicology*, Saunders, Philadelphia.

Thilly, W. G. and Liber, H. L. (1980). Genetic toxicology. In: *Casarett and Doull's Toxicology*, J. Doull, C. D. Klaaseen and M. O. Amdur (Eds), Macmillan Publishing Co., New York.

Truhaut, R. (1977). Ecotoxicology: objectives, principles and perspectives. *Ecotoxicol. Environ. Safety*, **1**, 151–73.

Truhaut, R. and Ferrando, R. (Eds) (1978). *Toxicology and Nutrition* (Symposium Alfort France), Karger, Basel/New York.

UNEP (1978). Report of the United Nations Conference on the Human Environment. In: *Compendium of Legislative Authority*, Pergamon Press, Oxford.

Vettorazzi, G. (1972). The formation and enzymatic oxidation of 5-hydroxytryptamine in *Musa* spp. Ph.D. thesis, Louisiana State University, Baton Rouge (Order No. 72-17, 818).

Vettorazzi, G. (1974). 5-Hydroxytryptamine content of banana and banana products. *Food Cosmet. Toxicol.*, **12**, 107–13.

Vettorazzi, G. (1975). The safety evaluation of food additives: the dynamics of toxicological decisions. *Lebensm.-Wiss. Technol.*, **8**, 195–201.

Vettorazzi, G. (1978). Tossicologia di regolamentazione. *Riv. Soc. Ital. Sci. Alim.*, **7**(1), 31–46.

Vettorazzi, G. (Ed.) (1980). *Handbook of International Food Regulatory Toxicology*. Vol. 1, *Evaluations*, SP Medical and Scientific Books, New York.

Vettorazzi, G. (Ed.) (1981). *Handbook of International Food Regulatory Toxicology*. Vol. 2, *Profiles*, SP Medical and Scientific Books, New York.

Vettorazzi, G. (1982). Lead as a food contaminant, *Rev. Ital. Sci. Alim.*, **11**(3), 303–10.

Vettorazzi, G. (1983a). Quantification in food regulatory toxicology. In: *Health Evaluation of Heavy Metals in Infant Formula and Junior Food*, E. H. F. Schmidt and A. G. Hildebrandt (Eds), Springer-Verlag, Berlin.

Vettorazzi, G. (1983b). Trends towards a real food safety policy. In: *La Nutrizione dell'Uomo verso una Reale Sicurezza*, Vignoli Ed., Modena, Italy.

Vettorazzi, G. and Kouthon, G. (1981). *JECFA: Past, Present and Future.*

Background Paper No. 2 for the Twenty-fifth Meeting of the Joint FAO/WHO Expert Committee on Food Additives, Geneva, Switzerland (unpublished document; copies are available from the authors).

WHO (1978). *Evaluation of Certain Food Additives and Contaminants*, 22nd report, Wld Hlth Org. Techn. Rep. Ser., No. 631.

WHO (1982). *Evaluation of Certain Food Additives and Contaminants*, 26th report, Wld Hlth Org. Techn. Rep. Ser., No. 683.

WHO (1983). *Evaluation of Certain Food Additives and Contaminants*, 27th report, Wld Hlth Org. Techn. Rep. Ser., No. 696.

WHO (1984). *Evaluation of Certain Food Additives and Contaminants*, 28th report, Wld Hlth Org. Techn. Rep. Ser., No. 710.

WHO (1986). *Evaluation of Certain Food Additives and Contaminants*, 29th report, Wld Hlth Org. Techn. Rep. Ser., No. 733.

WHO (1987a). *Principles for the Safety Assessment of Chemicals in Food*, International Programme on Chemical Safety, World Health Organization, Geneva, EHC 70.

WHO (1987b). *Pyrrolizidine Alkaloids*, International Programme on Chemical Safety, World Health Organization, Geneva, in press.

WHO/EURO (1984). *Workshop on Manpower Development and Training Report*. WHO/EURO Interim Document 18; IPCS Joint Seminar 9; CEC/EUR 9619, WHO Regional Office for Europe, Copenhagen, Denmark.

WHO/FAO (1961). *Evaluation of the Carcinogenic Hazards of Food Additives*, 5th report, Wld Hlth Org. Techn. Rep. Ser., No. 220.

WHO/FAO (1965). *Specifications for the Identity and Purity of Food Additives and Their Toxicological Evaluation: Food Colours and Some Antimicrobials and Antioxidants*, Wld Hlth Org. Techn. Rep. Ser., No. 309.

WHO/FAO (1971). *Evaluation of Food Additives*, 15th report, Wld Hlth Org. Techn. Rep. Ser., No. 462.

WHO/FAO (1972). *Evaluations of Certain Food Additives and the Contaminants Mercury, Lead and Cadmium*, 16th report, Wld Hlth Org. Techn. Rep. Ser., No. 505.

WHO/FAO (1974). *Evaluation of Certain Food Additives*, Wld Hlth Org. Techn. Rep. Ser., No. 557.

WHO/FAO (1975). *Evaluation of Certain Food Additives*, 19th report, Wld Hlth Org. Techn. Rep. Ser., No. 576.

WHO/FAO (1978). *Evaluation of Certain Food Additives*, 21st report, Wld Hlth Org. Techn. Rep. Ser., No. 617.

Chapter 2

REGULATORY ASPECTS OF FOOD ADDITIVES

A. MALASPINA

The Coca-Cola Company, Atlanta, Georgia, USA

INTRODUCTION

In most countries of the world food additives are regulated by government statute. This is usually achieved by the publication of permitted lists and purity criteria for each food additive; often the lists contain limitations of permitted levels in certain food products.

In this chapter, the regulatory framework within which food additives are approved will be examined from an international perspective, using as examples the United States, Japan, the EEC and some key international

17

agencies. The scientific principles related to safety assessment and some of the pertinent issues will be reviewed. Some important classes of ingredients are discussed as examples of the regulatory decision-making process.

US APPROACH

Food and Drug Administration
In the United States the primary agency concerned with the regulation of food additives became known in 1930 as the Food and Drug Administration (FDA) and is now a component of the Department of Health and Human Services (formerly the Department of Health, Education and Welfare).

The agency is charged with the responsibility for safeguarding the health and welfare of the public by ensuring the purity, safety, and proper labeling of foods, drugs, cosmetics, and therapeutic devices. The legislative branch of the US government (Congress) develops legal statutes and the FDA must work within them.

In 1938, the Food, Drug and Cosmetic Act (FD&C Act) was enacted. The act contains specific criteria which define adulteration, and bars from interstate commerce any adulterated, misbranded, or harmful food, drug, or cosmetic. Labeling requirements were made more specific in order to provide more information for the consumer. Under the FD&C Act, the addition of any chemical preservatives to foods must be declared on the label, and the addition of poisonous ingredients that may render the food injurious to health is illegal. The addition of any flavoring or coloring to make a product appear better is illegal and fraudulent unless the fact is stated on the label. The use of uncertified colors (colors without a certificate of acceptability issued by FDA on a batch-to-batch basis) is illegal. The act also prohibits traffic in food prepared under unsanitary conditions, authorizes factory inspections, and provides for procurement of transportation records. Under the FD&C Act of 1938, the FDA had the legal responsibility for demonstrating that a food substance was 'unsafe' (Hui, 1979; Hutt, 1984; Hutt and Hutt, 1984).

In 1958 Congress passed the Food Additives Amendment which fundamentally changed the regulation of intentional additives (Middlekauff, 1984; Ziporyn, 1985). First, it placed the legal burden to prove that an additive is 'safe' on the petitioner for the additive. Under this amendment, new additives that are not already generally recognized by the scientific community to be safe cannot be used in food until it has been demonstrated to FDA's satisfaction, on the basis of competent scientific evidence, that the substance is safe. Second, because Congress recognized the impossibility of proving the absolute safety of an additive under any conditions of use, it provided that 'safe' means a 'reasonable certainty' that no harm will result from the intended use of the food additive. This is often referred to as the 'general safety standard' for food additives. It is a rigorous, but not zero risk, safety standard. Third, because of particular concerns about cancer, the US Congress established a special rule for carcinogens. It enacted the Delaney clause (Fed. FD&C Act, 1958), whereby 'no additive shall be deemed to be safe if it is found to induce cancer when ingested by man or animal, or if it is found, after tests which are appropriate for the evaluation of the safety of food additives, to induce cancer in man or animal'.

In 1960, Congress passed the Color Additives Amendments to the FD&C Act (Marmion, 1979; Noonan and Meggos, 1980). These amendments established uniform rules for all permitted colors in foods, drugs and cosmetics and provided for the listing of color additives which must be certified and those exempt from certification (Noonan and Meggos, 1980; Ziporyn, 1985). The term 'natural colors', formerly applied to the uncertified color additives (which are synthetic as well as of natural origin), was also eliminated, and the Secretary of Health, Education and Welfare was given the authority to decide which colors must undergo batch-by-batch certification (for compliance with purity specifications) and which could be exempted from certification. This law also includes a clause similar to the Delaney clause for food additives stating, among other things, that a color additive cannot be listed for any use that might result in ingestion if it is found to induce cancer when ingested by man or animal (Noonan and Meggos, 1980).

Another important section of these amendments permitted the provisional listing or the continued use of existing color additives pending the completion of scientific investigations needed to determine whether these materials were acceptable for permanent listing. The provisional listing of the color additives had an original closing date of 2½ years after passage of the amendments. However, the Secretary of Health, Education and Welfare was given the power to grant extensions of the closing dates; this power has been exercised many times (Noonan and Meggos, 1980). The present status of some of the color additives is discussed later in this chapter.

Within the FDA, the Center for Food Safety and Applied Nutrition (formerly the Bureau of Foods) receives petitions for the use of food additives. In general, a petition contains the following types of information:

(1) The name of the additive, its chemical structure and/or formula
(2) Manufacturing process
(3) Physical-chemical properties and purity
(4) Methods of analysis in foods
(5) Functionality/technological need
(6) All data on short-term, sub-chronic study in non-rodent species and long-term toxicity/carcinogenicity in two species, mutagenicity, reproduction (including teratogenicity) and metabolic studies
(7) Environmental assessment statement
(8) Consumption data.

When the FDA determines that a petition is complete, a notice of filing is published in the Federal Register, and FDA then has 180 days to make a decision. During this review period, anyone may comment on the petition, including private citizens. If FDA determines that the additive has been shown to be safe, the final regulation is published and the additive is allowed.

Except for carcinogens, FDA's approach to the safety assessment of food additives is similar to that taken by other countries and international bodies. It derives 'acceptable daily intakes' (ADIs) for food additives by applying a 'safety factor' to the established 'no observed effect level' (NOEL) obtained from the required, appropriate animal toxicity studies. The resulting figure, expressed on the basis of mg of the chemical per kg of body weight, is (when possible) compared with the expected human exposure to the additive.

The reliance on animal data means that safety assessment is a judgmental and inferential process. The 100-fold safety factor, arrived at somewhat arbitrarily and lacking scientific justification, is nevertheless widely accepted. In actual practice, this safety factor is typically larger than 100, because the actual daily intake of a specific additive is usually much lower than estimated.

The Delaney clause made it impossible in the US to use the safety factor approach in evaluating food additives that induced tumors in experimental animals. When the Delaney clause was enacted in 1958, only a few compounds were known to produce tumors. Since then, many more chemical substances have been found to induce tumors in experimental animals, due to the increased quantity, intensity and sensitivity of toxicity testing. Parallel with this development, dramatic advances in analytical chemistry have enabled scientists to detect these chemical substances in the food supply more frequently, albeit at levels that are extraordinarily low. For instance, while in the 1960s the detection of ppm (mg/kg) was considered sophisticated, the detection of 1 ppb (μg/kg) and ppt (ng/kg) is becoming common. These two developments mean that the approach taken in the early 1960s, viz. to forbid absolutely the use of all compounds that induce tumors in animals, is no longer tenable. It would result in a substantial disruption of the food supply that is not justified by a commensurate gain in public health protection.

More recently, methods of quantitative risk assessment have been developed which enable scientists to calculate, on the basis of animal data, the probable upper limit of human risk. Conservative assumptions, designed to overestimate the risk, are used in these assessments (Rodricks and Taylor, 1983). FDA has calculated the risk from certain food colors to be well below one in one million over a lifetime of the exposed population, and in certain cases even as low as one in one billion. These figures mean that a person has no greater than a one in one million or one in one billion (or lower) chance of getting cancer over a lifetime as a result of ingesting the color additive on a daily basis.

Under long-established principles of US law, regulatory agencies are authorized to interpret the statutes they administer in a way that will accomplish the basic objectives of Congress without imposing results that defy common sense. Acting under this principle, FDA has developed new approaches to interpreting and applying the Delaney clause that are more compatible with contemporary scientific reality in order to avoid banning substances found to cause cancer in animals when it can be demonstrated that the risks posed to humans under intended conditions of use are insignificant, i.e. the substance is 'safe'.

One new approach is the 'constituents policy' which addresses the fact that some non-carcinogenic food and color additives contain trace amounts of carcinogenic contaminants or impurities. In order to avoid banning such additives when the risks they pose are trivial, FDA has interpreted the Delaney clause as applying to the additive as a whole and not to its individual constituents (FDA, 1982c). The additive is then evaluated under the general safety standard, where, using risk assessment, FDA can judge whether the additive is safe for human consumption, taking into consideration any risk posed by the carcinogenic constituents. FDA has used this approach to clear FD&C Yellow No. 5 (1985a) and 6 (1986a) and D&C Green No. 5 (1982d) and 6 (1982b), as well as important packaging materials such as acrylonitrile (DC Circuit Court, 1979) and vinyl chloride

(FDA, 1986*b*). FDA's constituents policy has been upheld by the courts in the case of D&C Green No. 6.

Another approach taken recently by FDA is the *de minimis* approach (FDA, 1985*b*; Middlekauff, 1985). Under general principles of law, regulatory agencies have some discretion to interpret their statutory mandates where necessary to avoid absurd results (DC Circuit Court, 1968). Under the *de minimis* doctrine, they need not act to address problems or risks that are so trivial as to be unworthy of government concern. FDA has applied this doctrine to the Delaney clause and has concluded that, as a legal matter, it is not required to ban substances under the Delaney clause when the risks are extremely small. Thus, even if the additive as a whole induces cancer, FDA is now prepared to approve it if the increased risk over a lifetime is no greater than one in one million (Middlekauff, 1985). FDA has applied this policy to the use of methylene chloride for decaffeinating coffee (FDA, 1985*b*) and is considering its application to certain colors. FDA's legal interpretation of the Delaney clause is controversial and may be challenged in court, but the policy embodied in the *de minimis* doctrine enjoys broad support (Middlekauff, 1985):

FDA has always operated under certain generally accepted principles for toxicity testing, but until 1982 had not developed written guidelines and criteria for the quality and quantity of testing that must be done in order to demonstrate the safety of an additive. As toxicological testing and the safety assessment process became more complex, both FDA and the regulated industry in the US felt the need for carefully devised, written guidelines in this area. In 1982, FDA responded by releasing a document entitled Toxicological Principles for the Safety Assessment of Direct Food Additives and Color Additives Used in Food, which has come to be known as the FDA Red Book (FDA, 1982*f*). In this document, FDA explains the special considerations that apply to the safety assessment of direct food additives and the criteria that should govern selection of required toxicity tests for particular substances. FDA adopted a 'principle of commensurate effort' which states that the amount of testing required for a substance should reflect the 'level of concern' that a substance poses in terms of safety. Substances that pose a higher level of safety concern are to be tested more thoroughly than substances that pose a lesser degree of safety concern.

The Red Book defines three levels of safety concern, based on anticipated human exposure to the substance and the substance's chemical structure. FDA concluded that very general inferences can be drawn about the toxic potential of substances by comparing their chemical structures with those of compounds whose toxic potential is already known. Three structure categories were adopted: those likely to be of low (I), intermediate (II) or high (III) toxic potential. FDA considers structure analysis, in conjunction with exposure data, to be adequate for determining initial requirements for toxicity testing. The Concern Level for a substance may be increased or decreased as more information becomes available about either the toxic properties or exposure levels. The Red Book prescribes the tests that FDA will generally require for substances at each Concern Level.

For Concern Level I compounds, FDA typically requires a short-term feeding study (at least 28 days in duration) in a rodent species and mutagenicity tests as screening tests for carcinogenic potential.

For Concern Level II compounds, FDA ordinarily requires: a short-term (also called subchronic) feeding study (at least 90 days in duration) in a rodent and one in a non-rodent species; a multi-generation reproduction study (minimum of two generations) including a teratology phase in a rodent species; and mutagenicity tests.

The most intensive testing is reserved for Concern Level III compounds. For these, FDA requires: carcinogenicity studies in two rodent species; a short-term (subchronic) study of at least one year duration in a rodent species (this study is ordinarily performed in combination with one of the carcinogenicity studies); a short-term (subchronic) feeding study of at least one year in duration in a non-rodent species; a multi-generation reproduction study (minimum of two generations) including a teratology phase in a rodent species; and mutagenicity tests.

The Red Book is intended to be a guide to toxicity testing and not an absolute standard. FDA recognizes that toxicity testing of each chemical substance should be considered on a case-by-case basis. The agency thus reserves the right to require additional tests, and is willing to discuss alternative approaches if sound arguments are made that some facet of the prescribed battery of tests is inappropriate for a particular situation.

Other US Initiatives toward Harmonization of Testing Procedures

The National Toxicology Program (NTP) was established in 1978 under the Department of Health, Education and Welfare to coordinate activities and resources concerned with determining the toxicological potential of chemicals and to establish dialogue among scientists so that toxicological research and regulatory needs would be better integrated. A wide range of chemical substances is evaluated in various test systems (teratology, toxicity, mutagenicity, carcinogenicity) that have become an integrated program in studying chemicals for various end points (NTP, 1984a; 1985).

In 1983 the Ad Hoc Panel was established to review the basic biology and chemistry of carcinogens and to recommend methods that NTP should use for the detection and evaluation of chemical carcinogens. The Panel submitted its report in 1984; conclusions were presented as a series of recommendations to the NTP Board (NTP, 1984b). It is expected that, as the NTP program evolves, protocols will be modified to reflect an increased understanding of the biochemical process of carcinogenesis. This will allow a better interpretation of the results of the tests.

An additional attempt to provide a coordinated framework for the development of regulation of carcinogens in the US was a report published in 1985 by the Office of Science and Technology Policy (OSTP), which is part of the Executive (presidential) Branch of the government. OSTP invited government and non-government scientists to submit comments defining principles which could be used by various regulatory agencies in the safety assessment process. The document presents a consensus of opinion based on current scientific information, but states that improvements will be made as scientific knowledge continues to evolve (OSTP, 1985). The preparation of the OSTP report signaled the recognition, at the highest level of the government, that a regulatory approach that is more flexible than the Delaney clause should be adopted for animal carcinogens.

JAPANESE APPROACH

The first Japanese food law was enacted in 1900. The Law for the Control of Foods and Things Related to Food was a general nationalized approach to food sanitation. Subsequently, more specific enforcement regulations were promulgated, targeted towards 'poisonous coloring materials', artificial sweetening agents, and preservatives.

In 1947 the Food Sanitation Law was adopted. The law defined food additives as 'synthetically obtained'. Therefore, regulations apply only to synthetic compounds; all natural compounds are permitted in foods. An important amendment, enacted in 1957, was the Standards of Food Additives provision, in which the limits for impurities, use restrictions and standards for labeling were defined.

In the same amendment, the Minister of Health and Welfare was given the authority to prepare standards for food additives, and the Food Sanitation Investigation Council was established to investigate methods of food poisoning prevention, preparation of Standards for Food Additives, and other related subjects. The 1957 amendment also established a Committee on Japanese Standards for Food Additives within the Food Sanitation Investigation Council. The first edition of standards was published in 1960, and included specifications for 198 food additives (Japan Food Hygiene Association, 1960). Supplements and new editions have been issued since then, with the last major edition released in 1986 (Japan Food Additives Association, 1986).

There are four basic standards which are considered when a petition for a new food additive is reviewed: (1) it must be shown to be of sufficient safety; (2) it must be advantageous to consumers in some way; (3) it must be demonstrated that the additive is useful or superior to similar registered food additives; (4) food additives must be able to be chemically estimated in the finished food product. The petitioner must include information about the physical-chemical, technological, and biological properties of the proposed additive.

The requirements for safety assessment in Japan are similar to those described for the USA and the EEC. The battery of tests includes acute, short-term, and long-term toxicity/carcinogenicity tests; mutagenicity, reproduction including teratogenicity tests, and metabolic studies.

Guidelines for the conduct of carcinogenicity studies have been published (Odashima, 1976). The Food Sanitation Investigation Council will also consider the estimated intake of the additive in light of the safety data generated by the toxicity tests.

Unlike the United States with its Delaney clause, the Food Sanitation Investigation Council and the Minister of Health and Welfare are not required by law to prohibit the use of animal carcinogens. Potential carcinogenic risk to humans is certainly considered, but a finding of carcinogenicity in animals does not automatically result in a negative regulatory decision.

THE EUROPEAN ECONOMIC COMMUNITY

If one envisions that US federal agencies have a difficult time regulating 50 states that have a common language, common currency, and common national government, one can only imagine the problems associated with the harmonization of 12 national governments, with 12 different currencies and 9 different languages.

The European Economic Community (EEC) in Brussels is trying to meet this challenge. Created in 1957, the EEC is now comprised of 12 member countries (Belgium, Germany, France, The Netherlands, Ireland, Denmark, Luxemburg, Italy, Greece, United Kingdom, Spain and Portugal) bound together by the Treaty of Rome (McGowan, 1981).

The founders of the EEC created permanent institutions on which real, if limited, powers have been conferred. The most important of these institutions are the Council of Ministers, the European Parliament, the Court of Justice, the Commission and the Economic and Social Committee.

The EEC has as its primary task to develop a United Market within its boundaries so that the circulation of commodities is not hindered between the various member states. The EEC is trying to achieve this by harmonizing the national legislations of its member states (McGowan, 1981).

The EEC food law harmonization is being carried out through 'directives'. The two most important types of directives are the 'horizontal directives' and the 'vertical directives'. The horizontal directives deal with food additives (positive lists) such as colors and emulsifiers. The vertical directives deal with standards for specific food commodities such as meat, wine, soft drinks and fruit juices, and specify the food additives which are permitted by those standards. Within the directives, food additives are controlled by requiring that only substances that are permitted and thus have been assigned an 'E' number may be used (Haigh, 1978b,c).

Although the Common Market has been in existence for almost 30 years, only a limited number of directives has been adopted. For example, the horizontal directives that have been adopted include: coloring matters (1962); preservatives (1963); preservatives (purity criteria) (1965); preservatives (control measures for citrus fruit) (1967); antioxidants (1970); certain sugars (1973); emulsifiers, stabilizers, etc. (1974); materials in contact with foods (1976); food labeling (1978); and antioxidants (purity criteria) (1978) (Haigh, 1978c).

The vertical directives that have been adopted include: cocoa and chocolate (1973); honey (1974); milk (1974); condensed milk (1975); fruit juice and similar products (1975); foods for particular nutritional uses (1976); coffee and chicory extracts (1977); jams and jellies (1979); quality of water for human consumption (1980); and mineral waters (1980) (Haigh, 1978c). In addition, most of these directives have undergone many amendments to make them consistent with scientific and technological progress.

As noted above, the overall aim of the directives is to permit the free circulation of commodities within the member states. In practice, a certain commodity can be marketed in any EEC country if it complies with either the EEC standards or the national standards of the member states. In the absence of a Common Market directive, national legislation prevails in each country. However, an important court decision in 1979 has had an impact on the EEC, especially in the area of food law harmonization.

This was the case of Cassis de Dijon, a blackcurrant liqueur exported from France into Germany. The product was legally manufactured and sold in France, but did not meet the requirements of the German law. The case was brought before the Court of Justice and, in the absence of relevant EEC regulations, the Court of Justice ruled that Article 30 of the Treaty of Rome prohibited quantitative differences in food standards from hindering trade between member states, and that this particular liqueur could be freely sold throughout the member states. In October 1980 the EEC Commission announced that it would support this kind of export. If a product is legal in the country of manufacture, it can be freely sold in all other EEC countries unless there are health reasons for restricting it nationally (*Food Chemical News*, 1985). Understandably, this decision is affecting the concept of food law harmonization, especially the vertical regulations which pertain to commodity standards.

In addition to the published directives, there are several in various stages of preparation, but each will undergo many drafts, and comments will be made by interested groups before a final draft directive is agreed upon. Directives that are being developed include: flavorings; acids, bases, solvents; claims in food advertising; irradiation of foodstuffs; methods of analysis; soft drinks; vinegar; quick frozen foods; tomato products; starches; pasta; oils and fats; butter; margarine; soups; condiment sauces; mustard; yeast; flour and biscuits; canned fruits and canned vegetables; low sodium dietary foods; egg products; and caseins and caseinates.

Within the EEC, it is the Scientific Committee for Food (SCF) that advises the Commission on the acceptability of food additives on the basis of the available toxicological information (Haigh, 1978a). Their advice is published periodically by the Commission of the European Communities in the Reports of the Scientific Committee for Food.

For the different EEC countries, toxicity testing of food additives and pesticides began in the late 1950s, based in part on procedures given by the Association of Food and Drug Officials of the United States (1959) in the FDA monograph on appraisals of the safety of chemicals in foods, drugs and cosmetics. The Netherlands (1964) published guidelines for toxicity testing which were based on both the FDA 'appraisals' and the procedures for the testing of intentional food additives to establish their safety in use, published by the Joint FAO/WHO Expert Committee on Food Additives (JECFA) (WHO/FAO, 1958). (The work of this committee is discussed in Chapter 7.) The required toxicity data resembled in principle the same toxicity data the FDA requires, viz. acute, short-term and long-term carcinogenicity studies, multigeneration reproduction (teratogenicity and mutagenicity were not known at that time) and metabolism studies.

However, from the beginning it was accepted that the requirements for toxicity data could be modified by factors such as type of use, actual exposure levels, chemical structure and toxicity data available from related compounds. In other words, as recorded in the US FDA Red Book, the toxicity testing of each chemical substance had to be considered as a separate scientific problem.

As early as the late 1960s, the countries of the EEC recognized that the induction of tumors in animal experiments varies from one chemical to another. For example, today it is recognized that many factors determine whether or not tumors will occur, including biological differences between humans and laboratory animals. Some of these inherent differences are genetic variability, lifespan, body size, sex/hormonal status, type of diet, exposure levels and patterns, pharmacokinetics, metabolism and repair of DNA. Furthermore, certain animal strains are genetically prone to tumors of specific organ systems. As a result of this, these animal strains may be overly resistant or susceptible to toxicological effects.

Other factors to be considered in safety assessment are the relevance of an increased incidence of the induction of benign tumors, an increase of rare tumors, a decrease in latency time, negative trends in tumor incidence in animal bioassays and dose–response relationships.

Dietary and other lifestyle factors may modify the induction of tumors. Certain food factors inhibit, while others promote, tumor formation. All relevant data should be considered in the process of hazard identification, and when the regulatory system allows some flexibility, as in the EEC countries, this can be done.

The SCF of the Commission also recognized the importance of describing the requirements for toxicity testing, and in 1977 published a guideline for the toxicological evaluation of a substance for materials and articles intended to come into contact with foodstuffs (packaging materials) (CEC, 1977). This was followed in 1980 by a guideline for the safety assessment of food additives (CEC, 1980). As with the FDA Red Book, deviation from the EEC guidelines is possible in certain circumstances.

ORGANIZATION FOR ECONOMIC
CO-OPERATION AND
DEVELOPMENT

The Organization for Economic Co-operation and Development (OECD) was set up under a convention signed in 1960 by 25 countries: Australia, Austria, Belgium, Canada, Denmark, Finland, France, Germany, Greece, Iceland, Ireland, Italy, Japan, Luxemburg, Netherlands, New Zealand, Norway, Portugal, Spain, Sweden, Switzerland, Turkey, United Kingdom and the United States, with Yugoslavia having special status. Under the auspices of the OECD, an OECD Chemicals Testing Program was launched in November 1977, and is comprised of six Expert Groups under the leadership of individual member countries (OECD, 1981). The Step Systems Group draws upon the work of the other Expert Groups which examine various aspects of chemicals (physical-chemical properties; effects on biotic systems other than man; degradation/accumulation; short-term health effects; and long-term health effects) and is currently developing an integrated stepwise approach to testing and assessment of chemical hazards to man and his environment. An important outcome of the work of the Step Systems Group is the OECD Minimum Pre-marketing set of Data (MPD). The MPD lists some 35 individual data components that normally would be sufficient to provide a meaningful first assessment of the potential hazard of a chemical.

The Chemicals Testing Program published the official OECD guidelines for testing of chemicals as adopted by the OECD Council (OECD, 1981). The OECD Test Guidelines contain procedures for the laboratory testing of a property or effect of a chemical deemed important for the evaluation of health and environmental hazards of that chemical. The guidelines include all the essential elements that will enable an investigator to carry out the required test, assuming good laboratory practices are followed. The guidelines are not designed to serve as rigid test protocols. They are designed instead to allow flexibility for expert judgment and adjustment to new developments. In 1981, the OECD Updating Programme for test guidelines was established in consultation with the Commission of the European Communities. The aim is to ensure that OECD Test Guidelines will not become outdated.

The purpose of the OECD Test Guidelines is to harmonize testing methods in the OECD countries. Whenever testing of chemicals is contemplated, the OECD Test Guidelines should be consulted. Since the test guidelines have been endorsed by the OECD member countries, their use in the generation of data provides a common basis for the acceptance of data internationally, together with the opportunity to reduce direct and indirect costs to governments and industry associated with testing and assessment of chemicals.

While harmonization of safety assessment protocols and data interpretation is an important goal, it will probably be some time before it is achieved.

EXPERT COMMITTEES CONCERNED WITH THE EVALUATION OF FOOD ADDITIVES

Food Additive Safety Assessment by JECFA

In 1954, the Joint FAO/WHO Expert Committee on Nutrition briefly reviewed the problem of food additives and proposed that a special conference should be convened by FAO and WHO (WHO/FAO, 1955). Accordingly, a joint FAO/WHO conference on food additives took place in September 1955, and in 1956 the Joint FAO/WHO Expert Committee on Food Additives (JECFA) established the general principles governing the use of food additives (WHO/FAO, 1957). An important conclusion was: "Safety for use is an all-important consideration. While it is impossible to establish absolute proof of the non-toxicity of a specified use of an additive for all human beings under all conditions, critically designed animal tests of the physiological, pharmacological and biochemical behavior of a proposed additive can provide a reasonable basis for evaluating the safety of use of a food additive at a specified level of intake."

At the second meeting of JECFA in 1957, a rather detailed description of the data that were considered necessary to evaluate the acceptability of a food additive was given (WHO/FAO, 1958). The requirements included data on chemical and physical identification, acute short-term and long-term toxicity, metabolism, biochemical and other special investigations. The committee had already decided that the problems of chemical carcinogenesis and mutagenic actions were important enough to merit further consideration at a later date (see also Chapter 1). Like the US Congress, the committee believed that no proven carcinogen should be considered suitable for use as a food additive in any amount. At that time they did not realize that the problem would be to define 'proved carcinogen' and 'any amount'. Because absolute proof of non-toxicity could never be provided, it was inescapable that some arbitrary factor had to be applied in order to provide an adequate margin of safety, and that some type of risk assessment was necessary. Since then many food additives and unintentional contaminants have been evaluated and ADIs established by the FAO/ WHO Expert Committee.

The data described in 1957 by JECFA as necessary for the evaluation of food additives (and pesticides) have been critically reviewed and updated several times (WHO/FAO, 1958, 1961, 1967, 1974a). JECFA is now in the process of developing new guidelines for toxicity testing.

International Agency for Research on Cancer (IARC)

Since 1971, 660 chemical substances and groups of chemicals have been evaluated for their carcinogenic potential by IARC. IARC publishes its assessment of carcinogenic risk of human exposure to environmental chemicals as a continuing monograph series (IARC, 1984).

Preparation of the IARC monographs involves two main steps: (1) collection of published data relevant to assessing the carcinogenic risk of exposure to chemicals in human populations (unpublished data are not used; this may be a drawback because often important studies are not used in the evaluation); (2) critical analysis and evaluation of these data by international working groups of experts in chemical carcinogenesis and related disciplines and experts in the field of epidemiology.

Chemical substances and complex mixtures (and occasionally chemical analogues) are evaluated on the basis of two principal criteria: (1) whether there are data suggesting carcinogenicity in experimental animals *and* humans; (2) whether there is evidence of human exposure to the chemical. Also taken into consideration are: the extent and duration of human exposure, including the persistence of a chemical in the environment; the existence of specific populations at risk, when applicable; the amount produced and pattern of use; and results of short-term tests (IARC, 1984).

EXAMPLES OF FOOD ADDITIVE REGULATORY DECISIONS

Antioxidants

This group of important compounds has been used for many years to prolong shelf life by preventing fats and oils from undergoing oxidation and becoming rancid during storage. Oxidation occurs when lipid molecules, activated by heat and light or other catalyzing agents, react with oxygen to form peroxides, and subsequently, aldehydes, ketones, acids, alcohols, etc. Once initiated, the oxidation process proceeds at accelerated rates, with trace metals such as iron and copper serving to catalyze or promote the oxidation. Consequently, the use of compounds such as the antioxidants which segregate the trace metals is necessary to retard or reduce the rate of oxidation.

Tocopherols

The presence in natural fats of minute amounts of compounds which protect them from oxidation has been recognized for a long time. However, the identity of all of these compounds is still not entirely known. The first compounds identified that possessed antioxidant properties were the tocopherols, the vitamins E. Four different tocopherols (α, β, γ, δ) occur naturally, and are readily oxidized and thereby protect fats and oils from oxidation (ILSI-NF, 1984e). Other naturally occurring antioxidants include ascorbic acid, erythorbic acid, citric acid and lecithin. Since tocopherols are naturally occurring as a form of vitamin E, few standard toxicity studies have been conducted on these compounds.

Tocopherols are approved for use in the US as antioxidants and nutrient supplements in non-alcoholic beverages, herbs, seeds, spices, seasonings, blends, extracts and flavorings. α-Tocopherol is also used to inhibit nitrosamine formation in pump-cured bacon. Tocopherols are also cleared for the purpose of retarding rancidity development in rendered animal fat (ILSI-NF, 1984e).

In addition to the naturally occurring tocopherols, several compounds have been developed synthetically that have very good antioxidant properties. Two classes of antioxidants are widely favored for many commercial uses; these are phenols and their derivatives and amines and their derivatives.

Of the many synthetic compounds with antioxidant properties, this chapter will discuss only BHT, BHA, the gallates and tertiary butylhydroquinone, which are the most widely used antioxidants in food (Andres, 1985). Sometimes antioxidants show a synergistic effect; two antioxidants may be more effective than would be expected from the sum of their activities. BHA and BHT are frequently combined with other antioxidants.

Although extensive evaluation and research work was performed before approval of the antioxidants, scientists and regulators continue to evaluate them.

BHT

Butylated hydroxytoluene (BHT) was first evaluated by JECFA in 1961 (WHO/FAO, 1962). JECFA concluded that a temporary ADI of 0–0·5 mg/kg body weight could be established and requested further long-term studies, with particular reference to the effect of BHT on lipid metabolism and the relationship between the dietary fat load and toxicity. They also requested metabolic studies in humans.

Subsequently, reproduction studies in a variety of species, including non-human primates, indicated effects on the offspring (decreased body weight of pups) at dose levels above 1000 mg/kg in the diet. Mutagenicity studies showed conflicting results. The results of lifetime feeding studies in mice showed a significant and dose-related increase in lung tumors in one experiment, but in another study the increase was not dose-related. Also, in three rat studies no increase in tumors was found. On the basis of these results, JECFA concluded that there was no indication that BHT was carcinogenic. Therefore, in 1983 JECFA reconfirmed the temporary ADI of 0–0·5 mg/kg body weight for BHT (sum of BHT, BHA and TBHQ) (WHO/FAO, 1983). In 1986, JECFA established a temporary ADI of 0–0·125 mg/kg body weight for BHT alone (WHO/FAO, 1986), due to additional studies as reported below.

In a study conducted in Denmark by Olsen and co-workers (1983), increased incidence of hepatocellular carcinomas in males and hepato-cellular adenomas in both sexes of the F_1 generation rats at a dose level of 250 mg/kg body weight was observed. No increase in tumor incidence was found at the lower dose levels (25 and 100 mg/kg body weight). An interesting observation in this study was that no tumors were seen before 111 weeks, the usual termination point for the other long-term studies, and survival of the controls was markedly poorer than that of the high dose group.

Studies on promotion and inhibition of carcinogenesis indicate that BHT, like other antioxidants, can exert both promoter and inhibitor activity depending on the time of administration (in relation to the administration of the carcinogen), the type of carcinogen and the target organ affected (ILSI-NF, 1984b).

BHA

Another antioxidant that is widely used is butylated hydroxyanisole (BHA). This antioxidant, which is chemically similar to BHT, was first evaluated by JECFA in 1962 (WHO/FAO, 1962). In 1983 JECFA decided to retain the temporary ADI of 0–0·5 mg/kg body weight (sum of BHA, BHT and TBHQ) (WHO/FAO, 1983), although studies performed by Ito and co-workers in Japan indicated that BHA induced the formation of tumors in the forestomach of rats when BHA was fed at a high level (Ito, 1982; Ito et al., 1982, 1983, 1985). (These and other studies are described in detail in a following chapter.) The publication of Ito's study led to the formation of the Four Nation Working Group composed of representatives from the US, Japan, the United Kingdom and Canada (FDA, 1982a). This group examined all the available data and concluded that there was insufficient evidence to require a ban on BHA. However, additional information on the mechanism of hyperplasia in the rat forestomach and studies performed in animals without a forestomach were requested.

Since the initial finding by Ito, additional studies on mutagenicity and carcinogenicity have been conducted. Studies by Williams and co-workers (1984) have demonstrated that BHA is not genotoxic, and studies by Clayson and co-workers (Iverson et al., 1985a, b) have shown that animals such as the cynomolgus monkey which has no forestomach do not develop hyperplasia as a result of the ingestion of BHA. Unpublished feeding studies using BHA in the diet of dogs sponsored by the US FDA are also negative (ILSI–NF, 1984a). Studies in the rat and hamster by Grünow (1984) and Altmann and co-workers (1985) have shown that the effects are reversible in animals with a forestomach.

In addition, Ito repeated his earlier study in the rat using dose levels of 2·0, 1·0, 0·5% and control animals. This study produced a clear dose response with the NOEL at 0·5%.

In summary, a variety of studies with different animal species has been carried out to elucidate the mechanism of tumor formation in the rat forestomach. It is clear from these studies that BHA causes tumor formation in animals with a forestomach. Altmann and co-workers (1985) reported a NOEL in rats of 0·125% BHA in the diet. Effects, such as hyperplasia and hyperkeratosis, are reversible, but the recovery period is long. The longer the exposure to BHA and the higher the dose level, the longer the recovery period. The esophagus is not affected.

The same changes were induced in the forestomachs of hamsters (Ito et al., 1984) and mice. However, in the dog and monkey (animals without a forestomach) no effects were seen; no esophageal involvement was observed.

From the currently available results it is likely that the effect of BHA is species-specific, and that animals without a forestomach are not susceptible to the effect. This fact suggests that the finding in rodents is not relevant to humans. However, in 1986 JECFA established a temporary ADI of 0–0·3 mg/kg body weight for BHA alone (WHO/FAO, 1986).

In addition, a number of studies have been carried out to determine the interaction of BHA with known carcinogens. BHA has been shown to have both inhibitory and promotional effects on tumor yield resulting from treatment with known carcinogens (McCormick et al., 1984).

Gallates

Another class of antioxidants is the gallates which include propyl, octyl and dodecyl gallate. Propyl gallate was approved in the US in 1947 for use as an antioxidant (ILSI-NF, 1984c). JECFA in 1961 established a temporary group ADI of 0–0·2 mg/kg body weight for propyl, octyl and dodecyl gallate (WHO/FAO, 1962). This group ADI was reconfirmed and made permanent in 1980 (WHO/FAO, 1980). However, in 1986 JECFA reconsidered the gallates and did not assign ADIs for dodecyl and octyl gallate due to insufficient information, and established an ADI of 0–2·5 mg/kg body weight for propyl gallate (WHO/FAO, 1986). The EEC Scientific Committee for Food established an ADI of 0–0·2 mg/kg body weight as the sum of propyl, octyl and dodecyl gallate (CEC, 1976).

TBHQ

Tertiary butylhydroquinone (TBHQ) was approved by FDA in 1972 for retarding the development of rancid flavors and odor in many highly unstable unsaturated fats. It is approved for use alone or in combination with BHA and/or BHT (ILSI-NF, 1984d). In 1975 JECFA established a temporary ADI of 0–0·75 mg/kg body weight for TBHQ (WHO/FAO, 1976a), and in 1977 the ADI was made permanent at a level of 0–0·5 mg/kg body weight (WHO/FAO, 1978). However, in 1986 JECFA lowered the ADI to a temporary value of 0–0·2 mg/kg body weight (WHO/FAO, 1986). TBHQ is not permitted in the EEC countries because the SCF concluded that the available toxicity data are inadequate to meet today's standards.

Sweeteners

Alternatives to sucrose and other carbohydrate sweeteners are being used increasingly in the food supply. Compounds which provide sweetness without requiring insulin for their metabolism are useful for individuals with diabetes mellitus. The so-called 'intense sweeteners' contribute no or minimal calories to the diet, either because they are not metabolized or because they are used in foods in minute amounts. In addition, many of these sweeteners are not utilized to any great extent by oral bacteria, and can therefore be considered non-cariogenic.

Polyol Sweeteners

'Bulk sweeteners' are those with a sweetness intensity similar to sucrose. Examples are the polyol sweeteners (mannitol, lactitol, maltitol, sorbitol and xylitol). In comparison with other food additives, they are quantitatively significant components of food, and have been used in candies, jams, jellies, chewing gum, baked goods and frozen dairy desserts.

The polyol sweeteners provide an example of somewhat unique issues in food safety evaluation, both in terms of testing protocols and 'adverse effects'. The 'adverse effects' produced by some of the polyol sweeteners are flatulence and laxation. They are incompletely absorbed from the intestine, which may result in an osmotic diarrhea. The amount of sweetener necessary to produce this effect varies with the type of sweetener, whether it is consumed in a bolus or spread throughout the day, the length of time since the previous meal, and individual differences in susceptibility. Sensitive individuals may experience the laxative effect after ingesting 10 g of the compound, while others can tolerate 90 g without adverse effects. The majority of individuals are affected after consuming about 50 g (Allison, 1979). Young children tend to be more susceptible because they weigh less than older children or adults. The nature of this adverse effect is clearly different from most other end points of safety assessment.

The incorporation of inherently non-toxic substances into experimental diets at maximum tolerated doses in an attempt to establish a dose–response relationship may produce dietary imbalances which may affect the interpretation of the data. Thus, the safety of dietary components such as bulk sweeteners cannot be evaluated in the same manner as additives which are present in foods at the ppm level. As additional modified food ingredients are introduced, the experimental approaches to safety evaluation will have to be developed and verified.

Scientific and regulatory review of the safety data on polyol sweeteners has led to their approval by many agencies. The EEC has given 'acceptable' evaluations to lactitol, maltitol, mannitol, sorbitol and xylitol (CEC, 1985). No ADI has been set, because the polyols cannot be evaluated in animal feeding studies at the level traditionally desired. The EEC has stated that laxation may be observed, but that 20 g/day is unlikely to cause symptoms.

Xylitol and sorbitol are permitted in the United States. Xylitol is permitted in foods for special dietary use (Code of Federal Regulations, 1985b), and sorbitol has been affirmed as a GRAS (generally recognized as safe) substance, with limits on permitted levels in specific foods. In the US, the label of foods whose consumption may result in a daily intake of 50 g or more of sorbitol must bear the statement 'Excess consumption may have a laxative effect' (Code of Federal Regulations, 1985d).

Sorbitol is approved for use in Japan, within the limits of good manufacturing practice. JECFA has assigned a temporary ADI of 50 mg/ kg body weight for mannitol (WHO/FAO, 1976b). The ADI for xylitol and sorbitol is not specified (WHO/FAO, 1983). JECFA recommends that national authorities consider the potential laxative effect when making decisions about the use of polyol sweeteners.

Intense sweeteners make no significant contribution to food bulk, because they are used in very low levels to achieve the desired technical effect. They can be tested in a traditional safety evaluation protocol.

Cyclamate

Cyclamate is a sweetener which has undergone extensive testing, and for which different regulatory bodies have reached different conclusions about its safety for humans. It was approved by the US FDA in 1951, and placed on the GRAS list in 1961. In 1969, preliminary results of a carcinogenicity study (Price et al., 1970) were released. Although the experimental design and results of the study generated extensive scientific debate, FDA banned all uses of cyclamate in food in 1970, using the general safety standard as the basis for its decision (although the FDA Commissioner referred to the Delaney clause in announcing the ban) (FDA, 1969a). A petition to reapprove the sweetener was submitted in 1973, and in 1980 the FDA upheld its ban, concluding that cyclamate had not been shown *not* to cause cancer or heritable genetic damage (FDA, 1980). Another petition was submitted in 1982, citing new evidence for its safety, and in 1984 the Center for Food Safety and Applied Nutrition's Cancer Assessment Committee (CAC) concluded that cyclamate was not a carcinogen and that no newly discovered toxic effects would likely be revealed by additional studies (FDA, 1984). In order to confirm their evaluation, FDA contracted with the National Academy of Sciences (NAS) to review the data and the CAC's conclusions. (This is an example of the increasing use by regulatory agencies of third party review groups.)

The NAS Committee on the Evaluation of Cyclamate for Carcino-genicity, in its report (NAS/NRC, 1985), agreed that cyclamate and its major metabolite cyclohexylamine (CHA) are not carcinogenic, but it recommended additional work on cyclamate's possible co-carcinogenic or 'promoting' effect. It also recommended further studies to detect possible DNA damage and gene mutation.

The studies which the committee cited as suggesting promotion activity (Hicks et al., 1975; Hicks and Chowaniec, 1977) have not been replicated in other laboratories (Green et al., 1980). FDA scientists have stated that attempting to include promotional effects in testing protocols is fraught with difficulty. Promoters may be organ-, species-, and chemical-specific; the permutations and combinations of tests required for comprehensive safety evaluation number in the tens of thousands. This situation clearly poses a problem for regulatory agencies. FDA has commissioned a review of the broad questions related to bladder promotion studies. In order to address the mutagenicity question raised by the committee (even though the vast majority of the tests already done have been negative), FDA proposed that the petitioner sponsor additional tests. These tests have been completed and were negative.

Another question raised about cyclamate (but not addressed by the NAS committee) is the evidence that high doses of CHA produce testicular atrophy in rats (Oser *et al.*, 1976), an effect not observed in mice (Hardy *et al.*, 1976). Cyclamate is metabolized in the gut by intestinal microflora to CHA. Cyclamate feeding studies in humans have demonstrated that conversion to CHA does not occur at a constant rate. The degree of conversion depends on the individual, with over 80% of the population converting less than 1% of ingested cyclamate to CHA. Only about 10% of the population will convert more than 1% of ingested cyclamate to CHA (Renwick, 1985). Regardless of the CHA production rate, it is clear that CHA is responsible for the testicular atrophy observed in rats given doses of 200 mg/kg body weight/day of the metabolite. In addition, data from recent studies suggest that the rat metabolizes CHA differently from man and the mouse (Roberts and Renwick, 1985*b*). In any event, regulatory agencies have considered the testicular effect when evaluating cyclamate's safety.

The EEC (CEC, 1985) and JECFA have established an ADI (temporary and permanent, respectively) for cyclamate at 0–11 mg/kg body weight (expressed as cyclamic acid) (WHO/FAO, 1982). This value is based on a rat study which showed a NOEL of 100 mg/kg body weight with respect to testicular atrophy. Should further research demonstrate that testicular atrophy is not relevant to humans, the ADI levels may be increased.

Cyclamate is an approved food additive in 34 countries, as a tabletop sweetener and/or a food ingredient. Its regulatory fate in the US is still uncertain, but most observers expect that it will eventually be reapproved by the FDA.

Saccharin

Like cyclamate, saccharin has had a stormy regulatory history. Discovered in 1879, it has been subject to scientific scrutiny ever since. The FDA banned it in 1912, but the ban was lifted during World War I when sugar supplies were low. In 1977, FDA again proposed to ban saccharin, citing studies in which high doses were associated with bladder tumors in male rats. FDA invoked the Delaney clause as the basis for the ban (FDA, 1977b).

Because saccharin was the only artificial sweetener approved for use in the US in 1977, the public outcry against the ban was loud and clear. Congress intervened and passed the Saccharin Study and Labeling Act, which has since been referred to as the 'moratorium'. This act prohibited the FDA from banning saccharin for 18 months, required that all products containing it carry a warning label stating that saccharin causes cancer in laboratory animals, and mandated (1) additional research on saccharin, (2) a study on its health benefits, and (3) a study of US regulatory policy. Since the original passage of the 'moratorium', Congress has extended it three times, most recently to May 1, 1987.

About 200 studies on saccharin have been published since 1977. A rat-feeding study conducted by the International Research and Development Corporation (IRDC) indicated that a dose–response relationship existed at levels of 3% or greater. The NOEL for carcinogenicity was 1% saccharin (Schoenig et al., 1985). Based on these results, an expert panel convened to evaluate the IRDC study concluded that the present level of exposure to saccharin through its use as a food additive is unlikely to present a cancer risk to humans (Saccharin Report, 1985).

Another recent study was conducted by the National Center for Toxicological Research (NCTR) in the United States. NCTR examined the potential promoting effect of saccharin when a known carcinogen, N-methyl-N-nitrosourea, was applied directly to the bladders of experimental rats. A dose–response effect was observed, although there were inconsistent results at the highest saccharin dose (5% of the diet) (West et al., 1986).

Because saccharin has been used for more than 80 years, many epidemiological studies to determine whether saccharin use is associated with bladder cancer have been done. Most studies have been negative. In 1979, the National Cancer Institute (NCI) completed the most extensive epidemiological study ever conducted, using a population group of about 9000 individuals. NCI concluded that artificial sweetener consumption (both cyclamate and saccharin, since frequently they had been used in combination) was not associated with bladder cancer in the general population (Hoover and Strasser, 1980). However, the study identified some groups as being at higher risk, although the possibility that these latter associations represented chance variations could not be ruled out.

The biological effects of saccharin are species-, sex- and dose-related.

Studies are currently being conducted to elucidate the mechanism of saccharin's effect on the rat urothelium. Preliminary results suggest that the sodium salt of saccharin exerts a unique effect, since the calcium salt and acid saccharin produce different biological effects (Hasegawa and Cohen, 1986). Preliminary results indicate the effect of saccharin is nonspecific and is related to changes in the physiologic milieu of the urothelium. These profound biochemical and physiological changes do not occur at levels consumed by man (Roberts and Renwick, 1985a).

JECFA and the EEC have set a temporary ADI for saccharin at 0–2·5 mg/kg body weight (WHO/FAO, 1984; CEC, 1985). Some of the countries around the world which permit its use in foods, soft drinks and as a tabletop sweetener are Australia, Austria, Federal Republic of Germany, Ireland, Italy, Japan, New Zealand, Norway, the Philippines, Sweden, Switzerland, the United Kingdom, and the United States. Other countries limit its use to selected categories. In all, 65 countries allow the use of saccharin, at least in one of the applications.

Extraction Solvents
Solvents and gases (unintentional food additives) are used in food processing for a variety of purposes. Some are used solely as extraction solvents or as carrier solvents; however, many solvents serve dual functions. Solvents used only for extraction purposes are typified by the chlorinated hydrocarbons such as dichloromethane. Their main application is the extraction of fats and oils from fish and other meals and for the decaffeination of coffee and tea. Once they have fulfilled their function, they are removed from the final product. The use of carrier solvents extends mainly to dissolving and dispersing a wide variety of food ingredients, e.g. nutrients, antioxidants and flavoring substances. Carrier solvents may occur at higher levels in food than extraction solvents.

In assessing the risk for consumers from the low levels of solvents in food, some of the toxicological issues that should be considered are the toxicity of the solvent residues themselves and the toxicity of impurities, additives and stabilizers.

In 1981 the EEC attempted to harmonize the use of extraction solvents, and the SCF was asked to evaluate the relevant toxicological issues (CEC, 1981). The SCF took the approach of classifying solvents into three categories: (1) when toxicological data provide a more than ample margin of safety or when consideration of the points listed above raises no concern, limitation of residues to the minimum levels attainable with appropriate technology appears to be an adequate safeguard for the health of the consumer; (2) when the results of the toxicological information are such that limitations are required for reasons of safety, it was considered appropriate to establish an ADI, or discourage the use of the substance; (3) when the available information was adequate to support continued use in food on a temporary basis, and no hazard to health was considered to arise from this use, additional studies have been required to permit a re-evaluation within a certain time period.

In their review, SCF evaluated 42 solvents of different classes: gases used as extraction solvents such as propane, butane, carbon dioxide and nitrous oxide; alcohols; hydrocarbon solvents such as cyclohexane, light petroleum and toluene; ethers; aldehydes; ketones; halogenated hydro-carbon solvents such as chloroform, carbon tetrachloride, trichloro-ethylene, dichloromethane and freon; and esters.

In considering these compounds, two groups of compounds were of major concern: the hydrocarbons, especially 2-nitropropane, and the halogenated hydrocarbons. All the others were acceptable or could be classified. In many cases an ADI was established, or a status of 'temporarily acceptable' was given, with the requirement to provide additional information (CEC, 1981).

The hydrocarbon solvent 2-nitropropane was considered not acceptable because the compound produced hepatocellular carcinomas in rats after exposure for 6 months by inhalation. The halogenated hydrocarbon solvents (chloroform, 1,2-dichloroethane, carbon tetrachloride, *cis* and *trans* 1,2-dichloroethylene) were considered not acceptable. The first three of the halogenated hydrocarbon compounds were considered unaccept-able because of conflicting results concerning carcinogenicity. The two dichloroethylene isomers were considered unacceptable due to lack of toxicological data, and because the substances are suspected of carcinogenic properties.

Dichloromethane (methylene chloride) was considered temporarily acceptable, because the available toxicological evidence was insufficient to establish an ADI. Based on available data, the SCF concluded that residues in the food as consumed should not exceed 10 mg/kg food (CEC, 1981).

Data provided by a recent NTP inhalation bioassay demonstrated that methylene chloride is a carcinogen in mice and rats (FDA, 1985*b*). A dose-dependent increase in liver and lung adenomas and carcinomas was induced in mice. Methylene chloride also produced a dose-related increase in mammary gland fibroadenomas, and subcutaneous fibromas were induced. The tumors observed in the NTP bioassay are consistent with the types of tumors observed in several other carcinogenicity studies of methylene chloride. Two epidemiological studies of workers in plants using the solvent were insufficient to assess cancer mortality. Mutagenicity data indicate that the solvent has the potential of inducing gene mutations in exposed human cells.

Methylene chloride is metabolized into metabolically active intermediates which are theoretically capable of combining with DNA and other cellular macromolecules. There is evidence that at high dose levels the metabolic pathway may become saturated. More studies are necessary to elucidate its metabolism in different animal species before a conclusion can be drawn about the carcinogenic potential of methylene chloride. When considering the use of methylene chloride as an extraction solvent in foods, a risk assessment may give some guidance about consumer risk.

The US FDA proposed in December 1985 that the *de minimis* policy be applied to methylene chloride in decaffeinated coffee (FDA, 1985b). The agency's risk assessment resulted in a calculated risk between one in 1 million and one in 100 million. Given such a low level of risk, FDA concluded that there would be no harm to the public from this use of methylene chloride.

Sulfiting Agents

Sulfiting agents present an interesting case for regulatory agencies, because they are compounds which present a known medical risk to a subset of the population but are safe for the vast majority. The issue has received high visibility primarily in the US.

Sulfiting agents make a significant contribution to the stability of the food supply. In their various forms, they are used in foods and beverages as antimicrobial agents, antioxidants, to control both enzymatic and non-enzymatic browning reactions, and as enzyme inhibitors.

Until July 1986 the US FDA listed sulfiting agents (sulfur dioxide, potassium bisulfite, potassium metabisulfate, sodium sulfite, sodium bisulfite, sodium metabisulfite) as GRAS (generally recognized as safe) substances, except for meats or other foods that are significant dietary sources of thiamin (Code Fed. Reg., 1985c). Except for potassium bisulfite, they are also permitted in the EEC, which also allows the use of calcium sulfite and calcium bisulfite. JECFA has established an ADI of 0–0·7 mg/kg body weight, expressed as SO_2 (WHO/FAO, 1974a).

In 1982, the FDA proposed to affirm the GRAS status of potassium metabisulfite, sodium bisulfite, sodium metabisulfite and sulfur dioxide, while proposing not to affirm the use of potassium bisulfite and sodium sulfite as GRAS (FDA, 1982e). Following the publication of this proposal, additional information became available, and the issues were re-examined by the Federation of American Societies for Experimental Biology (FASEB) Ad Hoc Panel on Reexamination of the GRAS Status of Sulfiting Agents. On the basis of their review, the panel concluded, while sulfiting agents presented no hazard for the majority of the population: 'For the fraction of the public that is sulfite sensitive, there is evidence in the available information . . . that demonstrates or suggests reasonable grounds to suspect a hazard of unpredictable severity to such individuals when they are exposed to sulfiting agents in some foods at levels that are now current and in the manner now practiced' (FASEB, 1985).

The medical and scientific issues surrounding sulfiting agents have been reviewed recently by Walker (1985) and Emerson and Johnson (1985). Briefly, sulfiting agents are clearly implicated in the induction of asthmatic attacks in sensitive individuals. Several sulfite-related deaths have been reported, and were associated with the consumption of restaurant food (particularly fruits and vegetables from the salad bar) that had been treated with sulfites. Of the non-fatal reactions that have been reported to the FDA, 80% were associated with restaurant foods, with the remainder related to consumption of packaged foods in the home. As a consequence of the pattern of reported adverse reactions, the US National Restaurant Association in 1983 requested its members to discontinue the use of sulfites at the retail level.

Original estimates of the population at risk for adverse reactions were placed at 5–10% of the 10 million asthmatics in the US (Simon et al., 1982). However, Taylor (1985) suggests that sulfite sensitivity is limited to 5–10% of the steroid-dependent asthmatic patients, bringing the overall sensitivity rate to 1–2% of the total asthmatic population. The response may also vary depending on the route of sulfite administration (Allen, 1985; Schwartz and Chester, 1984; Walker, 1985). Additional work must be done to define more accurately the at-risk population.

On the basis of the conclusions of the FASEB Ad Hoc Review Panel, in July 1986 the FDA published a regulation clarifying the circumstances under which the presence of sulfiting agents must be declared on the label of packaged foods (FDA, 1986c). Prior to this the law required that, when sulfiting agents are added to perform a specific technical effect, they must be declared on the ingredient label as 'intentional additives'. The purpose of the new regulation was to provide standards for the identification of sulfiting agents when they are present as 'unintentional additives', i.e. those which are present as 'carry-over' from other, intentional additives. In the regulation, FDA clarified its position that *any* detectable amount of sulfiting agent is 'significant', and must be declared, effective January 9, 1987. The detectable amount was defined as 10 ppm or greater, based on the Monier–Williams (AOAC) method of analysis (AOAC, 1984).

The use of an analytical method, rather than a biological parameter, to determine an 'insignificant' amount, has been questioned. First, the Monier–Williams method does not distinguish between free and bound sulfites. This is a critical point, because it is only the free sulfite that has been related to adverse reactions. In addition, the quantitative sensitivity of the accepted method may not be appropriate for all foods. Moreover, the amount of food consumed is not considered.

Secondly, Taylor has reported that foods with residual sulfite levels of less than 100 ppm seem unlikely to produce adverse reactions. Thus, he has suggested that the amount which triggers ingredient labeling should be increased from 10 to 25 or 50 ppm (Taylor, 1985). This solution would still serve the primary objective of alerting sensitive individuals to the presence of sulfites.

In July 1986 FDA published a regulation which revoked the GRAS status of sulfiting agents for use on fruits and vegetables sold or served raw (FDA, 1986*d*). FDA is still expected to publish a separate proposal regarding the GRAS status of the use of sulfites in potatoes and other foods.

The use of sulfites as food preservatives must be given careful thought by regulatory agencies. Sulfite sensitivity is a medical problem, one for which there are still many unanswered questions. Sulfite-sensitive individuals would be best served by regulations that reflect biological thresholds rather than mere analytical capabilities, and those that do not require the identification of sulfites in foods that in fact pose no risk.

Colors

Colors are substances added to foods and beverages to impart, preserve or enhance the color or shading of a food.

As a condition for continued provisional listing of the certified color additives, in February 1977 the US FDA set a closing date of January 31, 1981, for submission of data from chronic toxicity studies (FDA, 1977*a*). FDA required these new studies because the older toxicity studies (prior to 1977) that had been submitted in support of listing the color additives were deficient in light of the contemporary, more rigorous scientific standards that had since evolved.

The chronic testing of the key food colors that the FDA required in 1977 is now complete (Pearce and Hume, 1983). FDA has issued final rules on

14 of the 23 color additives that were the subject of the 1981 order. The remaining colors (including food, drug and cosmetic colors) have not received final approval due to objections by consumer groups, and the closing dates for these color additives have been extended to permit time to resolve the issues. Of the 9 color additives pending court decisions, 3 are food color additives: FD&C Blue No. 2, FD&C Red No. 3 and FD&C Yellow No. 6.

FD&C Blue No. 2 (Indigotine) was the subject of a hearing on a challenge by the Health Research Group (a consumer activist group) to FDA's final rule for its permanent listing. In early 1983 FDA published a final ruling proposing the permanent listing of Blue No. 2 (FDA, 1983). However, the Health Research Group filed objections and requested a hearing, stating that the long-term feeding study in rats does not support a finding that Blue No. 2 is safe, and that the brain gliomas observed in the high dose (2%) Blue No. 2 male rats were treatment-related. The FDA commissioner had ruled that, taken as a whole, there was no evidence to support any conclusion other than that FD&C Blue No. 2 has been shown not to be a carcinogen and that the increased number of tumors among male rats in the high dose group was not related to treatment. The administrative law judge upheld the FDA commissioner's conclusion. The final rule is still pending.

In the chronic studies on FD&C Red No. 3 (Erythrosine), there was an increased incidence of thyroid follicular cell carcinomas, adenomas and hyperplasia in male rats that were fed at the highest (4·0%) dose level. It has been asserted that these tumors were the result of a secondary mechanism and thus were not caused by Red No. 3. The results of new short-term tests suggest that iodine released by the color additive causes thyroid hormone imbalances that lead to an increased incidence of tumors. The evidence also suggests that when the color is ingested at lower levels the hormone levels are not affected and tumors are not induced.

The FDA commissioner has asked a color additives scientific review panel to evaluate the available data and other information. The report of this panel has been completed and is being peer reviewed by a number of non-panel scientists. In order to allow time to make a reasoned evaluation and decision on the safety of this color additive, the closing date for Red No. 3 has been extended until November 3, 1987 (FDA, 1986e). However, FDA has stated that perhaps only a new chronic study will resolve the secondary mechanism issue. In that case, FDA is prepared to extend the provisional listing of Red No. 3 for 6 years beyond the closing date to permit the necessary testing, if an interested party agrees to sponsor the research.

Chronic studies in both mice and rats were conducted using FD&C Yellow No. 6 (Sunset Yellow FCF). Based on the results of the chronic mouse toxicity study, FDA determined that Yellow No. 6 is not carcinogenic to Charles River CD-1 mice. However, the chronic toxicity/ carcinogenicity study in Sprague-Dawley rats revealed an increased incidence of renal tubular adenomas in female rats that received 5·0% Yellow No. 6 in the diet for 28 months following *in utero* exposure. There was also a dose-related increase in the incidence and severity of chronic nephropathy and tubular mineralization in these rats.

FDA requested NTP to conduct a peer review on Yellow No. 6. NTP completed its review in January 1986, and concluded that Yellow No. 6 is not a carcinogen.

On November 19, 1986 FDA published a regulation which would permanently list FD&C Yellow No. 6 and at the same time require its presence to be listed in the ingredient statement by November 19, 1987 (FDA, 1986a). Objections to the labeling requirement were filed, and FDA announced a postponement of the closing date until April 6, 1987 (FDA, 1987). This announcement had the effect of staying the final rule permanently listing this color additive and the labeling requirement.

FD&C Yellow No. 5 was permanently listed for food and drug use in 1969 (FDA, 1969b), and its labeling was required on food and drugs from July 1, 1981 (FDA, 1979): the first color required to be labeled in the US. The continued listing of FD&C Yellow No. 5 was not questioned due to problems of safety but was related to the specifications, namely, that the proposed specified method for detecting trace level impurities was not ready for use in the ppb range. On October 30, 1986 FDA confirmed the effective date for two final rules that amended the color additive regulations on the use of FD&C Yellow No. 5 (FDA, 1986f). One of these final rules affected a small change in the identity of FD&C Yellow No. 5 in the regulation listing this color additive for use in externally applied drugs and cosmetics (FDA, 1986g). The other final rule amended the identity and specifications in the listings of FD&C Yellow No. 5 for use in food and ingested drugs (FDA, 1986g).

All four of these food color additives have been given ADIs by JECFA and the SCF (WHO/FAO, 1965, 1974b, 1982, 1984; CEC, 1983). They are all permitted in the EEC countries and many other countries throughout the world (CEC, 1983; Parker, 1984).

Flavorings
Flavorings are chemical substances added to food to impart or help impart a taste or aroma. They can be natural, artificial or nature-identical

(synthetic compounds which are found in natural and traditional foods consumed by man). However, the concept of nature-identical is not recognized in the US. Natural and artificial flavoring substances are regulated by positive lists found in 21CFR 172, 182 and 189 (Code Fed. Regulations, 1985a).

After the FDA published the Generally Recognized as Safe (GRAS) list, the Flavor and Extract Manufacturers Association (FEMA) took the initiative for evaluating flavoring substances. FEMA established a panel of non-industry scientists who have subsequently published 14 FEMA GRAS Lists on Flavorings. In addition to the names of the flavorings, these lists also contain their uses and use levels. The FDA has expressed both explicit and tacit approval of the decisions of the FEMA expert panel. Information on safety of the artificial flavorings has been published in the form of Scientific Literature Reviews (SLRs). This type of safety evaluation has been based primarily on chemical structure of flavorings and existing knowledge about toxicity and metabolic pathways.

In the US, a committee of FASEB has been retained to establish criteria to judge the safety of flavoring materials. This committee is known as the Select Committee on Flavor Evaluation Criteria (SCOFEC). To determine use levels of flavorings in the US, the National Academy of Sciences/ National Research Council (NAS/NRC) sponsored a survey of the entire user industry. Information resulting from this survey is published (NRC, 1979, 1982).

That the safety evaluation of flavoring substances is different from the safety evaluation of food additives in general has been recognized by JECFA, which stated in its 17th report (WHO/FAO, 1974a) that the problem of evaluating flavoring substances is one that cannot be solved simply by adopting the procedures traditionally used to evaluate other types of food additives. In its 20th report, JECFA considered the vast number of flavoring substances and agreed to establish an order of priority for their evaluation (WHO/FAO, 1976b). Among the factors to be considered in proposing priorities for flavoring substances, the most important are the following:

— the total amount of each substance likely to be consumed by the average person;
— the similarity of the chemical structure with that of substances of known toxicological and biochemical properties;
— the nature and source of the substance.

FEMA, the International Organization of the Flavor Industry (IOFI) (1976), and the British Extract Manufacturers' Association have sponsored 90-day studies on several artificial flavoring substances which are representative of categories or groups of flavorings. None of these testing programs overlaps. The reason for testing representative samples from groups of similar flavorings is that it would take too long and be too costly to test every single flavoring substance. Instead, some priority setting is needed to handle the enormous numbers (several thousands) of synthetic flavorings.

An approach to priority setting of flavorings has been suggested by Cramer and co-workers (1978). This would involve using the FEMA 'decision tree' (series of decisions to be made on a compound based on structure, metabolism and toxicity), the ratio of the average quantitative intake of a flavoring material as a component of natural and traditional foods with the average intake of the same material as a food additive [the consumption ratio (CR)] (Stofberg and Kirschman, 1985), and the Red Book approach (described earlier in this chapter). Since most flavorings used by the food industry today occur widely in natural and traditional foods, a high CR means that the priority ranking for testing these flavorings should be no higher than that for testing the complete foods in which they occur.

IOFI is also active in the field of flavor regulation and safety evaluation of flavoring substances, and has adopted the mixed or combined system approach (IOFI, 1976). According to this scheme, any substance which occurs naturally in the diet may be used unless explicitly prohibited or restricted (restrictive list), whereas substances not yet found to occur in the human diet may not be used unless explicitly permitted (positive list). These restrictive and positive lists are enforceable by regulatory agencies because the number of substances listed is limited and their properties are known. Analytical methods for their determination are for the most part available.

In the area of public health, a Council of Europe *ad hoc* working party on flavors has published a 'blue' book containing a list of flavoring substances and their sources (Council of Europe, 1981). This list is not legally binding on any member state, but the book has received widespread attention. A fourth edition of this book is being developed.

The EEC has also drafted a proposed flavoring directive which, when finalized, will be binding on the member states. In its present form, the directive provides for the following classifications of flavors: (1) natural; (2) nature-identical; (3) artificial; (4) process flavoring; and (5) smoked flavoring. However, the commission does not feel that the term nature-identical is appropriate for labeling purposes. For labeling of flavorings not intended for sale to the final consumer, the categories of flavorings present have to be listed in order of the proportion by weight which each category contributes to the total. The word 'natural' can only be used for flavorings containing exclusively natural materials. When 'nature-identical' or 'artificial' flavorings are present, the label must read 'flavoring'.

The overall concept of the directive is a positive list for everything, including: artificial flavorings, nature-identical flavorings, source materials for the production of natural flavorings, lists of additives necessary for the production and storage of flavorings, lists of products used for dissolving and diluting, and of processing aids and extraction solvents. However, it has become evident that such lists are extremely difficult to compile, and if only substances with a full safety testing profile are on the list then it would be far too short to benefit the food industry. This directive is still being discussed.

In the US, flavorings are beginning to be included in the National Toxicology Program (NTP) bioassay program and in the National Cancer Institute (NCI) program. Since there are thousands of flavorings, priority setting for their evaluation is a crucial issue, one that must be resolved before any large-scale testing is undertaken.

CONCLUSION

The regulation of food additives is a complex process, and includes both scientific and legal considerations. Requirements for testing protocols are generally similar in the US, Japan, the EEC and JECFA, but minor differences do exist. Similarly, regulatory agencies and other bodies concerned with food additives may reach different conclusions about the data generated by toxicological studies.

The US FDA's experience with the Delaney clause is an example of how legal statutes can affect safety assessment. Although other countries and international bodies are appropriately quite sensitive to concerns about the carcinogenicity of food additives, no other jurisdiction in the world has adopted an absolute legal prohibition like that embodied in the Delaney clause. On the contrary, elsewhere in the world scientists and regulatory officials have some flexibility in their approach to assessing the human safety of chemical substances that induce tumors in animals.

In the future, more attention will be paid to functionality and tech-nological need of food additives. There is a tendency among regulatory agencies to minimize the number of food additives approved for each functional effect. However, many scientists believe that, if more than one food additive were available for each functional category, the daily intake of each food additive would decrease and the risk of exceeding the ADI for that additive would be minimized. Regulatory agencies will continue to require that food additives be adequately tested to ensure that public health is protected.

There is a great need to harmonize both the requirements for safety testing and the interpretation of toxicological data. Movement toward harmonization depends on the recognition that absolute safety can never be guaranteed, and that data from animals challenged with very high doses of a test substance may not be relevant to human exposure. Recent efforts to achieve international harmonization are encouraging, but more progress must be made if we are to have a food supply which is considered 'safe' in all countries around the world.

REFERENCES

Allen, D. H. (1985). Asthma induced by sulphites. *Food Technol.* (Australia), **37**, 506–7.

Allison, R. G. (1979). *Dietary Sugars in Health and Disease, III. Sorbitol*, Life Sciences Research Office, FASEB, Bethesda, Maryland.

Altmann, H. J., Wester, P. W., Matthiaschk, G., Grünow, W. and van der Heijden, C. A. (1985). Induction of early lesions in the forestomach of rats by 3-tert-butyl-4-hydroxyanisole (BHA). *Food Chem. Toxicol.*, **23**, 723–31.

Andres, C. (1985). Antioxidants: 'quality protectors'. *Food Processing*, February, 37–41.

Association of Food and Drug Officials of the United States, Division of Pharmacology, Food and Drug Administration, Department of Health, Education and Welfare (1959). *Appraisal of the Safety of Chemicals in Foods, Drugs and Cosmetics*, edited and published by the Editorial Committee, Baltimore, Maryland.

Association of Official Analytical Chemists (1984). *Official Methods of Analysis*, 14th edn, Assoc. Off. Anal. Chem., Washington, DC.

Code of Federal Regulations (1985a). Title 21, Parts 172, 182, 189. Office of the Federal Register National Archives and Records Administration (revised as of April 1, 1985), Washington, DC.

Code of Federal Regulations (1985b). Title 21, Part 172.395. Office of the Federal Register National Archives and Records Administration (revised as of April 1, 1985), Washington, DC.

Code of Federal Regulations (1985c). Title 21, Parts 182.3616, 182.3637, 182.3739, 182.3766, 182.3798 and 182.3862. Office of the Federal Register National Archives and Records Administration (revised as of April 1, 1985) Washington, DC.

Code of Federal Regulations (1985*d*). Title 21, Part 184.1835. Office of the Federal Register National Archives and Records Administration (revised as of April 1, 1985), Washington, DC.

Commission of the European Communities (1976). *Reports of the Scientific Committee for Food* (Second Series).

Commission of the European Communities (1977). *Reports of the Scientific Committee for Food* (Third Series).

Commission of the European Communities (1980). *Reports of the Scientific Committee for Food* (Tenth Series) (EUR 6892).

Commission of the European Communities (1981). *Reports of the Scientific Committee for Food* (Eleventh Series) (EUR 7421 EN).

Commission of the European Communities (1983). *Reports of the Scientific Committee for Food* (Fourteenth Series) (EUR 8752 EN).

Commission of the European Communities (1985). *Reports of the Scientific Committee for Food* (Sixteenth Series) (EUR 10210 EN).

Council of Europe (1981). *Flavouring Substances and Natural Sources of Flavourings*, 3rd edn, Council of Europe, Strasbourg.

Cramer, G. M., Ford, R. A. and Hall, R. L. (1978). Estimation of toxic hazard: a decision tree approach. *Food Cosmet. Toxicol.*, **16**, 255–76.

District of Columbia Circuit Court (1968). District of Columbia v. Orleans. *Federal Reporter Second*, **406**, 957.

District of Columbia Circuit Court (1979). Monsanto v. Kennedy. *Federal Reporter Second*, **613**, 947.

Emerson, J. L. and Johnson, J. L. (1985). Adverse reactions to sulphites: an overview. *Food Technol.* (Australia), **37**:11 (Suppl.), 37, i–v.

Federal Food, Drug, and Cosmetic Act (1958). *Section 409(c)(3)(A)*, HHS Publication No. (FDA) 86–1051.

Federation of American Societies for Experimental Biology (1985). *The Reexamination of the GRAS Status of Sulfiting Agents*, Life Sciences Research Office, Bethesda, Maryland.

Food and Drug Administration (1969*a*). Exemption of certain food additives from the requirement of tolerances; cyclamic acid and its salts. *Federal Register*, **34**, 17063–4.

Food and Drug Administration (1969*b*). FD&C Yellow No. 5; confirmation of effective date of order listing for food and drug use. *Federal Register*, **34**, 11542.

Food and Drug Administration (1977*a*). Part 8. Color additives, subpart provisional regulations, postponement of closing dates. *Federal Register*, **42**, 6992–8.

Food and Drug Administration (1977*b*). Food additives; saccharin and its salts. *Federal Register*, **42**, 19996–20010.

Food and Drug Administration (1979). FD&C Yellow No. 5; labeling in food and drugs for human use. *Federal Register*, **44**, 37212–21.

Food and Drug Administration (1980). Cyclamate (cyclamic acid, calcium cyclamate, and sodium cyclamate); commissioner's decision. *Federal Register*, **45**, 61474–530.

Food and Drug Administration (1982*a*). *Four Nation Working Group Report on the Evaluation and Safety of Antioxidants. A. Chemistry Working Group Report. B.*

Pathology Working Group Report. C. Toxicology and Metabolism Antioxidants Working Group Report, FDA, Washington, DC.

Food and Drug Administration (1982*b*). D&C Green No. 6; listing as a color additive in externally applied drugs and cosmetics. *Federal Register*, **47**, 14138–48.

Food and Drug Administration (1982*c*). Policy for regulating carcinogenic chemicals in food and color additives; advance notice of proposed rulemaking. *Federal Register*, **47**, 14464–9.

Food and Drug Administration (1982*d*). D&C Green No. 5. *Federal Register*, **47**, 24278–86.

Food and Drug Administration (1982*e*). Sulfiting agents; proposed affirmation of GRAS status with specific limitations. Removal from GRAS status as direct human food ingredient. *Federal Register*, **47**, 29956–63.

Food and Drug Administration (1982*f*). *Toxicological Principles for the Safety Assessment of Direct Food Additives and Color Additives Used in Food*, FDA, Washington, DC.

Food and Drug Administration (1983). FD&C Blue No. 2. *Federal Register*, **48**, 5252–61.

Food and Drug Administration (1984). *Scientific Review of the Long-term Carcinogen Bioassays Performed on the Artificial Sweetener, Cyclamate*, Cancer Assessment Committee, FDA, Washington, DC.

Food and Drug Administration (1985*a*). FD&C Yellow No. 5. *Federal Register*, **50**, 35774–83.

Food and Drug Administration (1985*b*). Cosmetics; proposed ban on the use of methylene chloride as an ingredient of aerosol cosmetic products. *Federal Register*, **50**, 51551–9.

Food and Drug Administration (1986*a*). Permanent listing of FD&C Yellow No. 6. *Federal Register*, **51**, 41765–83.

Food and Drug Administration (1986*b*). Proposed uses of vinyl chloride polymers. *Federal Register*, **51**, 4177–88.

Food and Drug Administration (1986*c*). Food labeling; declaration of sulfiting agents. *Federal Register*, **51**, 25012–20.

Food and Drug Administration (1986*d*). Sulfiting agents; revocation of GRAS status for use on fruits and vegetables intended to be served or sold raw to consumers. *Federal Register*, **51**, 25021–26.

Food and Drug Administration (1986*e*). Provisional listing of FD&C Red No. 3 in cosmetics and externally applied drugs and of its lakes in food and ingested drugs; postponement of closing date. *Federal Register*, **51**, 39856–7.

Food and Drug Administration (1986*f*). Confirmation of effective date for FD&C Yellow No. 5; identity and specifications. *Federal Register*, **51**, 39653–5.

Food and Drug Administration (1986*g*). FD&C Yellow No. 5; identity and specifications. *Federal Register*, **51**, 24517–24.

Food and Drug Administration (1987). Provisional listing of FD&C Yellow No. 6, D&C Red Nos. 8 and 9; postponement of closing date. *Federal Register*, **52**, 3224.

Food Chemical News (1985). EEC acceptance may be simplified, Fondu says. December 23, 18–19.

Green, U., Schneider, P., Deutsch-Wenzel, R. and Brune, H. (1980).

Syncarcinogenic action of saccharin or sodium cyclamate in the induction of bladder tumors in MNU-pretreated rats. *Food Cosmet. Toxicol.*, **18**, 575–9.

Grünow, W. (1984). Short-term studies with BHA. Transcript, Toxicology Forum Meeting, Washington, DC.

Haigh, R. (1978*a*). The activities of the Scientific Committee for Food of the Commission of the European Communities. In: *Chemical Toxicology of Food*, C. L. Galli, R. Paoletti and G. Vettorazzi (Eds), Elsevier/North-Holland Biomedical Press, Amsterdam/New York/Oxford, pp. 81–8.

Haigh, R. (1978*b*). Harmonization of legislation on foodstuffs, food additives and contaminants in the European Economic Community. *J. Food Technol.*, **13**, 255–64.

Haigh, R. (1978*c*). Harmonization of legislation on foodstuffs, food additives and contaminants in the European Economic Community. II. Achievements and programme. *J. Food Technol.*, **13**, 491–509.

Hardy, J., Gaunt, I. F., Hooson, J., Hendy, R. J. and Butterworth, K. R. (1976). Long-term toxicity of cyclohexylamine hydrochloride in mice. *Food Chem. Toxicol.*, **14**, 269–76.

Hasegawa, R. and Cohen, S. M. (1986). The effect of different salts of saccharin on the rat urinary bladder. *Cancer Lett.*, **30**, 261–8.

Hicks, R. M. and Chowaniec, J. (1977). The importance of synergy between weak carcinogens in the induction of bladder cancer in experimental animals and humans. *Cancer Res.*, **37**, 2943–9.

Hicks, R. M., Wakefield, J. St J. and Chowaniec, J. (1975). Evaluation of a new model to detect bladder carcinogens or co-carcinogens; results obtained with saccharin, cyclamate and cyclophosphamide. *Chem.-Biol. Interact.*, **11**, 225–33.

Hoover, R. N. and Strasser, P. H. (1980). Artificial sweeteners and human bladder cancer; preliminary results. *Lancet*, **i**, 837–40.

Hui, Y. H. (1979). *United States Food Laws, Regulations and Standards*, John Wiley and Sons, New York.

Hutt, P. B. (1984). Government regulation of the integrity of the food supply. *Ann. Rev. Nutr.*, **4**, 1–20.

Hutt, P. B. and Hutt, P. B., II (1984). A history of government regulation of adulteration and misbranding of food. *Food Drug Cosmetic Law J.*, **39**, 2–73.

International Agency for Research on Cancer (1984). *Chemicals and Exposures to Complex Mixtures Recommended for Evaluation in IARC Monographs and Chemicals and Complex Mixtures Recommended for Long-term Carcinogenicity Testing*. IARC Internal Technical Report No. 84/002.

International Life Sciences Institute-Nutrition Foundation (1984*a*). *Butylated Hydroxyanisole (BHA): A Monograph*, ILSI-NF, Washington, DC.

International Life Sciences Institute-Nutrition Foundation (1984*b*). *Butylated Hydroxytoluene (BHT): A Monograph*, ILSI-NF, Washington, DC.

International Life Sciences Institute-Nutrition Foundation (1984*c*). *Propyl Gallate: A Monograph*, ILSI-NF, Washington, DC.

International Life Sciences Institute-Nutrition Foundation (1984*d*). *Tertiary Butyl Hydroquinone (TBHQ): A Monograph*, ILSI-NF, Washington, DC.

International Life Sciences Institute-Nutrition Foundation (1984*e*). *Tocopherol: A Monograph*, ILSI-NF, Washington, DC.

International Organization of the Flavour Industry (1976). *Basic Features of Modern Flavour Regulation*, IOFI, Geneva, Switzerland.

Ito, N. (1982). *Carcinogenicity of Butylated Hydroxyanisole in F-344 Rats*, prepared for Japanese Food Sanitation Council.

Ito, N., Hagiwara, A., Shibata, N., Ogiso, T. and Fukushima, S. (1982). Induction of squamous cell carcinoma in the forestomach of F344 rats treated with butylated hydroxyanisole. *Gann*, **73**, 332–4.

Ito, N., Fukushima, S., Imaida, K., Sakata, T. and Masui, T. (1983). Induction of papilloma in the forestomach of hamsters by butylated hydroxyanisole. *Gann*, **74**, 459–61.

Ito, N., Hirose, M., Kurata, Y., Ikawa, E., Mera, Y. and Fukushima, S. (1984). Induction of forestomach hyperplasia by crude butylated hydroxyanisole, a mixture of 3-tert and 2-tert isomers in Syrian golden hamsters is due to 3-tert-butylated hydroxyanisole. *Gann*, **75**, 471–4.

Ito, N., Fukushima, S. and Tsuda, H. (1985). *Carcinogenicity and Modification of the Carcinogenic Response by BHA, BHT and Other Antioxidants*, CRC Crit. Rev. Toxicol., Vol. 15, Cleveland, Ohio.

Iverson, F., Lok, E., Nera, E., Karpinski, K. I. and Clayson, D. B. (1985*a*). 13-Week feeding study of butylated hydroxyanisole: the subsequent regression of the induced lesions in male Fischer 344 rat forestomach epithelium. *Toxicology*, **35**, 1–11.

Iverson, F., Truelove, J., Nera, E., Wong, D., Lok, E. and Clayson, D. B. (1985*b*). 85-Day study of butylated hydroxyanisole in the cynomolgus monkey. *Cancer Lett.*, **26**, 43–50.

Japan Food Hygiene Association (1960). *The Japanese Standards of Food Additives*, 1st edn, Tokyo.

Japan Food Additives Association (1986). *The Japanese Standards of Food Additives*, 5th edn, Tokyo.

Marmion, D. M. (1979). *Handbook of U.S. Colorants for Foods, Drugs, and Cosmetics*, John Wiley and Sons, New York.

McCormick, D. L., Major, N. and Moon, R. C. (1984). Inhibition of 7,12-dimethylbenz(a)anthracene-induced rat mammary carcinogenesis by concomitant or postcarcinogen antioxidant exposure. *Cancer Res.*, **44**, 2858–63.

McGowan, G. (1981). *The Formulation of Foodstuffs Legislation*, European News Agency, Brussels.

Middlekauff, R. (1984). Risk analysis and the interface of science, law and policy. *Food Technol.*, **38**, 97–100, 152.

Middlekauff, R. (1985). Delaney meets de minimis. *Food Technol.*, **39**, 62–9.

National Academy of Sciences/National Research Council (1985). *Evaluation of Cyclamate for Carcinogenicity*, NAS/NRC, National Academy Press, Washington, DC.

National Research Council/National Academy of Sciences (1979). *The 1977 Survey of Industry on the Use of Food Additives*, PB80-113418, Parts 1, 2, 3, US Department of Commerce, NTIS, Washington, DC.

National Research Council (1982). *Poundage Update of Food Chemicals*, PB84-162148, US Department of Commerce, NTIS, Washington, DC.

National Toxicology Program (1984*a*). *Annual Plan for Fiscal Year 1984* (NTP-84-023), US Department of Health and Human Services, Washington, DC.

National Toxicology Program (1984b). *Report of the Ad Hoc Panel on Chemical Carcinogenesis Testing and Evaluation*, US Public Health Service, Washington, DC.

National Toxicology Program (1985). *Annual Plan for Fiscal Year 1985* (NTP-85-055), US Department of Health and Human Services, Washington, DC.

Netherlands (1964). *Toevoegingen van Hulpstoffen en Voedingsmiddelen Voor de Mens*, Verslagen, Adviezen, Rapporten Ministerie Voor Volksgezondheid en Milieuhygiene.

Noonan, J. E. and Meggos, H. (1980). Synthetic food colors. In: *CRC Handbook of Food Additives*, Vol. 2, Cleveland, Ohio, pp. 339–83.

Odashima, S. (1976). *Guidelines for the Test Method for Carcinogenicity of Chemical Substances*, Japanese Ministry of Health and Welfare, Tokyo.

Office of Science and Technology Policy (1985). Chemical carcinogens; a review of the science and its associated principles, *Federal Register*, 50, 10372–442.

Olsen, P., Bille, N. and Meyer, O. (1983). Hepatocellular neoplasms in rats induced by butylated hydroxytoluene. *Acta Pharmacol. Toxicol.*, 53, 433–4.

Organization for Economic Co-operation and Development (1981). *OECD Guidelines for Testing of Chemicals*, Report No. ISBN 92-64-12221-4, OECD, Paris.

Oser, B. L., Carson, S., Cox, G. E., Vogin, E. E. and Sternberg, S. S. (1976). Long-term and multigeneration toxicity studies with cyclohexylamine hydrochloride. *Toxicology*, 6, 47–65.

Parker, L. E. (1984). Regulation of food colours. *Food Flavourings, Ingredients, Packaging and Processing*, 6, 23–9.

Pearce, A. and Hume, A. F. (1983). Synthetic food colours today. *Food Flavourings, Ingredients, Packaging and Processing*, 5, 26–9.

Price, J. M., Biava, C. G., Oser, B. L., Vogin, E. E., Steinfeld, J. and Ley, H. L. (1970). Bladder tumors in rats fed cyclohexylamine or high doses of a mixture of cyclamate and saccharin. *Science*, 167, 1131–2.

Renwick, A. G. (1985). The fate of intense sweeteners in the body. *Food Chem.*, 16, 281–301.

Roberts, A. and Renwick, A. G. (1985a). The effect of saccharin on the microbial metabolism of tryptophan in man. *Food Chem. Toxicol.*, 23, 451–5.

Roberts, A. and Renwick, A. G. (1985b). The metabolism of ^{14}C-cyclohexylamine in mice and two strains of rat. *Xenobiotica*, 15, 477–83.

Rodricks, J. and Taylor, M. R. (1983). Application of risk assessment to food safety decision making. *Regulatory Toxicol. Pharmacol.*, 3, 275–307.

Saccharin: current status (1985). Report of an expert panel. *Food Chem. Toxicol.*, 23, 543–6.

Schoenig, G. P., Goldenthal, E. I., Geil, R. G., Frith, C. H., Richter, W. R. and Carlborg, F. W. (1985). Evaluation of the dose response and in utero exposure to saccharin in the rat. *Food Chem. Toxicol.*, 23, 475–90.

Schwartz, H. J. and Chester, E. H. (1984). Bronchospastic responses to aerosolized metabisulfites in asthmatic subjects: potential mechanisms and clinical implications. *J. Allergy Clin. Immunol.*, 74, 511–3.

Simon, R. A., Green, L. and Stevenson, D. D. (1982). The incidence of ingested metabisulfite sensitivity in an asthmatic population. *J. Allergy Clin. Immunol.*, 69, 118.

Stofberg, J. and Kirschman, J. C. (1985). Consumption ratio of flavouring materials: a mechanism for setting priorities for safety evaluation. *Food Chem. Toxicol.*, **23**, 857–60.

Taylor, S. L. (1985). The sulfite story. *Assoc. Food and Drug Officials Quart. Bull.*, **49**, 185–93.

Walker, R. (1985). Sulfiting agents in foods: some risk/benefit considerations. *Food Additives and Contaminants*, **2**, 5–24.

West, R. W., Sheldon, W. G., Gaylor, D. W., Haskin, M. G., Delongchamp, R. R. and Kadlubar, F. F. (1986). The effects of saccharin on the development of neoplastic lesions initiated with N-methyl-N-nitrosourea in the rat urothelium. *Fundam. Appl. Toxicol.*, **7**, 585–600.

WHO/FAO (1955). *Joint FAO/WHO Expert Committee on Nutrition*, Fourth Session, WHO Tech. Rep. Ser., No. 97, Geneva.

WHO/FAO (1957). *General Principles Governing the Use of Food Additives*, First Report, WHO Tech. Rep. Ser., No. 129, Geneva.

WHO/FAO (1958). *Procedures for the Testing of Intentional Food Additives to Establish Their Safety for Use*, Second Report, WHO Tech. Rep. Ser., No. 144, Geneva.

WHO/FAO (1961). *Evaluation of the Carcinogenic Hazards of Food Additives*, Fifth Report, WHO Tech. Rep. Ser., No. 220, Geneva.

WHO/FAO (1962). *Evaluation of the Toxicity of a Number of Antimicrobials and Antioxidants, Sixth Report*, WHO Tech. Rep. Ser., No. 228, Geneva.

WHO/FAO (1965). *Specifications for the Identity and Purity of Food Additives and Their Toxicological Evaluation: Food Colours and Some Antimicrobials and Antioxidants*, Eighth Report, WHO Tech. Rep. Ser., No. 309, Geneva.

WHO/FAO (1967). *Procedures for Investigating Intentional and Unintentional Food Additives*, Report of WHO Scientific Group, WHO Tech. Rep. Ser., No. 348, Geneva.

WHO/FAO (1974*a*). *Toxicological Evaluation of Certain Food Additives with a Review of General Principles and of Specifications*, Seventeenth Report, WHO Tech. Rep. Ser., No. 539, Geneva.

WHO/FAO (1974*b*). *Evaluation of Certain Food Additives*, Eighteenth Report, WHO Tech. Rep. Ser., No. 557, Geneva.

WHO/FAO (1976*a*). *Evaluation of Certain Food Additives: Some Food Colours, Thickening Agents, Smoke Condensates, and Certain Other Substances*, Nineteenth Report, WHO Tech. Rep. Ser., No. 576, Geneva.

WHO/FAO (1976*b*). *Evaluation of Certain Food Additives*, Twentieth Report, WHO Tech. Rep. Ser., No. 599, Geneva.

WHO/FAO (1978). *Evaluation of Certain Food Additives*, Twenty-first Report, WHO Tech. Rep. Ser., No. 617, Geneva.

WHO/FAO (1980). *Evaluation of Certain Food Additives*, Twenty-fourth Report, WHO Tech. Rep. Ser., No. 653, Geneva.

WHO/FAO (1982). *Evaluation of Certain Food Additives and Contaminants*, Twenty-sixth Report, WHO Tech. Rep. Ser., No. 683, Geneva.

WHO/FAO (1983). *Evaluation of Certain Food Additives and Contaminants*, Twenty-seventh Report, WHO Tech. Rep. Ser., No. 696, Geneva.

WHO/FAO (1984). *Evaluation of Certain Food Additives and Contaminants*, Twenty-eighth Report, WHO Tech. Rep. Ser., No. 710, Geneva.

WHO/FAO (1986). *Summary and Conclusions*, Thirtieth Report, unpublished, Geneva.

Williams, G. M., Shimada, T., McQueen, C., Tong, C. and Ved Brat, S. (1984). Lack of genotoxicity of butylated hydroxyanisole (BHA) and butylated hydroxytoluene (BHT). *The Toxicologist*, **4**, 104.

Ziporyn, T. (1985). The Food and Drug Administration: how those regulations came to be. *J. Am. Med. Assoc.*, **254**(15), 2037–46.

Chapter 3

SOME ASPECTS OF FOOD TOXICOLOGY: A PERSONAL VIEW

FRANCIS J. C. ROE

Consultant in Toxicology, London, UK

DEFINITIONS

'One man's food is another's poison!' So what is food? And what is toxicity?

If a medieval monarch's dog keeled over and died on being fed a scrap of food or a splash of wine, it would not be unreasonable for the owner to sniff assassination in the air. But if he lived to the age of 70 and died of colon cancer although God had designed him to live to 75 and die of heart failure, it is most unlikely that anyone would suspect that his premature death was due to what he feasted on during his prime. At the time of his feasting, his high protein, high fat, diet would have been regarded as safe by his courtiers and an object of envy by peasants for whom undernutrition and malnutrition were major threats. So what is food safety? And how does nutritional inadequacy relate to toxicity?

Unquestionably, certain widely held concepts of food safety and food toxicology are utterly wrong. There is a tacit assumption that traditional

59

foodstuffs of natural origin are safe and that the possibility of poisoning stems only from departures from the natural. Thus, many people imagine that they are much more at risk from food additives than from food and that man-made pesticides are more dangerous than 'Nature's pesticides' as Ames (1983) has termed them. The truth of the matter is quite the contrary. Worldwide, natural poisons in natural foodstuffs cause far more cancers and far more evidence of toxicity than food additives or residues of man-made pesticides in processed food. Indeed, it has been argued that the people nowadays at greatest risk from food poisoning are those whose fanatic belief that 'natural' means 'safe' is unmatched by knowledge of the traditional folklore which enabled their grandparents and great grandparents to avoid the numerous hazards associated with natural and traditional foodstuffs.

Be that as it may, for the purposes of the present chapter, the following definitions have been adopted.

Toxicity: ability to cause adverse effects or to hasten the onset and/or rate of development of adverse age-related changes in the tissues of animals or man

Safety: lack of evidence of toxicity, where appropriate observations and tests have been made

Food: any material which, after ingestion, may act as a source of energy

Cause: increase in the age-standardized risk of developing the disease in question under defined conditions

DOSE–RESPONSE

'A little of what you fancy does you good.' So what is 'a little'? And what is 'good'?

A man who cites these words while sipping his tenth double whisky is distinguishable from the sober judge accepting his first. The latter is living in the realm of pharmacology and the former in the realm of toxicology. This would be evident by looking at biopsies of their livers and maybe by comparing their blood pressures. The point I am making is that a wholesome food, namely ethanol, can become a toxin as a consequence of overindulgence. In other words, it is often not sensible to apply the word 'toxic' to a substance without defining the dose and the circumstances.

For those who regard ethanol as an 'evil' anyway, let me pick lactose as an alternative example. Here we have the sugar of mother's milk, a nutrient of fundamental importance throughout the mammalian kingdom. However, a minority of babies are deficient in the gut enzyme lactase needed for the hydrolysis of lactose to glucose and galactose which are the absorbable products of lactose which act as sources of energy within the body. Those same babies cannot tolerate milk. In fact, the incidence of lactase deficiency increases with age among individuals who start life with enough intestinal lactase to cope with a milk-based diet. Lactase deficiency in later life is a common source of abdominal discomfort and flatulence. For lactase-deficient infants and adults, lactose fulfils the definition of 'toxin'. However, if we were simply to list lactose as a toxin without defining the special circumstances in which it gives rise to manifestations of toxicity, we would be in danger of rendering the whole concept of toxicity meaningless.

Unfortunately, this is what has already happened in the case of one particular manifestation of toxicity, namely 'carcinogenicity'.

For no sound scientific reason, carcinogenicity has long been regarded by many as something essentially different from toxicity. Fear of cancer as a disease has fostered the distinction, yet many progressive varieties of degenerative disease, such as atherosclerosis, Altzheimer's disease and osteoarthritis are, in reality, no more reversible and no more benign than cancer. Because carcinogenicity has been hived off from other forms of chronic toxicity, and has been subjected to far more research, a special rubric has been developed around it. Into this rubric has crept the concept that, if an association between a high level of exposure and an increased risk of developing a particular form of cancer can be demonstrated, then it should be assumed that exposure to a lower dose will carry a qualitatively similar risk at a proportionately lower level. Irrespective of whether or not this is true, it is surely no less likely to be true for environmental factors which cause other degenerative diseases? Heavy exposure to sunlight causes age-related changes in skin which may progress to skin cancer, but lower levels of exposure to sunlight are not without similar effects in lesser degree.

Returning to lactose, it is now clear that heavy exposure of rats to lactose disturbs the calcium balance of the animals and predisposes them to the development of adrenal medullary neoplasia (Roe and Baer, 1985). The same is true for vitamin A analogues such as retinyl acetate (Kurokawa *et al.*, 1985). There is no evidence that a 'sensible' level of exposure to these materials has any adverse effect on the adrenal medulla of rats. Is it, then, reasonable to label such substances as 'carcinogens' with all the stigma that is associated with the use of that term?

RELATIONSHIP BETWEEN MUTAGENICITY
AND CARCINOGENICITY

I once asked the Nobel laureate Peyton Rous a complex question which, in effect, cast doubt on the simplicity of the two-stage hypothesis of carcinogenesis which his earlier work had put onto the map. My question was long, tortuous and apologetic, but his reply was brief. The gist of it was that one of the most important aspects of research is to know when a working hypothesis has outlived its usefulness.

Following the development of logical, inexpensive and rapid *in vitro* test systems for mutagenicity during the 1960s, the attractively simple hypothesis spread like wildfire that positive results in such tests accurately predicted the tumour-initiating and, therefore, carcinogenic potential of chemicals. We now know that the hypothesis is, to say the least, oversimplistic, for there are important human carcinogens, such as asbestos dust, which are not mutagens, and *seemingly* numerous *in vitro* mutagens which are not carcinogenic in animals or man. Of course, 'seemingly' is the operative word. Maybe such substances are very weak carcinogens the activity of which has not yet been revealed by animal tests or by epidemiological studies. So the question arises: Have they been adequately tested for carcinogenicity? The next question is: What does 'adequate' mean in this context? However, irrespective of whether there is any qualitative correlation, one thing seems to be quite clear: there is no obvious quantitative correlation between the apparent potency of mutagens in *in vitro* tests and their apparent potency in *in vivo* tests for carcinogenicity.

The strength of the relationship between mutagenicity in *in vitro* tests and potential carcinogenicity is still a matter for debate and argument. However, most authorities nowadays are not especially worried about positive results for mutagenicity in *in vitro* test systems, if the results of sensitive *in vivo* tests for clastogenicity and mutagenicity are negative. Nevertheless, for chemicals to which man is likely to be exposed in high dosage or over prolonged periods, even a combination of negative *in vitro* and negative *in vivo* mutagenicity test data may not provide sufficient reassurance of lack of carcinogenic potential. For such chemicals, life span *in vivo* carcinogenicity tests in one or two species of animals (mice, rats, hamsters) with exposure by a realistic route may be deemed necessary.

It was against this cautious approach that the paper by Ames (1983) came as a breakthrough. For me it was a welcome blast of fresh air, but for others it was a kind of bombshell which exploded myths that they had been perpetuating for years. After all, it was the Ames test based on the use of various tester strains of *Salmonella typhimurium* which more than any other test system had demonstrated the mutagenicity of thousands of chemicals and thereby brought them under suspicion of possessing carcinogenic potential. As a result of the availability of tests such as the Ames test, we had moved from the 1940s, when it was possible to believe that most chemicals are carcinogenically safe and only a few are carcinogenically dangerous, to the 1970s when a sizeable proportion of the chemicals in everyday use had come to be suspected of carcinogenicity because they are mutagens. The chemical industry was under serious attack because they were thought to be exposing their workforce to carcinogens during manufacturing processes and the general public through contamination of the atmosphere, water and products. Pesticide manufacturers were accused of polluting the environment with carcinogens, and food manufacturers were suspected of adding carcinogens to food during processing.

Historically, there was another significant event that I must mention. Two years before Ames dropped his 1983 bombshell came the review by Doll and Peto (1981) in which they estimated the likely contributions of various environmental factors to the overall human cancer burden in the United States. Their best estimates for the contribution of food additives was less than 1% compared with a 35% contribution from diet, 3% from alcohol, and 30% from tobacco. Pollution came out at 2%, industrial products at less than 1%, occupation at 4%, medicine and medical procedure at 1%, and reproductive and sexual behaviour at 7%.

This list was maximally at variance with the priorities for safety/toxicity testing demanded the world over by regulatory authorities. More than 95% of the tests required related to drugs, food additives, pesticides, industrial products and chemicals to which people are exposed at work. Virtually none of the testing related to diet or food ingredients *per se*.

NATURE'S PESTICIDES

It was this admirably strategic review by Doll and Peto which set Ames thinking and led him to produce his 1983 bombshell paper. The latter begins with sixteen examples of groups of mutagens and putative carcinogens in natural foodstuffs. The list included; safrole in root beer; piperine and safrole in black pepper; various hydrazines in mushrooms; photocarcinogens in celery and parsnips; various flavenoids such as quercetin present in many plant-derived foodstuffs; mutagenic anthraquinones in rhubarb; caffeic acid in coffee; theobromine in cocoa and tea; various pyrrolizidine alkaloids which are present in numerous 'edible' plant species; allyl isothiocyanate in mustard and horseradish sauce; gossypol in cottonseed; sterculic and malvalic acid in cottonseed oil and in oils from related plants of the Malvaceal family; various sesquiterpene lactones in wild lettuce; and canavanine in alfalfa sprouts.

In addition to mutagens and carcinogens, tumour-promoting agents and potentially teratogenic agents abound naturally in plants. Thus, numerous tumour-promoting phenolic compounds such as catechol and its derivatives are present in food plants and some of the most potent tumour promoters known, namely various phorbol esters, are of plant origin. Potential teratogens include the cholinesterase-inhibiting glycoalkaloids solanine and chaconine found in potatoes, especially in wild varieties and when damaged or diseased edible potatoes are exposed to light. Theobromine has been reported to cause testicular damage in rats and severe developmental abnormalities have been seen in cattle allowed to forage on certain leguminous plants such as lupine. Certain pyrrolizidine alkaloids are teratogenic in addition to being mutagenic and carcinogenic.

Given choice, man tends to avoid mouldy foodstuffs. However, in hot humid climates where storage facilities are poor or lacking, fungal infection of stored cereals and of foodstuffs such as groundnuts may be unavoidable. Indeed, crops are apt to be attacked by moulds even before they are harvested. Many moulds produce toxins and some mould toxins, such as aflatoxin and sterigmatocystin, are potent mutagens and carcinogens.

By referring to this array of natural toxins as Nature's pesticides, and by estimating that humans are likely to consume at least 10 000 times more of Nature's pesticides each day then they consume of man-made pesticides, Ames sought to introduce an entirely new order of priorities into the safety and toxicity testing of food.

THE INFLUENCE OF COOKING

Man is the only species who regularly eats cooked food. Man is also the only species that is apt to suffer from a high incidence of cancers of the colon and rectum. Cancers arising at these sites are common in both sexes in North America and Western Europe, but 5 times *less* common in Japan where cancer of the stomach is 5 times *more* common. That dietary factors are mainly responsible for both these types of cancer is rendered virtually certain by the fact that, in Japanese who migrate to North America and adapt to a typical Western diet, colorectal cancer incidence rises dramatically and stomach cancer risk falls equally dramatically. Could it be that cooking destroys stomach carcinogens present in foods that the Japanese eat raw, but introduces colorectal carcinogens into the kinds of foods most commonly eaten in the West?

Two important clues to the answers to these questions are currently emerging. Firstly, it is clear that less meat is consumed in Japan than in the West. Secondly, ongoing research by Sugimura, Nagao and Sato and their colleagues in Japan is identifying several potent mutagens and animal carcinogens that are formed in meat and fish proteins when they are cooked, and particularly when they are grilled to the point of charring. Among the newly discovered mutagens/carcinogens are various heterocyclic amines capable of metabolic activation in the body by cytochrome P-448 to electrophilic N-hydroxy derivatives. The list includes various pyrido-indoles, pyrido-imidazoles and pyrido-carbazoles, and various quinolines and quinoxalines. These chemicals have been identified in the pyrolysates of individual amino acids such as tryptophan, glutamic acid and lysine, and in broiled meat and fish (Sugimura and Nagao, 1982). Recently, many of them have been proved to be potent carcinogens for the small and large bowel in mice and rats (Sato, 1985).

For several years epidemiological studies have been indicating a positive correlation between dietary fat intake and risk of colorectal cancer (e.g. Wynder and Shigematsu, 1967; Drasar and Irving, 1973; Armstrong and Doll, 1975) and a negative correlation between dietary fibre and colorectal cancer (Burkitt, 1971). Also it has been suggested that carcinogens or tumour promoters are formed in the lower bowel from bile acids, the secretion of which is stimulated by dietary cholesterol and fat (Reddy and Wynder, 1977). However, it now looks as though any contribution of fat *per se*, bile acid and secretion *per se*, or deficiency of fibre *per se* may be quite minor compared with a major contribution from carcinogens produced during the cooking of food.

In any case, the findings emerging from the ongoing research of Sugimura and his colleagues on the effects of cooking are pointing very strongly to the fact that governmental and international authorities who have the responsibility for ensuring the safety of food need as a matter of urgency to devote far more attention than they devote at present to the evaluation of 'food on the fork' as eaten (i.e. after appropriate cooking).

At present most of the available testing facilities for the safety evaluation of food are given over to tests on food additives rather than food constituents and to raw foodstuffs rather than cooked foods.

OVERNUTRITION: LABORATORY ANIMALS

Lack of fundamental training in biology is apt to leave even erudite chemists and statisticians with the wholly unrealistic view that healthy eating consists simply of introducing into the top end of a tube a mixture of non-toxic (and non-carcinogenic) nutrient chemicals. If, as often happens, such scientists reach positions of power in government food regulatory bodies, they are apt to see their main duty as making sure that enough nutrients but no toxins find their way into what goes into the top end of the tube. Only very recently have they begun to be concerned about the possibility that *too many* nutrients may be stuffed down the tube.

It has long been known, particularly from the pioneering work of Tannenbaum, that diet restriction may prolong the survival of, and reduce the incidence of neoplastic disease in, laboratory rodents (see Tannenbaum, 1945). However, 'diet restriction' tended to be regarded as 'malnutrition' and it simply did not occur to most investigators that the mere putting of too many nutrients down the tube might have toxicological consequences. The results of more recently published studies leave absolutely no room for doubt that *overnutrition* is a serious contributor to premature death from a variety of causes in laboratory rats and mice. In rats the kidneys and the endocrine system are usually most affected by overnutrition, whereas in the mouse the kidney is a less obvious target but increased incidences of lung, liver and lymphoreticular neoplasms are usually evident (Nolan, 1972; Roe and Tucker, 1973; Tucker, 1979; Conybeare, 1980; Roe, 1981; Harleman *et al.*, 1984).

Quite apart from general overnutrition (i.e. too much of everything going down the tube), nutrient imbalance may have dire consequences. Thus, as pointed out above, rats given a diet that contains 20% lactose develop enlargement of the caecum and toxicological changes secondary to excessive absorption of calcium from the gut. The latter include various forms of nephrocalcinosis and hyperplasia and neoplasia of the adrenal medulla (Roe and Baer, 1985).

It is not really clear why the endocrine system is such a clear target for overfeeding in the rat. Effects on the pituitary gland leading to hyperplasia and then neoplasia of prolactin-producing cells appear to constitute the earliest change. The resulting excessive output of prolactin secondarily increases the risk of development of mammary gland tumours, mainly benign fibroadenomas and adenomas but also adenocarcinomas. But these are not the only 'endocrine' targets in overfed rats, the incidences of islet-cell tumours of the pancreas, adrenal medullary tumours and C-cell tumours of the thyroid also tend to be increased. In addition, parathyroid hyperplasia and neoplasia secondary to progressive nephropathy are relatively commonly seen in overfed rats.

Focal hyperplasia and neoplasia of the exocrine cells of the pancreas occur in high incidence from time to time in overfed rats (Kociba et al., 1979). This may be simply a manifestation of general overfeeding. Alternatively, it might be a specific consequence of exposure to particular dietary ingredients. It is known that if rats are fed on diets containing high percentages of raw soy flour, their pancreatata undergo hypertrophy which tends to progress to focal hyperplasia of exocrine cells and then to benign and malignant tumour formation (Mackenzie et al., 1986). The effect is thought to be secondary to a component of raw soy that is a potent trypsin inhibitor. The presence of such activity in the lumen of the duodenum of rats leads to the secretion of excessive amounts of the regulatory peptide cholecystokinin (CCK). CCK exerts a trophic effect on the exocrine pancreas. According to Wormsely (personal communication, 1984) the anti-trypsin activity of raw soy flour is not entirely destroyed during the heat sterilization of animal feedstuffs containing it. This, Wormsely suggests, is the explanation of the high incidences of exocrine pancreatic tumours that are sometimes seen in untreated rats (usually males).

OVERNUTRITION AND DISEASE IN MAN

An obviously important question is: To what extent does overnutrition contribute to early death, degenerative diseases and/or cancer in man?

The diseases of obesity are well known to the family physician, and the difficulties and hazards of surgery in obese patients are well known to the general surgeon. Overeating is a major contributory factor in causation of diabetes, and the pharmaceutical industry makes a fortune from antacids for the relief of dyspepsia secondary to overeating. Life insurance companies are well aware of the fact that premature death is more common in overweight individuals. Coronary heart disease is a disease of affluence which is rare in parts of the world where meat and dairy products are not eaten in excess and where the people are slim and active. Some forms of cancer in man, e.g. breast, colon, prostate, are also associated with obesity, with high consumptions of animal fat and with general over-nutrition. However, the big differences seen between *ad libitum* fed and diet-restricted rats in the incidences of endocrine disturbances (other than diabetes) and endocrine neoplasia are not obvious in comparisons of overfed and non-overfed humans. Nor are the striking effects of diet restriction on the incidence of non-endocrine neoplasia in mice (Conybeare, 1980) easy to see in such comparisons. However, there are several reasons why effects of overeating on tumour risk may not be obvious in man even though they occur. The foodstuffs eaten in poor countries are more likely to contain, or be contaminated with, carcinogens than the foodstuffs eaten in excess in rich countries. Thus, the higher incidences of breast, colon and prostate cancer associated with overeating in rich countries are offset by higher incidences of liver cancer due to the consumption of hepatocarcinogens in poor countries. Another difficulty is that necropsy rates for humans are very low, so many early and more benign neoplasms of internal organs go unnoticed in man whereas detailed post-mortem examination reveals the presence of such neoplasms in animals.

For these and other reasons I suspect that general overeating is far more associated with excessive age-standardized cancer risk in humans than is presently obvious from the available data.

HOW USEFUL ARE LABORATORY STUDIES IN PREDICTING TOXIC AND CANCER RISKS FOR MAN?

In recent years, it has been generally assumed that laboratory studies, particularly long-term feeding studies in animals, are good predictors of toxic and cancer risks from food chemicals in man. However, this assumption does not bear very close analysis. There are many examples of adverse effects in man that have not been predicted by prior laboratory studies. In particular, true allergies and various idiosyncratic responses to extensively laboratory-tested food chemicals may be wholly unexpected until they are observed in humans. The situation with regard to 'toxic chemicals' (e.g. organophosphates, heavy metals) is much better, but even here there may be one or more orders of magnitude difference in susceptibility. Laboratory rats fed on ordinary laboratory diets can be exposed in the diet or drinking water to lead salts at levels far in excess of those which would be fatal for humans (Van Esch *et al.*, 1962). Exposed to these high levels of lead, male rats develop kidney cancers whereas, try as they may, epidemiologists have been unable to detect any evidence of an increased risk of renal cancer (or any other form of cancer) in humans as a consequence of exposure to lead (Dingwall-Fordyce and Lane, 1963; Moore and Meredith, 1979). If, however, rats are fed on a high milk diet, then their tolerance of ingested lead falls dramatically and they exhibit some of the same signs of acute lead poisoning as man (Kello and Kostial, 1973; Kostial and Kello, 1979). It seems that lead is poorly absorbed from the gastrointestinal tract of rats when they are fed on standard laboratory chow diets, but well absorbed when they are fed on a milk diet or on the kind of diets which humans eat.

This simple example raises two matters of importance, namely intraspecies and inter-species variation in response. Within a species, quite apart from genetically determined qualitative and quantitative differences between animals of different strains and between the two sexes, there may also be environmentally determined differences (e.g. laboratory chow versus typical human diet). Inter-species differences encompass not only the intra-species differences in both the species being compared (e.g. man and rat) but also a much bigger genetic gap than between sub-lines of a single species.

We have no right, therefore, to expect there to be a very close relationship between the responses of different species to a particular food chemical. Regulators think in terms of a ten-fold difference in susceptibility attributable to intra-species variation and a further ten-fold difference in susceptibility attributable to inter-species variation. In fact there is no solid basis for these figures and they may not be particularly conservative in the case of some chemicals.

Whether a chemical is toxic and, if so, its potency as a toxin depend on numerous variables—anatomical, physiological, metabolic, dietary, to identify just four. In a few cases differences in respect of these variables may be absolute between species and even between strains of the same species. More often they are merely quantitative such that if the dose is pushed up high enough in any species a similar manifestation of toxicity will be observed.

Partly because this is so, and partly in the hope of detecting the potential toxicity of weakly toxic agents, it is a normal requirement that chemicals are tested in animals at dose levels that exceed the anticipated human exposure by tenfold, hundredfold or thousandfold, or even higher. The results of studies in which animals are so exposed cannot be readily interpreted as far as risk to man is concerned without a mass of other information. To translate negative data from animal studies of this kind into 'safety factors' for human exposure, as is commonly done, has no firm scientific basis without, for instance, comparative pharmacokinetic and metabolic data.

Despite the huge limitations of predicting toxicity from laboratory studies, particularly studies in living animals, I firmly believe that some such studies are necessary for new food chemicals. The important thing is that they should not only be sensibly designed but also sensibly executed and interpreted, both by those who carry them out and by regulatory authorities.

At present we are falling down both in study design and in interpretation in the case of long-term animal tests. By overfeeding animals we are making them prone to all sorts of degenerative diseases and to high incidences of neoplasms. In the case of the rat, overfeeding predisposes to progressive kidney disease, cardiomyopathy, polyarteritis, degenerative changes in the cauda equina and to all manner of endocrine changes and endocrine tumours. Against this background of disease in untreated control animals it is often difficult to detect chronic toxicity. Also, it is impossible to interpret treatment-related changes in incidence of endocrine tumours.

CONCLUSIONS

1. Whether or not substance A gives rise to manifestations of toxicity in subject B depends not only on the identity of A but also on the exposure dose and the sensitivity of B.

2. Over-indulgence in almost any nutrient material (e.g. ethanol, lactose, fat, rhubarb) may cause manifestations of toxicity.

3. Nature's pesticides have as great a potential for causing toxic effects as man-made chemicals.

4. Food ingredients, and possibly carcinogens introduced into food as a consequence of mould growth or cooking, are responsible for far more human disease than residues of man-made pesticides in food and the addition to food of man-made chemicals during processing or for the purposes of preservation.

5. Overnutrition markedly increases cancer risk in laboratory rats and mice. In the case of rats, much of the increase in cancer risk is associated with a major disturbance of endocrine status.

6. The present custom is to conduct carcinogenicity tests in animals under conditions of overnutrition. In such tests, high incidences of tumours in control animals confuse the interpretation of the results, increasing the chances that both false negative and false positive results will be obtained.

7. Superimposed on this confused background there may be imposed gross disturbances of nutritional status or mineral balance associated with a requirement by regulatory authorities to test food ingredients at concentrations vastly in excess of those that would be encountered in Nature.

8. Overnutrition is associated with increased cancer risk in man but seemingly less so than has been observed in laboratory animals.

9. Inter-species and inter-individual differences in susceptibility to potential toxins are wide. Both genetic and environmental factors influence susceptibility. A comparison of the responses of man and rats to lead serves to illustrate these points.

10. There is an urgent need to define the laboratory conditions needed to maintain control animals in normal endocrine status and generally free from excessive cancer risk. Only when this has been done will the predictive value for man of tests conducted in rats and mice justify our confidence.

REFERENCES

Ames, B. N. (1983). Dietary carcinogens and anticarcinogens: oxygen radicals and degenerative diseases. *Science*, **221**, 1256–64.

Armstrong, B. K. and Doll, R. (1975). Environmental factors and cancer incidence and mortality in different countries, with special reference to dietary practices. *Int. J. Cancer*, **15**, 617–31.

Burkitt, D. P. (1971). Epidemiology of cancer of the colon and rectum. *Cancer*, **28**, 3–13.

Conybeare, G. (1980). Effect of quality and quantity of diet on survival and tumour incidence in outbred Swiss mice. *Food Cosmet. Toxicol.*, **18**, 65–75.

Dingwall-Fordyce, I. and Lane, R. E. (1963). A follow-up study of lead workers. *Brit. J. Ind. Med.*, **20**, 313.

Doll, R. and Peto, R. (1981). *The Causes of Cancer*, Oxford University Press, New York.

Drasar, B. S. and Irving, D. (1973). Environmental factors and cancer of the colon and breast. *Brit. J. Cancer*, **27**, 167–72.

Harleman, J. H., Roe, F. J. C. and Salmon, G. K. (1984). Life span and spontaneous lesions in rats. The effects of ad libitum versus controlled feeding. Proceedings of Joint Meeting of the European Society of Veterinary Pathology, The American College of Veterinary Pathologists and the World Association of

Veterinary Pathologists. Sept. 4–7, 1984, Veterinary Faculty, de Uithof, Utrecht, Netherlands.

Kello, D. and Kostial, K. (1973). The effect of milk diet on lead metabolism in rats. *Environ. Res.*, **6**, 355–60.

Kociba, R. J., Keyes, D. G., Lisowe, F. W., Kalnins, R. P., Dittenber, D. D., Wade, C. E., Gorzinski, S. J., Mahle, N. H. and Schetz, B. A. (1979). Results of a 2-year chronic toxicity and oncogenic study of rats ingesting diets containing 2,4,5-trichlorophenoxyacetic acid. *Food Cosmet. Toxicol.*, **17**, 205–21.

Kostial, K. and Kello, D. (1979). Bioavailability of lead in rats fed 'human' diets. *Bull. Environ. Contam. Toxicol.*, **21**, 312–4.

Kurokawa, Y., Hayashi, Y., Maekawa, A., Takahashi, M. and Kukubo, T. (1985). High incidences of Pehochromocytomas after long-term administration of retinol acetate to F344/DuCrj rats. *J. Nat. Cancer Inst.*, **74**, 715–23.

Mackenzie, K. M., Hauck, W. N., Wheeler, A. G. and Roe, F. J. C. (1986). Three-generation reproduction study in rats ingesting up to 10% sorbitol in the diet. *Food Chem. Toxicol.*, **24**, 191–200.

Moore, M. R. and Meredith, P. A. (1979). The carcinogenicity of lead. *Arch. Toxicol.*, **42**, 87–94.

Nolan, G. A. (1972). Effect of various restricted dietary regimes on the growth, health and longevity of albino rats. *J. Nutr.*, **102**, 1477.

Reddy, B. S. and Wynder, E. L. (1977). Metabolic epidemiology of colon cancer: fecal bile acids and neutral sterols in colon cancer patients with adenomatous polyps. *Cancer*, **39**, 2533–9.

Roe, F. J. C. (1981). Are nutritionists worried about the epidemic of tumours in laboratory animals? *Proc. Nutr. Soc.*, **40**, 57–65.

Roe, F. J. C. and Baer, A. (1985). Enzootic and epizootic adrenal medullary proliferative disease of rats: influence of dietary factors which affect calcium absorption. *Human Toxicol.*, **4**, 27–52.

Roe, F. J. C. and Tucker, M. J. (1973). Recent developments in the design of carcinogenicity tests on laboratory animals. *Proc. Eur. Soc. for Study of Drug Toxicity*, **15**, 171.

Sato, S. (1985). Papers entitled: The formation of mutagens and carcinogens during food processing; Carcinogenicity of mutagens formed during cooking. XIII Int. Congr. Nutrition, Brighton, UK, 18–23 August 1985.

Sugimura, T. and Nagao, M. (1982). The use of mutagenicity to evaluate carcinogenic hazards in our daily lives. In: *Mutagenicity: New Horizons in Genetic Toxicology*, J. A. Heddle (Ed.), Academic Press, New York, pp. 73–88.

Tannenbaum, A. (1945). The dependence of tumour formation on the composition of the calorie-restricted diet as well as on the degree of restriction. *Cancer Res.*, **5**, 616.

Tucker, M. J. (1979). Effect of long-term restriction on tumours in rodents. *Int. J. Cancer*, **23**, 803.

Van Esch, G. J., Van Genderen, H. and Vink, H. H. (1962). The induction of renal tumours by feeding of basic lead acetate to rats. *Brit. J. Cancer*, **16**, 289–97.

Wynder, E. L. and Shigematsu, T. (1967). Environmental factors of cancer of the colon and rectum. *Cancer*, **20**, 1520–61.

Chapter 4

PESTICIDES AND OTHER INDUSTRIAL CHEMICALS

MARY E. ZABIK

Department of Food Science and Human Nutrition, Michigan State University, East Lansing, Michigan, USA

INTRODUCTION

Use of pesticides and fertilizers makes possible modern agriculture which is necessary to produce food for the world's growing population. Nevertheless, the acute toxicity and long-range effects of pesticides have been of concern for a number of years. The United Nations Food and Agriculture Organization and the World Health Organization (FAO/WHO) meet yearly to increase the knowledge of the effects of these compounds, to develop or update recommended maximum residue limits for various commodities as well as to develop or update recommended maximum acceptable daily intakes for humans (ADIs). The latter is the maximum daily intake of a chemical which, during a lifetime, appears to be without appreciable risk.

Persistent industrial chemicals, although not manufactured to be used in direct contact with food or feed, can become general environmental contaminants through translocation by drift or aqueous transfer. Thus, as

73

societies become more industrialized, constant surveillance must be used to evaluate the levels of unintentional additives in the world food supply.

PESTICIDE RESIDUES: FDA MARKET BASKET SURVEY DATA

The United States Food and Drug Administration (US FDA) conducts 'total diet studies' to determine the dietary intake of selected pesticides and industrial chemicals. These studies involve the retail purchase and analyses of foods representative of a 14-day diet for infants, toddlers or adults. In the most recently published study, giving the results of data collected for food purchased from October 1979 to September 1980, foods were purchased in 20 cities representing all geographic areas of the continuous United States (Gartrell *et al.*, 1985c,d).

For the adult diet (Gartrell *et al.*, 1985d), dairy products were found to contain 8 chemical residues: αBHC, DDE, dieldrin, heptachlor epoxide, hexachlorobenzene, lindane, methoxychlor and octochlor epoxide. All average residue levels for the dairy products were <1 ppb. The meat, fish and poultry groups had 18 detectable chemicals. In addition to the 8 listed for dairy products were the following, with average ppb given in parenthesis for the few instances the residue level exceeded 1 ppb: 2–chloroethyl linoleate (14·5 ppb), DDT, diazinon, 2-ethylhexyl diphenyl phosphate (98·5 ppb), malathion, nonachlor (*trans*), pentachloroanisole, pentachlorophenol (8·4 ppb), polychlorinated biphenyls (2 ppb) and TDE. Meat, fish and poultry also had average values of 4·8 ppb of DDE and 3·3 ppb of dieldrin. Potatoes and leafy vegetables had some of the same residues with a total of 12 and 13 residues being detected, respectively. Common residues to these two groups were: chlorophopham (113·5 ppb for potatoes), DDE (1·7 ppb for leafy vegetables), DDT, diazinon, dicloran (1 ppb for potatoes), endosulfan I and endosulfan sulfate. Additional residues for potatoes included dieldrin, tecnazene, tetrachloroaniline, tetrachloroanisidine, and tetrachlorothioanisole, while leafy vegetables contained DCPA (1·6 ppb), demeton-S sulfone (2·8 ppb), endosulfan I, parathion, methyl parathion and toxaphene (2·5 ppb). All average residue concentrations were less than 1 ppb unless the value is given.

Grain and cereal products in the average adult American diet contained 13 chemical residues, with average values given in parenthesis if the level exceeded 1 ppb: αBHC, 2-chloroethyl linoleate (7·1 ppb), 2–chloroethyl palmitate (1·1 ppb), chloropropham, chloropyrifos, diazinon, dieldrin, penitrothion, fonofos, malathion (29·9 ppb), parathion, pentachloro-phenol and tri-n-butyl phosphate. Legume vegetables contained 5 residues: carbaryl (2 ppb), 2-chloroethyl linoleate (1·1 ppb), diazinon, parathion and toxaphene. Root vegetables contained 6 residues: DCPA, DDE (1·0 ppb), diazinon, dieldrin, ethion and linuron.

Garden fruits in the US adult diet contained 19 chemical residues while fruits had 20. Residues found for garden fruits included: αBHC, γBHC, carbaryl (2 ppb), chlorodane, chlorophopham, chloropyrifos, DCPA, DDE, diazinon, dieldrin (1·2 ppb), dimethoate, endosulfan I (1·0 ppb), endosulfan II (1·3 ppb), endosulfan sulfate, lindane, parathion, penta-chloroaniline, quintozene, and toxaphene (7·7 ppb). Fruits contained: captan, carbaryl (5 ppb), chlorobenzilate, chlorophopham, diazinon, dicloran (6·3 ppb), dicofol (3·8 ppb), dieldrin, dimethoate, endosulfan I, endosulfan II, endosulfan sulfate, ethion, malathion, methidathion, parathion, pentachloroanisole, perthane, o-phenylphenol (5 ppb) and phosalone.

The food groups fats and oils as well as sugars and adjuncts contained many of the same residues, with totals of 18 and 14 different residues, respectively. Common residues were: αBHC (1·1 ppm for sugar and adjuncts), DDE, diazinon, fonofos (1·5 ppb for fats and oils), hexachloro-benzene (1·5 ppb for fats and oils), malathion (16·7 ppb for fats and oils and 3·1 ppb for sugars and adjuncts), pentachloroaniline (8·3 ppb for fats and oils), pentachloroanisole (1·2 ppb for fats and oils), pentachloro-benzene (1·8 ppb for fats and oils), pentachlorophenol (3·2 ppb for fats and oils), pentachlorothioanisole (2·7 ppb for fats and oils) and quintozene (1·0 ppb for fats and oils). In addition, fats and oils had: 2–chloroethyl linoleate (92·5 ppb), 2-chloroethyl palmitate (4·7 ppb), dieldrin, 2-ethylhexyl diphenyl phosphate, hexachlor epoxide, and tecnazene (1·0 ppb). The food group sugar and adjunct also contained dicloran and lindane (1·3 ppb). No residues were found in the groups.

DDE and dieldrin were the most prevalent residues, with 50 or more samples in all groups having measurable values. Malathion and hexa-chlorobenzene levels were quantifiable in over 40 samples in all groups. Nevertheless, daily intakes of these residues in the adult diet as shown in the column identified as FY 1980 were very low and are well below the FAO/WHO acceptable daily intakes (Table 1). Residue levels have also been fairly constant since 1977 (Johnson *et al.*, 1984*b*; Podrebarac, 1984*b*; Gartrell *et al.*, 1985*b*; Gartrell *et al.*, 1985*d*).

Infant and toddler foods are monitored separately in the United States. The most recent publication (Gartrell *et al.*, 1985*c*) gives data for foods

TABLE 1
Daily Intake per Unit of Body Weight (μg/kg of body weight/day) of Pesticides and
Industrial Chemicals in Fiscal Years 1977–1980 (Gartrell *et al.*, 1985*d*)

Chemical	FAO/WHO Acceptable Daily Intake	FY 1977	FY 1978	FY 1979	FY 1980
BHC (total)		0·015	0·012	0·015	0·014
BHC, alpha		0·011	0·009	0·010	0·011
BHC, beta		<0·001	0·001	0·001	ND
BHC, delta		<0·001	<0·001	ND	<0·001
Lindane (BHC, gamma)	10	0·004	0·002	0·004	0·003
Captan	10	0·031	0·008	0·005	0·001
Carbaryl	10	ND	0·016	0·016	0·021
Chlordane (total)	1	0·004	0·004	0·004	0·003
Chlordane		0·001	0·001	ND	<0·001
Octachlor epoxide		0·003	0·003	0·004	0·003
Chlorbenzilate	20	ND	ND	ND	<0·001
2-Chloroethyl caprate		ND	0·009	ND	ND
2-Chloroethyl laurate		ND	0·056	ND	ND
2-Chloroethyl linoleate		0·078	0·228	0·079	0·197
2-Chloroethyl myristate		ND	0·023	ND	ND
2-Chloroethyl palmitate		0·010	0·023	0·005	0·012
Chlorpropham		0·310	0·144	0·300	0·268
Chlorpyrifos	10	ND	0·005	0·005	0·001
DCPA		0·001	0·001	0·001	0·002
DDT (total)	5	0·046	0·070	0·093	0·034
DDT		0·006	0·008	0·004	0·003
DDE		0·039	0·061	0·087	0·031
TDE		0·001	0·001	0·002	<0·001
DEF		ND	ND	<0·001	ND
Demeton-S sulfone		NA	NA	NA	0·002
Diazinon	2	0·006	0·004	0·010	0·004
Dicloran	30	0·056	0·033	0·030	0·023
Dicofol	25	0·004	0·005	0·007	0·012
Dieldrin	0·1	0·023	0·017	0·016	0·022
Dimethoate	20	NA	NA	NA	0·001
Endosulfan (total)	8	0·010	0·011	0·010	0·015
Endosulfan I		0·003	0·003	0·003	0·003
Endosulfan II		0·003	0·003	0·002	0·008
Endosulfan sulfate		0·004	0·005	0·005	0·004
Endrin	0·2	<0·001	<0·001	ND	ND
Ethion	1	0·018	0·001	0·005	0·001
2-Ethylhexyl diphenyl phosphate		ND	ND	ND	1·82
Fenitrothion	1	ND	ND	ND	0·001
Fenthion	1	ND	<0·001	ND	ND
Fonofos		ND	0·001	<0·001	0·002

TABLE 1—*contd.*

Chemical	FAO/WHO Acceptable Daily Intake	FY 1977	FY 1978	FY 1979	FY 1980
Heptachlor epoxide	0·5	0·007	0·008	0·006	0·007
Hexachlorobenzene		0·002	0·004	0·003	0·004
Leptophos		0·002	ND	ND	ND
Linuron		NA	NA	NA	<0·001
Malathion	20	0·154	0·142	0·265	0·203
Methidathion	5	NA	NA	NA	0·001
Methoxychlor		0·008	0·007	0·003	0·007
Nitrofen		ND	ND	<0·001	ND
Nonachlor, *trans*		0·002	0·001	<0·001	<0·001
Parathion	5	0·002	0·004	0·002	0·001
Parathion-methyl	1	0·001	ND	ND	<0·001
Pentachloroanisole		<0·001	0·001	0·001	0·002
Pentachlorobenzene		0·001	0·002	0·002	0·002
Pentachlorobenzonitrile		ND	<0·001	ND	ND
Pentachlorophenol		0·001	ND	0·006	0·040
Pertane		<0·001	0·005	0·003	0·001
o-Phenylphenol	20	0·004	0·038	0·046	0·015
Phosalone	6	0·001	0·017	0·003	0·004
Polychlorinated biphenyls		0·016	0·027	0·014	0·008
Quintozene (total)	7	0·002	0·003	0·005	0·013
Quintozene		0·001	0·001	0·001	0·001
Pentachloroaniline		0·001	0·001	0·003	0·009
Pentachlorothioanisole		<0·001	0·001	0·001	0·003
Ronnel		ND	ND	0·001	ND
Tecnazene	10	0·035	0·005	0·001	0·001
Tetrachloroaniline		0·005	0·002	<0·001	<0·001
Tetrachloroanisidine		0·003	0·001	0·001	<0·001
Tetrachloroanisole		<0·001	ND	ND	ND
Tetrachlorobenzene		0·005	<0·001	ND	ND
Tetrachlorothioanisole		ND	0·001	<0·001	<0·001
Toxaphene		0·080	0·107	0·003	0·015
Tri-n-butyl phosphate		NA	NA	NA	0·041
Vinclosolin		ND	ND	0·003	ND

The FAO/WHO ADIs are expressed here in μg/kg of body weight/day. The intake is presented as a total in cases in which the ADI is expressed as the sum of related residues. The intake is indicated as ND in cases in which the chemical was not detected but could have been if it had been present. It is listed as NA in cases in which the analytical methodology used was not capable of determining that chemical. The intakes for Fiscal Years 1977–1979 were reported previously (Johnson *et al.*, 1984a, b; Podrebarac, 1984b). Because trace level findings were assigned a value of zero in calculation of intakes prior to Fiscal Year 1978, the intakes shown for Fiscal Year 1977 may be slightly lower than if they had been calculated using an estimate of the level for trace findings.

collected for 1979–80. For infant and toddler diets, water was not found to contain any chemical residue. All other food groups were sources of some chemical residues.

For infants, whole milk was a source of the following 7 chemical residues: BHC, DDE, dieldrin, heptachlor epoxide, hexachlorobenzene, methoxychlor, and nonachlor epoxide. All of these residues had average concentrations of less than 1 ppb. Eight chemical residues were found in other dairy and dairy substitute foods of infant diets: αBHC, DDE, dieldrin, ethion, heptachlor epoxide, hexachlorobenzene, lindane and methoxychlor. Again, all the average concentrations for these food groups were less than 1 ppb.

Meat, fish and poultry foods for infants were found to contain 8 chemical residues, with only one occurring above 1 ppb: αBHC, DDE (1·4 ppb), diazinon, dieldrin, heptachlor epoxide, hexachlorobenzene, lindane and pentachlorophenol. Grain and cereal products were the source of 4 chemical residues in infant diets but two of these had average concentrations exceeding 1 ppb: lindane, malathion (23·6 ppb), pentachlorophenol and tri-n-butyl phosphate (8·6 ppb). Potatoes contributed 9 chemical residues to the total diet of infants, with two of these residues having average concentrations exceeding 1 ppb: chlorophopham (46·6 ppb), diazinon, dicloran (3·3 ppb), dieldrin, endosulfan sulfate, tecnazene, tetrachloroaniline, tetrachloroanisidine and tetrachloro-thioanisole.

Seven chemical residues were found in the vegetables of the total infant diet of 1980 but only the average concentration of one of these exceeded 1 ppb: captan (1·3 ppb), chlorophopham, DDE, diazinon, malathion, parathion and tetrachloroaniline. Fruit and fruit juices contributed 8 chemical residues: chlorobenzilate, dicloran, endosulfan II, endosulfan sulfate, parathion, perthane, phosalone and tri-(2-chloroethyl) phosphate. Beverages in the infant diets were found to have only 1 residue which was dicofol. All the residues in fruit and fruit juices and beverages had average concentrations of less than 1 ppb. Sugars and adjuncts in infant diets were found to contain carbaryl (50 ppb) and pentachlorophenol (<1 ppb).

Fats and oils in the infant diets contained both the greatest number of chemical residues and the greatest number with average concentrations exceeding 1 ppb: DDE, dicloran, dieldrin, fonofos (1·4 ppb), heptachlor epoxide, hexachlorobenzene, malathion (32·0 ppb), pentachloroaniline (5·0 ppb), pentachloroanisole (1·1 ppb), pentachlorobenzene (1·3 ppb), pentachlorophenol (2·1 ppb), pentachlorothioanisole (1·2 ppb), quinto-zene and toxaphene (8·6 ppb). Fats and oils were also the major sources of chemical residues in the toddler diet, with many of the average concentrations of these compounds exceeding 1 ppb: chlorodane, 2-chloroethyl linoleate (76·6 ppb), 2–chloroethyl palmitate (5·6 ppb), DDE, diazinon (1·6 ppb), dieldrin (1·7 ppb), fonofos, heptachlor epoxide, hexachlorobenzene (2·0 ppb), malathion (43·1 ppb), octochlor epoxide, pentachloroaniline (7·7 ppb), pentachloroanisole (2·3 ppb), pentachlorobenzene (2·9 ppb), pentachlorophenol (9·3 ppb), pentachlorothioanisole (3·3 ppb), quintozene (3·2 ppb) and toxaphene (42·6 ppb).

Meat, fish and poultry had the next highest number of chemical residues in the toddler total diet, with 5 of the 15 average concentrations exceeding 1 ppb: BHC, 2-chloroethyl linoleate (5·9 ppb), chloropyrifos, DDE (3·0 ppb), DDT, diazinon, dieldrin (1·7 ppb), 2–ethylhexyl diphenyl phosphate, heptachlor epoxide, hexachlorobenzene, lindane, octochlor epoxide, pentachlorophenol (3·2 ppb), TDE and toxaphene (5·0 ppb).

Whole milk contributed 7 chemical residues while other dairy and dairy substitutes (d/ds) contributed 9 chemical residues to the diets of US toddlers. None of the average concentrations for whole milk exceeded 1 ppb while over half of the average concentrations of the other group did. Common residues found in both groups were: αBHC (1·6 ppb in d/ds), DDE (1·5 ppb in d/ds), dieldrin (1·6 ppb in d/ds), heptachlor epoxide, hexachlorobenzene, methoxychlor (1·1 ppb in d/ds) and octochlor epoxide. In addition, other dairy and dairy substitutes contained: malathion and pentachlorophenol (1·4 ppb).

Six chemical residues were found in grain and cereal products in the US toddler diets, with half of these having average values greater than 1 ppb: chlorophopham, chloropyrifos, diazinon, malathion (22·4 ppb), pentachlorophenol (2·1 ppb) and tri-n-butyl phosphate (15·8 ppb). Potatoes had measurable levels of 9 chemical residues: chlorophopham (0·3 ppm), diazinon, dicloran, dieldrin, endosulfan sulfate, tecnazene, tetrachloroaniline, tetrachloroanisidine and tetrachlorothioanisole. Vegetables in the toddler diets had the following 8 chemical residues: DCPA, diazinon, dieldrin, endosulfan I, endosulfan II, endosulfan sulfate and malathion, while fruits and fruit juices had carbaryl (5 ppb), chlorobenzilate (1·2 ppb), dicloran (9·3 ppb), ethion, methidathion, methoxychlor (2·0 ppb) and perthane (2·6 ppb). Finally, sugar and adjuncts contributed residues from the following 8 compounds: αBHC (1·9 ppb), diazinon, 2-ethylhexyl diphenyl phosphate (33 ppb), lindane (2·9 ppb), malathion, pentachloroaniline, pentachlorophenol (2·6 ppb) and pentachlorothioanisole.

Daily intake levels of these compounds for infants and toddlers are very

TABLE 2

Daily Intake per Unit of Body Weight (μg/kg of body weight/day) of Pesticides and Industrial Chemicals in Fiscal Years 1977–1980 (Gartrell et al., 1985c)

Chemical	FAO/WHO Acceptable Daily Intake	Infant FY 1977	FY 1978	FY 1979	FY 1980	Toddler FY 1977	FY 1978	FY 1979	FY 1980
BHC (total)		0·037	0·037	0·034	0·029	0·035	0·034	0·035	0·036
BHC, alpha		0·031	0·034	0·033	0·028	0·025	0·029	0·029	0·028
BHC, beta		ND	ND	ND	ND	0·002	ND	ND	ND
Lindane (BHC, gamma)	10	0·006	0·003	0·001	0·001	0·008	0·005	0·006	0·008
Captan	10	ND	ND	ND	0·015	ND	ND	ND	ND
Carbaryl	10	<0·001	0·088	ND	0·060	ND	0·050	0·049	0·035
Chlordane (total)	1	0·001	0·010	<0·001	0·003	<0·005	0·032	0·003	0·005
Chlordane		<0·001	0·005	ND	ND	<0·001	0·024	ND	<0·001
Octachlor epoxide		0·001	0·005	<0·001	0·003	0·005	0·008	0·003	0·005
Chlorobenzilate	20	ND	ND	ND	ND	ND	ND	ND	0·008
2-Chloroethyl linoleate		ND	0·061	ND	ND	ND	0·418	0·198	0·145
2-Chloroethyl palmitate		ND	0·008	ND	ND	ND	0·015	0·009	0·007
Chlorpropham		0·051	0·007	0·060	0·025	0·225	0·034	0·238	0·726
Chlorpyrifos	10	ND	ND	0·002	ND	ND	ND	0·007	0·001
DCPA		ND	0·020	0·002	ND	ND	<0·001	<0·001	<0·001
DDT (total)	5	0·102	0·091	0·113	0·034	0·548	0·104	0·090	0·049
DDE		0·100	0·088	0·110	0·034	0·332	0·088	0·089	0·045
DDT		0·001	0·003	ND	ND	0·048	0·013	ND	0·002
TDE		0·001	ND	0·003	ND	0·168	0·003	0·001	0·002
Diazinon	2	0·014	0·002	0·002	0·004	0·007	0·007	0·004	0·011
Dicloran	30	0·013	0·016	0·127	0·010	0·085	0·106	0·088	0·099
Dicofol	25	ND	ND	ND	0·001	ND	ND	0·006	0·005
Dieldrin	0·1	0·041	0·045	0·048	0·033	0·042	0·039	0·036	0·046
Endosulfan (total)	8	ND	<0·001	0·013	0·005	0·002	0·015	0·074	0·008
Endosulfan I		ND	ND	0·001	ND	<0·001	0·005	0·037	0·001
Endosulfan II		ND	<0·001	0·005	0·001	0·001	0·006	0·037	0·002
Endosulfan sulfate		ND	<0·001	0·007	0·004	0·001	0·004	ND	0·005

Compound								
Endrin	0·2	ND	<0·001	ND	ND	ND	ND	<0·001	ND
Ethion	1	0·001	0·003	0·002	0·001	0·001	0·004	0·003	0·005
2-Ethylhexyl diphenyl phosphate		ND	ND	ND	ND	ND	ND	ND	0·307
Fenitrothion	1	ND	<0·001	ND	ND	ND	0·002	ND	ND
Fenthion	1	ND	ND	ND	ND	ND	<0·001	ND	ND
Fonofos		ND	ND	0·002	0·003	0·001	0·001	0·001	0·001
Heptachlor epoxide	0·5	0·013	0·023	0·021	0·019	0·018	0·019	0·018	0·020
Hexachlorobenzene		0·038	0·012	0·010	0·006	0·022	0·015	0·008	0·006
Malathion	20	0·064	0·331	0·126	0·191	0·209	0·299	0·259	0·234
Methidathion	5	NA	NA	NA	NA	NA	NA	NA	0·002
Methoxychlor		0·007	0·029	0·016	0·016	0·002	0·008	0·015	0·026
Nonachlor, *trans*		ND	ND	ND	ND	0·002	ND	ND	ND
Parathion	5	ND	ND	0·002	0·003	<0·001	ND	0·002	ND
Pentachloroanisole		0·011	0·005	0·003	0·003	0·003	0·003	0·003	0·002
Pentachlorobenzene		0·001	0·004	0·008	0·003	0·003	0·007	0·004	0·003
Pentachlorophenol		0·001	0·005	0·009	0·010	0·006	0·005	0·003	0·068
Perthane	20	ND	ND	0·026	0·008	ND	ND	ND	0·034
o-Phenylphenol		ND	0·012	0·061	ND	ND	0·014	0·086	ND
Phosalone	6	0·012	0·037	0·086	0·012	0·043	0·099	0·008	ND
Polychlorinated biphenyls		0·025	0·011	ND	ND	0·030	0·011	ND	ND
Quintozene (total)	7	0·008	0·016	0·035	0·017	0·014	0·003	0·013	0·016
Quintozene		0·001	0·005	0·003	0·002	0·003	0·004	0·001	0·004
Pentachloroaniline		0·005	0·004	0·022	0·012	0·008	0·004	0·008	0·008
Pentachlorothioanisole		0·002	0·007	0·010	0·003	0·003	0·004	0·004	0·004
Ronnel	10	ND	ND	ND	ND	ND	<0·001	ND	ND
Tecnazene		0·001	<0·001	0·008	0·001	0·003	0·001	0·028	0·002
Tetrachloroaniline		<0·001	ND	0·003	0·001	<0·001	ND	0·010	0·001
Tetrachloroanisidine		<0·001	<0·001	0·003	<0·001	0·001	<0·001	0·010	0·001
Tetrachloroanisole		<0·001	ND	ND	ND	0·001	ND	ND	ND
Tetrachlorobenzene		0·002	ND	<0·001	ND	ND	0·008	0·001	ND
Tetrachlorothioanisole		<0·001	ND	<0·001	<0·001	<0·001	ND	0·001	<0·001
Toxaphene		0·068	0·088	0·072	0·021	0·044	0·059	0·050	0·080
Tri-n-butyl phosphate		NA	NA	NA	0·051	NA	NA	NA	0·132
Tris-(2-chloroethyl) phosphate		ND	ND	0·016	0·004	ND	ND	0·009	ND

See footnote for Table 1.

low (Table 2). Generally, intake levels have been fairly stable since 1977 (Johnson *et al.*, 1984*a*; Podrebarac, 1984*a*; Gartrell *et al.*, 1985*a,c*). In general, the FAO/WHO acceptable daily intake is 100 to 1000 times higher than the intake level of US infants and toddlers established by the US FDA market basket survey, showing a wide margin of safety.

PESTICIDE DISAPPEARANCE FROM ANIMAL TISSUES

Another method of monitoring pesticide residue availability for human diets is to monitor residue levels in selected animal tissues. Frank *et al.* (1985) of the Ontario Ministry of Agriculture and Food reported levels of organochlorine residues in abdominal fats of chickens (broilers) slaughtered at provincially inspected abattoirs across Ontario between 1969 and 1982. Eggs were collected from either egg grading stations or producers over the same time period. The results of their analyses are summarized in Table 3. ΣDDT, dieldrin and PCB residues declined exponentially over the 13-year period and the observation was confirmed with frequency data. For example, the percentage of fat samples with less than 10 μg/kg ΣDDT increased from zero in 1969–70 to 94% in 1981–2. The authors regressed the log of concentration of ΣDDT, dieldrin and PCB to determine half residue disappearance for these residues (Table 4). The slightly longer disappearance time for eggs may be related to the age of the birds. Broilers (8 weeks) would be expected to have lower dietary accumulation of these residues than laying hens (14–36 weeks). Egg fat residue levels tended to be lower in abdominal fat, thus the slower redistribution from carcass fat to egg fat would increase the length of time necessary to reduce the residue level in egg fat.

PESTICIDE RESIDUE IN HUMAN MILK

Most contaminants found in human milk are fat-soluble substances which will be detected mainly in the fatty phase of the milk. Jensen (1983) stated: 'Low exposure to pesticide residues and other environmental contaminants can be reflected in human milk if these substances have a high degree of environmental and metabolic persistence which together with a high fat solubility and ability to be bioaccumulated in organisms and biomagnified through natural food chains'. Jensen summarized numerous studies reporting levels of organochlorine residues in human milk from

TABLE 3

Organochlorine Residues in Chicken Fat and Eggs Collected across Ontario between 1969 and 1982 (Frank *et al.*, 1985).

| Years | No. composite samples (eggs or carcasses) | Mean residue in extractable fat ($\mu g/kg$) | | | | | |
		ΣDDT	Dieldrin	Heptachlor epoxide	Chlordane	Lindane	PCB
Abdominal Fat							
1969–70	19(36)	391	28	<1	NM[c]	9	946
1971–72	21(81)	114	7·7	<1	NM	2	54
1973–74[a]	17(49)	35	6·3	14	NM	<1	195
1975–76	9(30)	139	20	6	22	<1	391
1979–80	21(102)	7·6	1·5	1·1	1·0	0·7	6·5
1981–82[a]	50(180)	2·3	0·7	4·6	4·6	0·4	4·8
Eggs							
1969–70[b]	30(102)	188	8·3	<1	NM	5	405
1971–72	31(124)	177	4·9	<1	NM	<1	209
1973–74	22(64)	137	10·5	<1	NM	<1	255
1979–80	4(10)	27	1·3	1·5	<1	2·4	126
1981–82	31(101)	3·9	<0·5	<1	<1	<1	<10

[a] Endosulfan and its metabolite found in 6% of abdominal fat samples at 160 $\mu g/kg$ (1973–74) and in 2% of samples at 5·4 $\mu g/kg$ (1981–82).
[b] Methoxychlor found in 3% of eggs in 1969 at a mean of 380 $\mu g/kg$ in the extractable fat.
[c] NM = not measured.

TABLE 4

Organochlorine Residue Disappearance Rates for Samples Collected in Ontario, Canada, 1969–1982 (Frank *et al.*, 1985)

Tissue	Contaminant	Half residue disappearance (years)
Abdominal fat	ΣDDT	1·8
	dieldrin	2·6
	PCB	1·8
Egg fat	ΣDDT	2·3
	dieldrin	3·0
	PCB	2·9

around the world. Ranges of values from these 1970 studies which were reported by Jensen are summarized in Table 5. Use patterns of pesticides are reflected in this bioaccumulation summary.

TABLE 5
Range of Halogenated Hydrocarbon Residues in Whole Human Milk (ppb)
Reported in the 1970s (summarized from Jensen, 1983)

Area	DDT	Dieldrin	Aldrin	Heptachlor and heptachlor epoxide	Chlordane and oxychlordane
Europe					
Central Europe	50–707	0·5–11·0	0·04–50	1·3–39	0·3
Scandinavia	24–280	0·7–16·0	21·8	1·6	—
Great Britain	75–170	2–6	—[a]	—	—
Americas					
Canada	39–77	2–5	1	1–3	1
United States	63–719	2–14	—	1–12	0–12
Central America	35–3 100	2–5	—	3–7	—
South America	61–258	32	—	—	—
Africa	29	—	—	0·5	—
Asia					
Japan	30–106	0·2–7	3	0·2–2	0·5
India	127–535	—	29·8	—	—
Australia	78–415	4–30	—	—	—

[a] Data unavailable.

FAO/WHO GUIDELINE FOR PESTICIDE RESIDUES IN FOODS

In 1961, the World Health Organization expert committee on pesticide residues held a joint meeting with the United Nations Food and Agriculture Organization panel of experts on the use of pesticides in agriculture and recommended that studies be undertaken to evaluate possible hazards to man arising from the occurrence of residues of pesticides in foods. Joint meetings have been held, with reports published for most years since 1965. During these joint meetings, the FAO working party reviews data on selected pesticides and their residues, proposes pesticide residue limits, and recommends methods of analysis, while the WHO expert committee reviews toxicological and other data and establishes, where possible, acceptable daily intakes for man for those residues. Thus, this yearly examination of data has brought international attention to the possible toxicological effects of pesticide residues, has coordinated efforts to develop and coordinate research projects necessary to provide data to determine the risks versus the benefits of pesticide use.

To meet the increasing need for food there has been a worldwide increase in use of pesticides in agriculture. Pesticides, even when applied with good agricultural practice, sometimes leave residues in foods. Thus, these two expert groups review the toxicological data, residue data, and establish maximum acceptable daily intake (ADI) levels as well as maximum (MRI) or guideline residue limits for selected commodities. The working of this joint meeting has focused attention on this important food safety question. Moreover, as additional data become available, ADIs and MDIs are revised appropriately.

In the 1984 report (FAO, 1985) acceptable daily intakes and/or maximum residue limits were established or updated for 43 compounds. Selected examples of these actions are summarized in Table 6. Guideline levels for 6 compounds which do not have established acceptable daily intakes were also given. Each year, FAO actions include a listing of previous actions for that pesticide so that a user can obtain a complete listing of maximum residue levels as well as follow any changes in recommendations over time (FAO, 1984, 1983, 1982, 1981, 1980, 1979, 1978*a,b*, 1976).

REDUCTION IN RESIDUE LEVELS VIA COOKING/PROCESSING

Fruits and Vegetables
Commercial processing and home preparation have been shown to reduce the level of many chlorinated hydrocarbon, organophosphate, and carbamate residues in fruits and vegetables (Tables 7–9). Much of the residue contamination has been found to be primarily on the surface, so that peeling *per se* has been found to be very effective in reducing residue levels in fruits and vegetables (Baldwin *et al.*, 1968; Elkins *et al.*, 1968; Lamb *et al.*, 1968*a,b*; Farrow *et al.*, 1968, 1969; Fahey *et al.*, 1969, 1970). Washing alone was found to be less effective. Residue reductions were found to be lower in vegetables with a larger amount of surface area, i.e. broccoli and spinach.

Elkins *et al.* (1972) studied the effect of heating *per se* during the processing of apricots (100°C) and spinach (115·5°C). Each was spiked with a number of pesticides just prior to processing. Heat processing at 100°C resulted in minimal heat destruction of chlorinated hydrocarbon pesticides spiked at levels shown on Fig. 1. Storage at ambient temperature (23°C) greatly increased the losses of spiked chlorinated hydrocarbon pesticides but the greatest loss occurred after storage at 37·7°C for 1 year.

TABLE 6
Selected FAO Acceptable Daily Intakes (ADIs) and Maximum Residue Limits (MRLs) (FAO, 1985)

Pesticide, CCN and years of previous evaluations	Recommended maximum ADI (mg/kg body weight)	Commodity	Recommended MRL or ERL (mg/kg)	Remarks
Captan CCN 007 1965, 1969, 1973, 1974, 1977, 1978, 1980, 1982	0·1	*Kiwi fruit	20	TADI replaced by ADI at higher level. TMRLs are for captan. Metabolites are not included
Carbaryl CCN 008 1965, 1966, 1967, 1968, 1969, 1970 1973, 1975, 1976, 1977, 1978	0·01	Bananas	5 (5 in the pulp)	MRLs are for carbaryl. Metabolites are not included
		Poultry meat	0·5 (0·5 for poultry in the edible portion)	
Chlordane CCN 012 1965, 1967, 1969 1970, 1972, 1974, 1977, 1982	0·001 (1986)	Almonds	0·02 (E) (0·05)	TADI extended at same level. TERLs are for the sum of cis- and trans-chlordane in plant commodities and for the sum of cis- and trans-chlordane and 'oxychlordane' in animal products
		Bananas	0·02 (E) (0·05)	
		Figs	0·02 (E) (0·05)	
		Guavas	0·02 (E) (0·05)	
		Mangoes	0·02 (E) (0·05)	
		Papayas	0·02 (E) (0·05)	
		Passion fruit	0·02 (E) (0·05)	
		Pecans	0·02 (E) (0·05)	
		Pineapples	0·02 (E) (0·05)	
		Pomegranates	0·02 (E) (0·05)	
		Rice (polished)	0·02 (E) (0·05)	
		Rye	0·02 (E) (0·05)	
		Strawberries	0·02 (E) (0·05)	
		Walnuts	0·02 (E) (0·05)	
		Wheat	0·02 (E) (0·05)	
Cypermethrin	0·05	Beans (with pod)	0·05	(0·05 for kidney beans (in pod))

	Commodity			Notes
CCN 118 1979, 1981, 1982	Beans (without pod)	0·05**		(0·05 for kidney beans (without pods))
	*Small fruits and berries	0·5		(1 for grapes; 0·05 for currants (black, red and white), gooseberries, raspberries and strawberries)
	*Legume oilseed	0·05**		(0·05 for soybeans; 0·02 for peanuts)
	*Tea	20		MRLs are for cypermethrin (sum of isomers). Metabolites are not included. The meeting agreed that 0·05 mg/kg should be regarded as the limit of determination for all commodities except milk
	Milk products	MRL withdrawn (0·2)		
DDT CCN 021 1965, 1966, 1967, 1968, 1969, 1978, 1979, 1980, 1983			0·02	Conditional ADI replaced by ADI at higher level
Parathion CNN 058 1965, 1967, 1969, 1970			0·005	The definition of the residue is changed to 'parathion'. Metabolites are not included
Parathion-methyl CCN 059 1965, 1968, 1972, 1975, 1978, 1979, 1980, 1982			0·02	The definition of the residue is changed to 'parathion-methyl'. Metabolites are not included

New, as distinct from amended, recommendations are identified by the symbol '*' *before* the commodity or *before* the ADI. Residue levels at or about the limit of determination are *followed* by the symbol '**'. Amended recommendations are followed by the previous recommendation in parentheses.

TABLE 7
Reduction of Chlorinated Hydrocarbon Residues in Fruits and Vegetables

Produce	Pesticide	Reduction (%) during:		Reference
		commercial preparation	home preparation	
Apples	Total DDT		32–51	Baldwin et al. (1968)
Green beans	DDT	61–99+		Carlin et al. (1966)
Green beans	DDT	79–83	55–80	Elkins et al. (1968)
Green beans	Total DDT		46–63	Hemphill et al. (1967)
Potatoes	DDT	96+	14–90	Lamb et al. (1968a)
Spinach	DDT	86–91	30–52	Lamb et al. (1968b)
Tomatoes	Aldrin	75		Powell et al. (1970)
	Dieldrin	50		
Tomatoes	DDT	99+	78–99+	Farrow et al. (1968)

TABLE 8
Reduction of Organophosphate Residues in Fruits and Vegetables

Produce	Pesticide	Reduction (%) during:		Reference
		commercial preparation	home preparation	
Broccoli	Parathion	3–39	—[a]	Farrow et al. (1969)
Cherries	Gardona	95		Fahey et al. (1970)
Corn	Gardona	100		Fahey et al. (1969)
Green beans	Guthion	87–92		Carlin et al. (1966)
Green beans	Malathion	94+	99+	Elkins et al. (1968)
Green beans	Azodrin	98		Fahey et al. (1969)
Green beans	Gardona	100		Fahey et al. (1969)
Peaches	Gardona	99+		Fahey et al. (1970)
Pears	Gardona	98+		Fahey et al. (1970)
Spinach	Parathion	58–64	11–39	Lamb et al. (1968b)
Tomatoes	Azodrin	90–98		Fahey et al. (1971)
Tomatoes	Gardona	96–98		Fahey et al. (1969)
Tomatoes	Malathion	99+	96–99+	Farrow et al. (1969)

[a] Increases of 5–95%.

Processing spinach at 115·5°C (Fig. 2) was more effective than processing apricots in reducing most of the spiked chlorinated hydrocarbon pesticides. Storage also increased the losses of these compounds from spinach.

Heat processing apricots at 100°C or spinach at 115·5°C (Elkins et al., 1972) resulted in similar high losses of most organophosphate pesticides

TABLE 9
Reduction of Carbamate Residues in Fruits and Vegetables

| Produce | Pesticide | Reduction (%) during: | | Reference |
		commercial preparation	home preparation	
Broccoli	Carbaryl	73–97	25–90	Farrow et al. (1969)
Green beans	Carbaryl	86–92	26–58	Elkins et al. (1968)
Spinach	Carbaryl	58–64	11	Lamb et al. (1968b)
Tomatoes	Carbaryl	98–99+	69–92	Farrow et al. (1969)

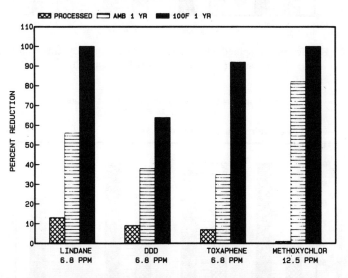

FIG. 1. Reduction of spiked chlorinated hydrocarbon pesticides during the processing (100°C) and storage of apricots.

(Fig. 3). Storage for 1 year resulted in virtually complete loss of all of the spiked organophosphates except trithion. The latter was reduced by 80%.

Elkins et al. (1972) also spiked their samples with carbamates. Heat processing apricots at 100°C resulted in modest reductions of 10–39% of the spiked carbamate residues. Storage did not greatly increase the

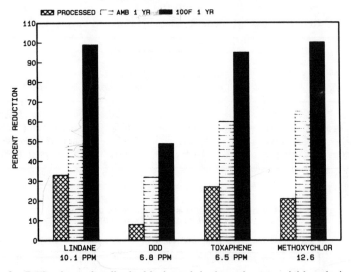

FIG. 2. Reduction of spiked chlorinated hydrocarbon pesticides during the processing (115·5°C) and storage of spinach.

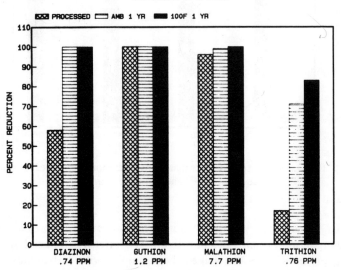

FIG. 3. Reduction of spiked organophosphate hydrocarbon pesticides during the processing (115·5°C) and storage of spinach.

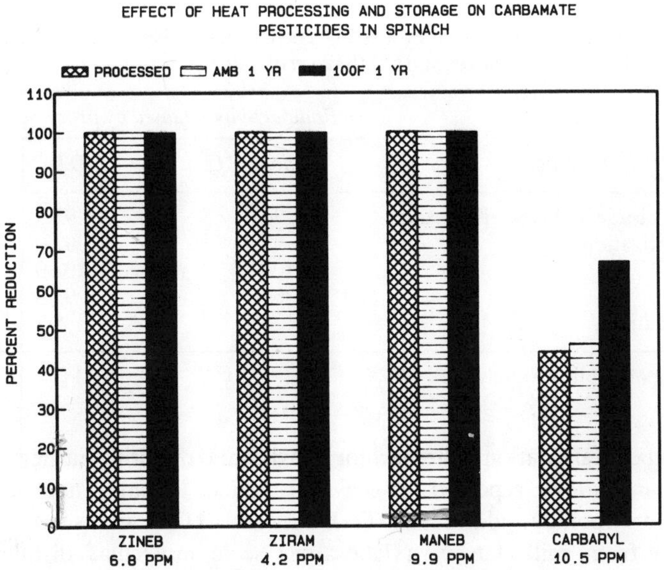

EFFECT OF HEAT PROCESSING AND STORAGE ON CARBAMATE
PESTICIDES IN SPINACH

FIG. 4. Reduction of spiked carbamate hydrocarbon pesticides during the processing (115·5°C) and storage of spinach.

reduction of these spiked carbamate residues. In contrast, heat processing spinach at 115·5°C naturally eliminates most of the carbamate residues (Fig. 4).

Cooking also has been found to substantially reduce ethylene dibromide (EDB) residues in rice (Clower *et al.*, 1985). Four samples of long and medium grain white rice containing 113, 295, 956 and 1568 ppb EDB were cooked according to package instructions. All levels of EDB in the cooked rice were <10 ppb. A second study involved the cooking of medium grain white rice containing 1600 ppb. After cooking, samples contained from 8 to 49 ppb, again showing major residue reduction.

Fats and Oils

Gooding (1966) reported the removal of numerous organochlorine pesticides from crude oil during commercial processing. Smith *et al.* (1968) studied this removal further and found that the deodorization step was primarily responsible for the reduction.

Kroger (1968) demonstrated that steam deodorization of butter oil at 180–195°C and 0·01–0·05 mm Hg for 5 h completely removed naturally

TABLE 10
Effect of Individual Commercial Processing Techniques on Residues in Rapeseed
Flakes and Oil (Saka *et al.*, 1970)

	% Radioactivity retained by processed oil[a]	
Operation	Lindane-[14]C	DDT-[14]C
Cooking rapeseed flakes with hexane	96·4	95·5
Desolventization	98·3	102·0
Refining	104·7	102·0
Bleaching	94·7	93·8
Deodorization	4·7	1·7

[a] Average of duplicate analyses.

occurring contamination of heptachlor epoxide and dieldrin. Earlier, Bills and Sloan (1967) reported 95–99% of added lindane, heptachlor, heptachlor epoxide, aldrin, DDT, DDE and TDE was successfully removed from milk fat by a laboratory scale molecular distillation apparatus. Saka *et al.* (1970) studied the effects of simulated commercial vegetable oil processing techniques on the removal of lindane and DDT residues from the rapeseed oil. Their data showed that alkali refining and bleaching had little or no effect on these residues but confirmed the effectiveness of deodorization for residue removal (Table 10).

Meat, Fish and Poultry
Liska *et al.* (1967) first reported the feasibility of removing selected chlorinated hydrocarbon pesticides by cooking. Simmering chicken at 88–93°C for 2–3 h reduced the level of DDT, dieldrin and heptachlor residue per gram of fat in white meat but the level of DDT and heptachlor per gram of fat in dark meat remained constant after the cooking period while the level of dieldrin slightly increased. Subsequent studies (McCaskey *et al.*, 1968) showed that all lindane, dieldrin, endrin, DDT, telodrin and chlorodane were rendered from hen carcasses after autoclaving at 15 psi for 3 h, whereas heptachlor epoxide, kelthane and oriex were resistant to removal even by this extreme heat treatment.

Ritchey *et al.* (1967a) reported the reduction of lindane, total DDT compounds, and kelthane in broilers cooked by baking or frying. These authors attributed most of the pesticide loss to removal of the pesticide associated with the leaching of the fat, which was substantiated in a second study (Ritchey *et al.*, 1967b).

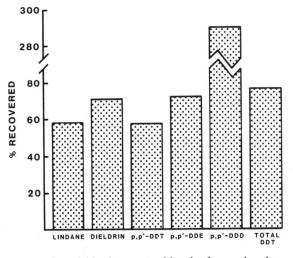

FIG. 5. Recovery of pesticides in meat and broth of stewed and pressure-cooked chicken.

Morgan *et al.* (1972) cooked stewing hens which had been fed for 5 weeks a standard laying ration contaminated with 25 ppm each of lindane, dieldrin, and p,p'-DDT. Breast pieces and drumsticks were cooked intact while thigh skin was separated from the meat and each was cooked separately. The chicken pieces were cooked by either stewing at 93°C for 2·5 h or pressure cooking at 10 psi (110°C) for 15 min. Both cooking methods were equally effective in reducing levels of these pesticides, showing an average loss from both the meat and broth of 41·9% for lindane, 27·6% for dieldrin, and 26·4% for total DDT compounds (Fig. 5). Lindane's higher vapor pressure probably contributed to its greater loss. Distribution patterns of the pesticides recovered in the meat and broth (Fig. 6) showed that the broth accounted for 66–80% of all the pesticides recovered, making the removal from the meat *per se* substantially higher.

Pan-frying, baking, and cooking with microwave has been found to reduce dieldrin levels (Fig. 7) in bacon baked to well done, i.e. 12 min in an oven at 204±1°C, or fried for 11 min with a surface temperature of 128°C, and sausage cooked to an internal temperature of 75°C by 42–72% (Yadrick *et al.*, 1971; Funk *et al.*, 1971). Cooking was effective equally in removing dieldrin from meat of control sows with very low levels of dieldrin and sows experimentally fed dieldrin (Fig. 8). Maul *et al.* (1971) braised, broiled, and cooked pork chops by microwave to well done

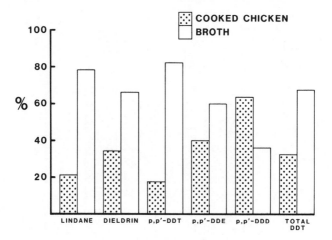

FIG. 6. Distribution of pesticides in cooked meat and broth of stewed and pressure-cooked chicken.

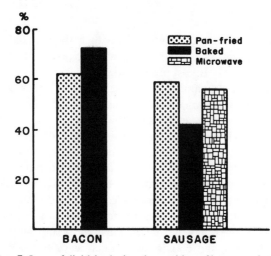

FIG. 7. Loss of dieldrin during the cooking of bacon and sausage.

81–90°C and roasted pork loins at 177±1°C to an internal temperature of 77°C. Because persons may choose whether to eat the fat associated with these cuts, the lean and fat portions were analyzed for dieldrin separately (Table 11). For this study, the more intense heating method of broiling and the longer heating time associated with baking appeared to be more

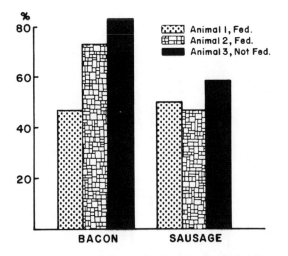

FIG. 8. Loss of dieldrin from control animals and animals fed during cooking of bacon and sausage.

TABLE 11
Dieldrin Reduction in Pork Chops and Pork Loins after Cooking (Maul *et al.*, 1971)

State	ppm (fat basis)		
	Lean	Fat	Drip
Raw	0·71	0·58	—
Cooked			
Braised	0·44	0·47[a]	0·43
Microwave	0·54	0·45	0·44
Broiled	0·07[b]	0·08[b]	0·43
Roasted	0·05[b]	0·41[a]	0·03

[a] Significantly less than raw ($p < 0.05$).
[b] Significantly less than raw ($p < 0.01$).

effective in reduction of the dieldrin residues in both the lean and fatty portions of the meat.

Although fat rendering has been considered to be the major mode of pesticide removal (Liska *et al.*, 1967; Ritchey *et al.*, 1967a), muscles dissected from the rounds of these pigs and roasted after all external fat had been trimmed (Yadrick *et al.*, 1972) exhibited 20–40% loss of dieldrin. Drip accounted for very low levels of the pesticide removal (Fig. 9).

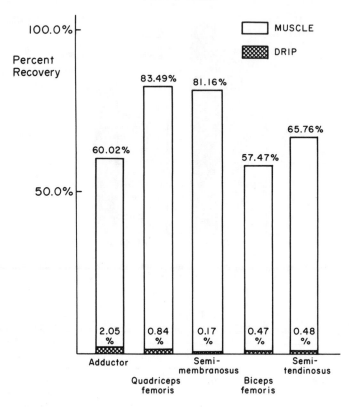

ȴIG. 9. Recovery in muscle and drip of dieldrin from trimmed muscles of pork rounds.

Muscles with greater surface area per unit of weight (i.e. adductor and biceps femoris) exhibited greater reduction in dieldrin than did the blockier quadriceps femoris or semimembranosus muscle. Thus, loss of environmental contaminants may be promoted by shaping cuts to have maximum surface area.

Stewing or pressure cooking breast and drumstick pieces, thigh meat, thigh skin, and adipose tissue from hens that had been fed a PCB mixture with 54% chlorination (Zabik, 1974), using cooking methods outlined earlier (Morgan *et al.*, 1972), showed that overall loss of PCBs ranged from 17% for the drumstick to 40% for the breast piece. Those overall losses were similar to levels seen for chlorinated hydrocarbon pesticides (Morgan *et al.*, 1972); however, the distribution patterns for all the meat pieces and thigh skin differed. Roughly half of the PCBs recovered were found in the meat and half in the broth.

The effectiveness of reducing PCBs from fish depends largely on the species and its fat content. Roasting, broiling, or cooking lake trout fillet by microwave to an internal temperature of 75°C reduced PCBs by 26–53% (Zabik *et al.*, 1979). Those fish averaged 25–29% fat and contained from 3·8 to 4·8 ppm PCBs in the raw edible fillet. In contrast, the level of PCBs in raw carp fillets (Zabik *et al.*, 1982) with an average fat content of 7·7±3·2% fat and 1·58±1·06 ppm PCBs was virtually unaffected by poaching, roasting, deep-fat frying, charbroiling, or cooking by microwave to the same end point temperature.

PBBs are members of the halogenated hydrocarbon class of compounds with structure, reactivity, use and toxicity similar to PCBs of high chlorination. Michigan Chemical Corporation manufactured a product called Firemaster BP-6. Those industrial compounds were used most commonly as fire retardants and plasticizers in business machines, electrical appliances and fabricated products. PBBs are not a general environmental contaminant and would not be of concern except for an incredible error in animal feed manufacture in Michigan in May 1973. The PBB compound Firemaster FF-1 was mistaken for magnesium oxide (trade name Nutrimaster) and mixed into high protein dairy pellets. Through this contamination and consequent cross-contamination of other feeds, dairy animals, poultry and swine in Michigan were affected. Contaminated meat and milk products exceeding the United States Food and Drug Administration tolerance of 0·3 ppm in the fat, set in November 1973, were destroyed. Moreover, starting in 1978, the State of Michigan purchased and destroyed all dairy animals having more than 20 ppb in their tail fat.

A study (Smith *et al.*, 1977) of pressure cooking breast pieces, drumsticks, thigh meat and thigh skin at 10 psi (110°C) for 15 min showed similar overall losses to that found for chlorinated hydrocarbon pesticides and PCBs, but 66% of the recovered PBBs were found in the meat. The bulkier size and high molecular weight of the PBBs may render them more difficult to remove with cooking out fat.

Because some Michigan dairy animals were thought to possibly contain low levels of PBBs, a second study (Zabik *et al.*, 1980) was undertaken to see the potential reduction of PBBs from beef rounds during cooking. Table 12 presents the average loss of PBBs compared to total cooking losses. For longer cooking times of roasting or high heat of broiling steak, the PBB loss exceeded the loss of fat and moisture. Total cooking losses and PBB losses were similar to braising steak, but total cooking losses

TABLE 12
Comparison of Polybrominated Biphenyls (PBB) Loss and Cooking Loss of Cuts
from Beef Rounds (Zabik *et al.*, 1980)

Beef cut	Cooking method	Internal temperature	PBB lost (%)	Total cooking loss
Sirloin tip	Roasted	65	45·7	25·8
Semimembranous steak	Broiled	77	71·2	41·6
	Braised	77	34·9	34·1
Adductor steak	Broiled	77	53·2	39·8
	Braised	77	37·2	33·7
Ground beef patties	Broiled	77	32·3	43·4
Hamburger patties	Broiled	77	31·5	42·1

exceeded PBB losses for broiling hamburgers or ground beef patties; the latter cooked in the shortest time. Moreover, the distribution of the PBB congeners differs significantly ($p < 0.01$) between raw and cooked samples for all cuts except hamburger.

Thus it has been shown that most pesticide residues are reduced during cooking and processing but the amount is related to the type of pesticide, the location of the residue and the type of process. Thus high heat processing is more likely to result in greater loss. Deodorization is the most effective step in reducing residues during the processing of oil. Removal of pesticide from meat is primarily due to removal when fat is rendered during cooking but loss also occurs during codistillation. In the latter case the ratio of surface area to weight is an important factor.

SUMMARY

Pesticides and chemical fertilizers are necessary to produce the quantities of food to meet the needs of the world population but their use should be integrated with other methods of pest management. Use of industrial chemicals can contribute safety, i.e. use of fire retardant for clothes, plastics etc., and make possible current life styles, but risk versus benefit always needs to be assessed and possible environmental impacts, especially as they affect the food chain, need to be evaluated. Generally residue levels are low but continual surveillance is needed to ensure the safe use of these compounds. Cooking and/or processing can be an additional safety factor as many residues in food are reduced if the food is eaten after cooking and/or processing.

WHO/FAO groups, as well as scientists in numerous countries, continually evaluate toxicological data as they become available and use the data in estimating maximum daily intakes of various compounds. These published values have changed over time and it is expected that further changes will be necessary as more data become available. Again, use of any pesticide or industrial chemical may result in some risk but the benefit of the compound in a particular setting must be carefully considered and its risk/benefit ratio determined before deciding whether the use is warranted.

REFERENCES

Baldwin, R. E., Sides, K. G. and Hemphill, D. D. (1968). DDT and its derivatives in apples as affected by preparative procedures: a pilot study. *Food Technol.*, **22**, 126–9.

Bills, D. D. and Sloan, J. L. (1967). Removal of chlorinated insecticide residues from milk fat by molecular distillation. *J. Agric. Food Chem.*, **15**, 676–8.

Carlin, A. J., Hibbs, E. T. and Dahm, P. A. (1966). Insecticide residues and sensory evaluation of canned and frozen snap beans field-sprayed with guthion and DDT. *Food Technol.*, **20**, 80–4.

Clower, M., McCarthy, J. P., Jr. and Rains, D. M. (1985). Effect of cooking on levels of ethylene dibromide residues in rice. *J. Assoc. Off. Anal. Chem.*, **68**, 710–11.

Elkins, E. R., Lamb, F. C., Farrow, R. P., Cook, R. W., Kawai, M. and Kimball, J. R. (1968). Removal of DDT, malathion and carbaryl from green beans by commercial and home preparative procedures. *J. Agric. Food Chem.*, **16**, 962–6.

Elkins, E. R., Farrow, R. P. and Kim, E. S. (1972). The effect of heat processing and storage on pesticide residues in spinach and apricots. *J. Agric. Food Chem.*, **20**, 286–91.

Fahey, J. E., Gould, G. E. and Nelson, P. E. (1969). Removal of Gardona and Azodrin from vegetable crops by commercial preparative methods. *J. Agric. Food Chem.*, **17**, 1204–6.

Fahey, J. E., Nelson, P. E. and Ballee, D. L. (1970). Removal of Gardona from fruit by commercial preparative methods. *J. Agric. Food Chem.*, **18**, 865–8.

Fahey, J. E., Nelson, P. E. and Gould, G. E. (1971). Removal of Azodrin residues from tomatoes by commercial preparative methods. *J. Agric. Food Chem.*, **19**, 81–2.

FAO (1976). *Pesticide Residues in Foods.* FAO Plant Production and Protection Series, No. 1, Rome, 45 pp.

FAO (1978a). *Pesticide Residues in Foods: 1977 Report.* FAO Plant Production and Protection Paper, 10 Rev., Rome, 81 pp.

FAO (1978b). *Pesticide Residues in Foods: 1977 Evaluations.* FAO Plant Production and Protection Paper, 10 Sup., Rome, 459 pp.

FAO (1979). *Pesticide Residues in Foods: 1978 Evaluations*. FAO Plant Production and Protection Paper, 15 Sup., Rome, 293 pp.

FAO (1980). *Pesticide Residues in Foods: 1979 Evaluations*. FAO Plant Production and Protection Paper, 20 Sup., Rome, 560 pp.

FAO (1981). *Pesticide Residues in Foods: 1980 Evaluations*. FAO Plant Production and Protection Paper, 26 Sup., Rome, 460 pp.

FAO (1982). *Pesticide Residues in Foods: 1981 Evaluations*. FAO Plant Production and Protection Paper, 35 Sup., Rome, 571 pp.

FAO (1983). *Pesticide Residues in Foods: 1982 Evaluations*. FAO Plant Production and Protection Paper, 49 Sup., Rome, 434 pp.

FAO (1984). *Pesticide Residues in Foods: 1983 Evaluations*. FAO Plant Production and Protection Paper, 56 Sup., Rome, 68 pp.

FAO (1985). *Pesticide Residues in Foods: 1984 Evaluations*. FAO Plant Production and Protection Paper, 62 Sup., Rome, 98 pp.

Farrow, R. P., Lamb, F. C., Cook, R. W., Kimball, J. R. and Elkins, E. R. (1968). Removal of DDT, malthion, and carbaryl from tomatoes by commercial and home preparative methods. *J. Agric. Food Chem.*, **16**, 65–71.

Farrow, R. P., Lamb, F. C., Elkins, E. R., Cook, R. W., Kawai, M. and Cortes, A. (1969). Effect of commercial and home preparation procedures on parathion and carbaryl residues in broccoli. *J. Agric. Food Chem.*, **17**, 75–9.

Frank, R., Rasper, J., Braun, H. E. and Ashton, G. (1985). Disappearance of organochlorine residues from abdominal and egg fats of chickens, Ontario, Canada, 1969–1982. *J. Assoc. Off. Anal. Chem.*, **68**, 124–9.

Funk, K., Zabik, M. E. and Smith, S. L. (1971). Dieldrin residues in sausage patties cooked by three methods. *J. Food Sci.*, **36**, 616–8.

Gartrell, M. J., Craun, J. C., Podrebarac, D. S. and Gunderson, E. L. (1985a). Pesticides, selected elements, and other chemicals in infant and toddler total diet samples. October 1978–September 1979. *J. Assoc. Off. Anal. Chem.*, **68**, 842–61.

Gartrell, M. J., Craun, J. C., Podrebarac, D. S. and Gunderson, E. L. (1985b). Pesticides, selected elements, and other chemicals in adult total diet samples. October 1978–September 1979. *J. Assoc. Off. Anal. Chem.*, **68**, 862–75.

Gartrell, M. J., Craun, J. C., Podrebarac, D. S. and Gunderson, E. L. (1985c). Pesticides, selected elements, and other chemicals in infant and toddler total diet samples. October 1979–September 1980. *J. Assoc. Off. Anal. Chem.*, **68**, 1163–83.

Gartrell, M. J., Craun, J. C., Podrebarac, D. S. and Gunderson, E. L. (1985d). Pesticides, selected elements, and other chemicals in adult total diet samples. October 1979–September 1980. *J. Assoc. Off. Anal. Chem.*, **68**, 1184–95.

Gooding, C. M. B. (1966). Fate of chlorinated organic pesticide residues in the production of edible vegetable oils. *Chem. and Ind.*, 344.

Hemphill, D. D., Baldwin, R. E., Deguzman, A. and Deloach, H. K. (1967). Effects of washing, trimming, and cooking on levels of DDT and derivatives in green beans. *J. Agric. Food Chem.*, **15**, 290–4.

Jensen, A. A. (1983). Chemical contaminants in human milk. *Residue Rev.*, **89**, 1–128.

Johnson, R. D., Manske, D. D., New, D. H. and Podrebarac, D. S. (1984a). Pesticide, heavy metal, and other chemical residues in infant and toddler total diet samples. III. August 1976–September 1977. *J. Assoc. Off. Anal. Chem.*, **67**, 145–54.

Johnson, R. D., Manske, D. D., New, D. H. and Podrebarac, D. S. (1984*b*). Pesticide, heavy metal, and other chemical residues in adult total diet samples. XIII. August 1976–September 1977. *J. Assoc. Off. Anal. Chem.*, **67**, 154–66.

Kroger, M. (1968). Effect of various physical treatments on certain organochloride hydrocarbon insecticides found in milk fat. *J. Dairy Sci.*, **51**, 196–8.

Lamb, F. C., Farrow, R. P., Elkins, E. R., Cook, R. W. and Kimball, J. R. (1968*a*). Behavior of DDT in potatoes during commercial and home preparation. *J. Agric. Food Chem.*, **16**, 272–5.

Lamb, F. C., Farrow, R. P., Elkins, E. R., Cook, R. W. and Kimball, J. R. (1968*b*). Removal of DDT, parathion and carbaryl from spinach by commercial and home preparative procedures. *J. Agric. Food Chem.*, **16**, 967–73.

Liska, B. J., Stemp, A. R. and Stadelman, W. J. (1967). Effect of method of cooking on chlorinated insecticide residues in edible chicken tissues. *Food Technol.*, **21**, 117–20.

Maul, R. E., Funk, K., Zabik, M. E. and Zabik, M. J. (1971). Dieldrin residues and cooking losses in pork loins. *J. Am. Dietet. Assoc.*, **59**, 481–4.

McCaskey, T. A., Stemp, A. R., Liska, B. J. and Stadelman, W. J. (1968). Residue in egg yolks and raw and cooked tissues from laying hens administered chlorinated hydrocarbon insecticides. *Poultry Sci.*, **47**, 564–9.

Morgan, K. J., Zabik, M. E. and Funk, K. (1972). Lindane, dieldrin and DDT residues in raw and cooked chicken and chicken broth. *Poultry Sci.*, **51**, 470–5.

Podrebarac, D. S. (1984*a*). Pesticide, heavy metal, and other chemical residues in infant and toddler total diet samples (IV). October 1977–September 1978. *J. Assoc. Off. Anal. Chem.*, **67**, 166–75.

Podrebarac, D. S. (1984*b*). Pesticide, heavy metal, and other chemical residues in adult total diet samples (XIV). October 1977–September 1978. *J. Assoc. Off. Anal. Chem.*, **67**, 176–85.

Powell, A. J. B., Stevens, T. and McCully, K. A. (1970). Effects of commercial processing on residues of aldrin and dieldrin in tomatoes and residues in subsequent crops grown on the treated plots. *J. Agric. Food Chem.*, **18**, 224–7.

Ritchey, S. J., Young, R. W. and Essary, E. O. (1967*a*). The effects of cooking on chlorinated hydrocarbon pesticide residues in chicken tissues. *J. Food Sci.*, **32**, 238–40.

Ritchey, S. J., Young, R. W. and Essary, E. O. (1967*b*). Cooking methods and heating effects on DDT residues in chicken tissues. *J. Food Sci.*, **34**, 569–71.

Saka, J. G., Nielsen, M. A. and Summer, A. K. (1970). Effect of commercial processing techniques on lindane- and DDT-^{14}C residues in rapeseed oil. *J. Agric. Food Chem.*, **18**, 43–4.

Smith, K. J., Polan, P. C., DeVries, D. M. and Coon, F. B. (1968). Removal of chlorinated pesticide from crude vegetable oils by simulated commerciial processing procedures. *J. Am. Oil Chem. Soc.*, **45**, 886–69.

Smith, S. K., Zabik, M. E. and Dawson, L. E. (1977). Polybrominated biphenyl levels in raw and cooked chicken and chicken broth. *Poultry Sci.*, **56**, 1289–96.

Yadrick, M. K., Funk, K. and Zabik, M. E. (1971). Dieldrin residues in bacon cooked by two methods. *J. Agric. Food Chem.*, **19**, 491–4.

Yadrick, M. K., Zabik, M. E. and Funk, K. (1972). Dieldrin levels in relation to total, neutral and phospholipid composition in selected pork muscles. *Bull. Environ. Contam. Toxicol.*, **8**, 289–93.

Zabik, M. E. (1974). Polychlorinated biphenyl levels in raw and cooked chicken and chicken broth. *Poultry Sci.*, **53**, 1785–90.

Zabik, M. E., Hoojjat, P. and Weaver, C. M. (1979). Polychlorinated biphenyls dieldrin and DDT in lake trout cooking by broiling, roasting or microwave. *Bull. Environ. Contam. Toxicol.*, **21**, 136–43.

Zabik, M. E., DeFouw, C. and Weaver, C. M. (1980). Polybrominated biphenyl congener levels and distribution patterns in raw and cooked beef. *Arch. Environ. Contam. Toxicol.*, **9**, 651–9.

Zabik, M. E., Merrill, C. and Zabik, M. J. (1982). PBCs and other xenobiotics in raw and cooked carp. *Bull. Environ. Contam. Toxicol.*, **28**, 710–15.

Chapter 5

HORMONES IN FOOD: OCCURRENCE AND HAZARDS

ENRICA QUATTRUCCI

Istituto Nazionale della Nutrizione, Rome, Italy

INTRODUCTION

It is well known that our food, whilst containing all the necessary nutrients, may also be the vehicle of undesirable substances either of natural or xenobiotic origin. In countries where agriculture and animal production are practised on a large scale, the use of chemicals to prevent or cure diseases, or to secure economic advantages, such as pesticides, veterinary drugs and anabolic hormones, is rapidly increasing. Therefore their residues may reach the consumers via food. Problems related to substances exerting hormonal activity will be especially emphasized in this chapter.

Components of food, either of vegetable or animal origin, possessing biological properties have been known for many years. In animals as well as in man these substances have a well-defined metabolic role and their formation and secretion are determined by a complex mechanism.

The possibility of controlling fertility both in humans and in animals using fruits, plants and plant extracts has also been recognized for a long

103

time. In the Orient, the pomegranate, for example, has been traditionally associated with fertility for over 2000 years.

Farnsworth *et al.* (1975) described over 300 plants which were able to initiate oestrus in animals. Those plants, i.e. legumes and fodders, which are consumed in substantial quantities, interfere with normal reproductive function causing infertility in livestock and may possibly be of some relevance to humans who consume them directly or through food of animal origin carrying residues of such plant oestrogens.

Since some protein/peptide and steroidal hormones act as anabolic agents, they have been used for the purpose of promoting growth of domestic animals. The protein and peptide hormones have little significance to man because they are denatured and biologically inactivated during the digestive process. In contrast, the steroidal hormones are readily absorbed from the gastrointestinal tract, maintaining their effectiveness until they are metabolized to inactive compounds. During the last few decades many other chemicals have been shown to possess hormonal activity and some of these have also been used both with the aim of controlling reproductive function in breeding animals and as anabolic agents. These compounds cannot be considered simply as 'hormones' and should be carefully studied not only in relation to their potential toxicological properties.

The presence in the diet of residues of either natural or xenobiotic hormones might present a risk, and recent misuse and illegal use of such compounds has led to serious concern about the consumer's health. This chapter reviews the advances in this area, taking into account the needs of modern biotechnology as well as the ethical standpoint of the public health.

OESTROGENIC ACTIVITY OF PLANT AND FUNGAL COMPOUNDS

Substances showing oestrogenic properties in the vegetable kingdom are well known although the potential hazard they represent to animals and to man has not yet been completely clarified. Oestrogenic activity has been detected in grasses and feedstuffs as well as in fruits, vegetables, cereals, and oils, e.g. apples, cherries, carrots, garlic, parsley, potatoes, barley, corn, oats, rice, wheat, and oils from soy, coconut, peanuts, olives, etc. Extensive reviews have been published by Verdeal and Ryan (1979), Stob (1983) and Price and Fenwick (1985).

The principal oestrogenic compounds present in plants are isoflavones, often in their glycosidic form, and coumestans which are biogenetically similar. In addition, consideration will be given to resorcylic acid lactones with oestrogenic activity which may be produced by moulds in moist stored cereals (Table 1).

Isoflavones and Coumestans

Among the large number of isoflavones isolated from plants only a few have been shown to possess oestrogenic properties of some relevance; these include daidzein and genistein, their glucosides daidzin and genistin, and their 4'-methyl ethers formononetin and biochanin A. Other isoflavones such as pratensein and prunetin are of limited occurrence and minor effectiveness. The general structure of isoflavones is shown in Fig. 1. The isoflavones occurring in the glycoside form are readily hydrolysed in animals and presumably in man. Isoflavones have lower biological activity than endogenous or synthetic oestrogens. In fact genistein, the most effective of them, first isolated from soya (Walz, 1931), exhibits only 10^{-5} of the activity of the synthetic powerful oestrogen diethylstilboestrol (Stob, 1973), but it has been shown to be high enough to interfere with animal breeding. Manifestations of this hormonal interference in grazing animals are infertility, dystocia and uterus prolapse (Bradbury and White, 1954). It has been found that isoflavones, and more generally many plant oestrogens, exhibit binding affinity to oestrogen receptor sites, displacing 17ß-oestradiol from uterine receptors (Shutt, 1967, 1976).

The magnitude of the hormonal effects is related not only to the dose but mainly to the different metabolic pathways of these compounds. Whereas genistein and biochanin A are inactivated, formononetin is converted mainly into the isoflavone equol, a compound affecting oestrus in animals (Shutt and Braden, 1968; Nottle and Beck, 1974).

Isoflavones exerting the highest hormonal activity have proved to be non-mutagenic in the salmonella/mammalian microsome assay (Bartholomew and Ryan, 1980).

Human foodstuffs often contain oestrogens of plant origin, their levels being much greater in diets of vegetarian subjects. It is difficult to evaluate the potential hazard they might represent, many factors being involved, such as time of exposure, gut microflora activity, intestinal transit time etc. In fact Axelson et al. (1982) found equol in human urine, excreted as glucuronide or sulphoconjugate. Soya proved to be an important source of isoflavones (Carter et al., 1955; Eldridge and Kwolek, 1983; Seo and Morr, 1984). Whereas Axelson et al. (1984) found a considerable increase of

TABLE 1
Source and Active Principles of Oestrogens Isolated from Some Edible Plants

Botanic name	Common name	Family	Plant part	Active principle
Allium sativum L.	garlic	Liliaceae	bulb	—
Avena sativa L.	oats	Gramineae	seeds	zearalenone[a]
Cicer aretinum L.	chick pea	Leguminosae	seeds	isoflavones
Daucus carota L.	carrot	Umbelliferae	root	isocoumarin deriv.
Hordeum vulgare L.	barley	Gramineae	seeds/embryo	zearalenone[a]
Pirus malus L.	apple	Rosaceae	fruit	oestrone
Prunus avium L.	cherry	Rosaceae	fruit	isoflavones
Prunus domestica L.	plum	Rosaceae	fruit	isoflavones
Oryza sativa L.	rice	Gramineae	seeds/embryo	zearalenone[a]
Phaseolus vulgaris L.	French bean	Leguminosae	seed/plant	oestradiol
Punica granatum	pomegranate	Myrtaceae	seed	oestrone
Secale cereale	rye	Gramineae	seed	zearalenone[a]
Soya hispida L.	soybean	Leguminosae	seed	isoflavones
Triticum aestivum	wheat	Gramineae	seed	zearalenone[a]
Zea mays	corn	Gramineae	seed	zearalenone[a]

[a] Produced by grain fungi (*Fusarium*).

Isoflavones

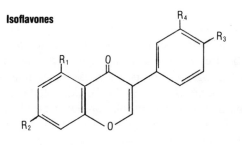

	R₁	R₂	R₃	R₄
Daidzein	H	OH	OH	H
Daidzin	H	O-Gluc	OH	H
Genistein	OH	OH	OH	H
Genistin	OH	O-Gluc	OH	H
Formononetin	H	OH	OCH₃	H
Biochanin A	OH	OH	OCH₃	H
Pratensein	OH	OH	OCH₃	OH
Prunetin	OH	OCH₃	OH	H

Coumestans

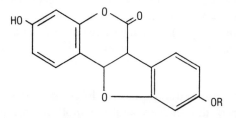

Coumestrol R = H
4-Methoxycoumestrol R = CH₃

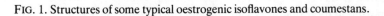

FIG. 1. Structures of some typical oestrogenic isoflavones and coumestans.

equol excretion in healthy subjects eating 40 g of texturized soya foods for 5 days, Setchell *et al.* (1984) observed much lower levels of this active metabolite under similar conditions.

Many coumestans have been isolated from plants, especially beans, alfalfa and other fodder crops, but only two of them, i.e. coumestrol (7,12-dihydroxycoumestan) and 4'-methoxycoumestrol, possess much greater oestrogenic activity than the isoflavones, to which they have a closely related structure, as shown in Fig. 1. Also coumestans exhibit a binding affinity to oestrogen receptors, which is greater in uterine cytosol of calf than in other species (Lee *et al.*, 1977). Cattle fed with alfalfa and other fodder crops may undergo serious breeding problems. It is not known if any potential risk to humans might arise from hormonal residues present in products from animals fed with oestrogenic pasture containing coumestans, or from soybeans, soybean sprouts and, more generally, 'health foods' often containing significant levels of coumestrol (Elakovich and Hampton, 1984). Coumestans, like isoflavones, have been shown to be non-mutagenic (Bartholomew and Ryan, 1980) but to be tumour promoters (Verdeal *et al.*, 1980).

Resorcylic Acid Lactones
Resorcylic acid lactones exerting oestrogenic activity are metabolic products of some fungal species, common field moulds, which may grow on seeds stored in moist conditions. Some of these organisms synthesize substances having toxic and/or hormonal effects such as the *Fusarium roseum* 'graminearum' (Gibberella zeae in its sexual stage) and *Fusarium tricinctum* which produce the resorcylic acid lactone zearalenone. Zearalenone, first isolated by Stob *et al.* (1962), was chemically identified by Urry *et al.* (1966) as 6-(10-hydroxy-6-oxo-*trans*-1-undecenyl)-β-resorcylic acid lactone (Fig. 2). Among a large literature on this subject, many important aspects of these moulds, such as production of mycotoxins, have been reviewed by Betina (1984) and Moss and Smith (1984).

Zearalenone and its reduced and hydrogenated derivatives 7β-zearalanol (taleranol) and 7α-zearalanol (zeranol) are the best known oestrogens of this group (Fig. 2). Zearalenone has been found in stored cereals, mainly corn. In different years 1% to 17% of the examined corn samples contained detectable quantities of zearalenone (Bennett and Shotwell, 1979). High levels, approaching 3000 ppm, have also been reported in food samples (Mirocha and Christensen, 1974).

Consumption of *Fusarium*-infected feeds by cattle, swine, and poultry resulted in serious pathological effects on the animals. Mouldy corn containing zearalenone caused hyperplasia of the uterus, infertility, reduced litter size and neonatal mortality (Kurtz *et al.*, 1969; Miller *et al.*, 1973; Chang *et al.*, 1979). McNutt *et al.* (1928) first described cases of

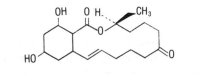

ZEARALENONE

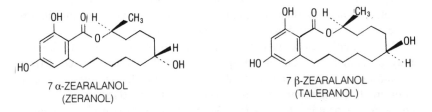

7 α-ZEARALANOL
(ZERANOL)

7 β-ZEARALANOL
(TALERANOL)

FIG. 2. Structures of oestrogenic resorcyclic acid lactones zearalenone, 7α-zearalanol (zeranol) and 7β-zearalanol (taleranol).

vaginal prolapse in sows related to the consumption of infected feed. The adverse effects depend on dose and time of exposure. In immature boars fed with corn containing 500–600 ppm zearalenone, growth and testis weight were considerably reduced (Christensen et al., 1972), whilst boars fed with 40 ppm zearalenone from 14 to 18 weeks of age were only temporarily affected by the treatment, i.e. reduced libido and testosterone concentration, returning to normality at 36 weeks of age (Berger et al., 1981).

Zearalenone is considered to be a mycotoxin (F-2 toxin) but a number of serious physiological disorders reported in livestock and poultry fed with *Fusarium*-infected rations may be attributed to the simultaneous presence of zearalenone and other more toxic mycotoxins such as the secondary metabolites trichothecenes, nivalenol, deoxynivalenol (DON), 3-acetyldeoxynivalenol (ADON), and diacetoxyscirpenol (Micco et al., 1986; Greenhalgh et al., 1986; Stob, 1983; Price and Fenwick, 1985; Lee et al., 1985; Tanaka et al., 1985a,b) (see following chapter).

Zearalenone was reported to be mutagenic in *Bacillus subtilis* (Ueno and Kubota, 1976), but not in *Salmonella typhimurium* (Wehner et al., 1978), the Ames reverse mutation test with and without mammalian S9 activation systems or the mouse lymphoma assay *in vivo*. However, only low-level exposures were tested in these systems.

It has been demonstrated that zearalenone, zearalanol and zearalenols bind to oestrogen receptor sites, inhibiting the binding of 17β-oestradiol to the rat uterine cytosolic and nuclear receptors (Kiang et al., 1978), and β-zearalenol proved to be most active. In rat, zearalenone binds to the uterine oestrogen receptors in the following order of affinity: coumestrol > zearalenone > isoflavones (Verdeal et al., 1980); in addition, zearalenone binds to the hepatic cytosolic receptors (Powell-Jones et al., 1981). cis-Zearalenone was shown to possess stronger uterotropic activity than the natural trans isomer, while no differences have been found between cis- and trans-zearalenols.

Contamination of cereal crops with Fusarium in wet temperate climates may be sometimes relevant. Eppley et al. (1974) found, in corn from contaminated areas in the USA, about 17% of the 223 samples examined contained zearalenone ranging from 100 to 5000 μg/kg. Levels of zearalenone peaking to 10 400 μg/kg have been measured in damaged corn (Stoloff et al., 1976). More recently Bennett and Shotwell (1979) reviewed the data on zearalenone levels found in various cereals and soya beans.

Many other cases of seriously contaminated crops have been detected in Canada (Andrews et al., 1981), in Australia (Blaney et al., 1984) and in the USA, in association with DON and aflatoxin B$_1$ (Hagler et al., 1984; Stoloff and Dalrymple, 1977), and in Korea co-existing with NIV and DON (Lee et al., 1985). In contrast, Osborne (1982) reported that virtually no contamination was detected in recent surveys of cereals and commercial flour in the UK.

Cereals are widely used for human consumption either directly or in processed foods. An extensive review of many surveys dealing with zearalenone contamination of human foods is reported in the above-mentioned papers by Price and Fenwick (1985). The results of surveys carried out mainly in southern Africa, where humidity facilitates the growth of Fusarium species, are summarized in Table 2.

It has been shown that zearalenone and, especially, zearalanol administered by subcutaneous implantation to farm animals have anabolic effects, increasing weight gain in different animal species (Hidy et al., 1977; Van Veerden et al., 1981; Roche, 1981). Zearanol, more commonly known by the synonym zeranol or the Ralgro trade name, is obtained from zearalenone produced in submerged culture of F. graminearum by Raney nickel reduction and hydrogenation yielding a mixture of 7β- and 7α-zearalanols. The commercial product or zeranol contains mainly (98%) the more powerful 7α diastereoisomer (Windholtz, 1976).

TABLE 2

Surveys on Natural Occurrence of Zearalenone in Food Commodities (μg/kg or litre)

Commodity	Mean level or range	Max level	Country	Reference
Barley (unpolished)	500–750	—	Scotland	in Bennett and Shotwell (1979)
(polished)	110	1 581	Korea	Lee et al. (1985)
flour	—	—	Korea	Lee et al. (1985)
	2[a]	4	Japan	Tanaka et al. (1985b)
malt (unpol.)	19	36	Korea	Lee et al. (1985)
Beer	920	4 600	Zambia	Lovelace and Nyathi (1977)
Beer	300	2 000	Lesotho	in Bennett and Shotwell (1979)
Maize	200–500	—	USA	Eppley et al. (1974)
Maize	280	800	Zambia	Lovelace and Nyathi (1977)
Maize	450–550	5 750	Transkei	Marasas et al. (1979)
Maize	200	—	Canada	in Bennett and Shotwell (1979)
Maize	73	670	N. Italy	Micco et al. (1986)
Maize malt	680	4 000	Zambia	Lovelace and Nyathi (1977)
Maize porridge, sour drinks etc.	800	5 300	Swaziland	in Bennett and Shotwell (1979)
Rye (polished)	2	4	Korea	Lee et al. (1985)
Wheat (polished)	5	40	Korea	Lee et al. (1985)
Wheat flour	3[a]	27	Japan	Tanaka et al. (1985b)

[a] Mean in positive samples.

The metabolism of zearanol has been studied in various species, using radiometric technique. When administered orally, most of the compound is absorbed and eliminated in the faeces and urine, the proportion between them being species-dependent. After administration of a single oral dose to rat, rabbit, dog, monkey and man (Migdalof *et al.*, 1983), the absorbed compound was oxidized and/or conjugated. The excretion was accomplished mainly via bile in all the species except man, where urinary and faecal excretions 120 h after dosing were 55% and 23% respectively. In both cases free and conjugated zeranol and free and conjugated zearalenone were found. In urine 19% was conjugated zeranol and 13% conjugated zearalenone. About 23% was a more polar unknown metabolite, presumably hydroxy-zeranol. Radioactivity in blood reached a peak after 1 h, practically disappearing in 72 h.

Growth promoters are mainly administered to farm animals, e.g. sheep, steers and oxen, calves etc., by implantation, usually in the ear region, so zeranol metabolism has been studied in these animals after implantation. In steers, implanted zeranol (72 mg) was slowly released and rapidly cleared from the plasma. Urinary excretion gradually increased, peaking at about 12 days and decreasing until 90 days, reaching 10% of the dose in total, while 45% was eliminated through faeces. Bile was shown to be the major excretory route (Sharp and Dyer, 1972).

It has been demonstrated that the oestrogenic properties of zeranol and its metabolites are far lower than those of 17β-oestradiol, stilbene and stilbene derivatives, depending on the age of the animals at administration and their species. In rat, experiments carried out on zearalenone by uterotropic assay have shown that this compound possesses less than 0·1% of the biological activity of 17β-oestradiol, while neonatal exposure produced sterility of a much higher potency, about 10% that of the natural compound (Kumagai and Shimizu, 1982). Pigs proved to be especially sensitive to zearalenone (Chang *et al.*, 1979). All the dose levels of zeranol used in long-term studies on rodents, dog and monkey showed hormonal efficacy (Roe, 1983). In rats and mice biological activity was still detectable at levels of 30–50 μg/animal/day.

Studies on fetotoxicity and teratogenicity of zeranol have been carried out on mice. Dose levels ranging from 300 to 1000 μg/kg/day resulted in a reduction in number of live litters. No significant teratogenicity was found at any level (Davis *et al.*, 1977).

No carcinogenic effects were seen in a life span study in rats at all dose levels, but toxic effects on liver were observed at all doses and haematological changes occurred at the highest doses (CEC report, 1982). Toxic effects on the haemopoietic system, increased weight of liver, kidney and adrenals, and hormonal effects on the reproductive system have been detected in female beagles. No evidence of carcinogenicity was found (CEC report, 1982). Haematological changes, alterations in liver function, and hormonal effects on reproductive organs have been detected in female rhesus monkeys receiving dose levels ranging from 15 to 75 mg/kg body weight; again no evidence of carcinogenicity was found (CEC report, 1982).

In man there are no epidemiological data clearly related to zeranol or zearalenone ingestion but it was suggested that *Fusarium* mycotoxins may be involved in the aetiology of tumours of the digestive tract and reproductive system (Martin and Keen, 1978; Schoental, 1979). Consumption of *Fusarium*-infected corn, containing high levels of zearalenone and DON, has been associated with a high incidence of oesophageal cancer (Marasas *et al.*, 1979).

The authors concluded that available information on chronic or synergistic activity of these substances is largely insufficient to evaluate their potentially harmful effects to health. This conclusion is even more true if we consider the possible residues in food of animal origin after zeranol treatment of farm animals. Presence and quantity of residues depend on many factors, e.g. hormone dose levels, appropriate withdrawal period before slaughtering, proper discarding of the application sites, types of organs and tissues examined, nature of metabolites and chemical impurities in the commercial products. So far it is difficult to evaluate and interpret results of studies carried out quite differently with respect to doses used, withdrawal period, sensitivity of detection methods and, last but not least, always on very few animals (Brown, 1973; Hoffmann and Karg, 1975; Roche, 1981). In general it might be assumed that there would be no significant accumulation of zeranol and/or its metabolites in edible tissues, apart from the implantation site, if appropriate time (usually 65 days) intervenes before slaughtering. Re-implantation every 90–100 days, used to increase the anabolic efficacy of zeranol, might increase the possible residues (Brown, 1983; Janski, 1983).

Is the presence of residues maintaining hormonal activity in food of animal origin safe? According to the point of view of many observers, the majority of sex hormones, both natural and synthetic, might be classed as tumour-promoting agents, making a distinction of tumour-initiating agents and complete carcinogens. Therefore it is necessary to determine a 'no hormonal effect level' (NHEL) when judging the safety of use of any anabolic agents.

In monitoring programmes for the presence and levels of anabolics in food, the availability of suitable detection methods is particularly important. Many procedures have been described based on biological, histological, chemical and immunological techniques. Biological methods have been carried out determining the increased weight of the uterus in immature female rats due to the treatment or evaluating the vaginal cornification promoted by the hormone in mature castrated mice (Umberger et al., 1958; Kroes and Huis in't Veld, 1975). Examination for histological changes in the prostate of male calves or in the Bartholin glands of female calves is also used (Kroes and Huis in't Veld, 1975).

Among the chemical methods the chromatographic techniques, widely used, have been reviewed by Gilbert (1984). For routine screening a thin-layer chromatography (TLC) procedure has been performed. In corn and corn derivatives, the detection limit for zearalenone in TLC has been reported to be 20 ppb (Scott et al., 1978) while a two-dimensional TLC method for zeranol in meat presents a detection limit of 10 ppb. Zeranol and zearalenone can be determined by HPLC, with a detection limit of 10 ppb, and zearalenone has been determined in corn products with a detection limit of 5 ppb (Scott et al., 1978).

Radioimmunological techniques have been proposed to quantify zeranol in biological fluids (Dixon, 1980; Dixon and Heitzman, 1981; Janski, 1983). These methods have been judged satisfactory for plasma and urine but not sufficiently sensitive for determining residues of zeranol in edible tissues (CEC report, 1982). More recently, sensitive HPLC methods for estimation of zeranol in muscle tissue have been developed (Medina and Sherman, 1986).

NATURAL SEX HORMONES AND THEIR RESIDUES IN FOOD OF ANIMAL ORIGIN

Natural sex hormones, whether exerting oestrogenic, androgenic or gestogenic activity, have the well known steroid chemical structure. The most effective of them likely to be used as growth promoters are shown in Fig. 3.

Steroid hormones are secreted by the gonads, the adrenals and the placentas of pregnant females, and control the proper function of sexual

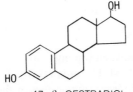

17 - β - OESTRADIOL

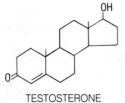

TESTOSTERONE

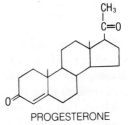

PROGESTERONE

FIG. 3. Natural sex hormones used as growth promoters.

physiology in man as well as in animals. The level of secretion is subject to a complex but well established feed-back mechanism. They are transported in plasma bound either to specific steroid binding proteins or to some non-specific serum albumins (Mercier-Bodard *et al.*, 1979; Rico *et al.*, 1981). These molecules exert their hormonal effects at target organs and tissues passing through the membrane into the cells. In the cytosol they interact with proteic receptors which are thus activated, changing their conformation. The hormone–receptor complex undergoes translocation to the nucleus where it binds to a large number of acceptor sites on chromatin and can modify expression of the genetic message. In this way, through specific RNA messengers, cellular protein synthesis is regulated (Katzenellenbogen *et al.*, 1980; Clark *et al.*, 1980).

It has been supposed that the few receptors in muscles might also be affected in this manner by some chemicals possessing hormonal androgenic activity (Heitzman, 1975). The presence of oestrogen receptors has been described also in liver cytosol of mammals (Eisenfeld *et al.*, 1980) including post-menopausal women (Duffy and Duffy, 1978).

Endogenous sex hormones are rapidly metabolized, mainly in liver, through various reductions and hydroxylations, then conjugated with glucuronic or sulphuric acid to form water-soluble compounds easily excreted in the bile. However, a small percentage of free and conjugated metabolites are found in liver, kidney and other tissues because of systemic circulation. When oxidation processes interfere, reactive intermediates might be formed, covalently binding to biological macromolecules. Correlations have been found between binding capacity and carcinogenic potency (Brookes and Lawley, 1964; Horning *et al.*, 1978; Taylor, 1981). Many workers have compared different carcinogens by their DNA-binding capacity using the covalent-binding index (CBI) (Lutz, 1979):

$$CBI = \frac{\text{mmol of bound product per mol of nucleotide}}{\text{mmal of administered product per kg of animal}}$$

Direct correlations between CBI and hepatocarcinogenicity have been found in rat (Lutz, 1979). Using the CBI parameter, Barraud *et al.* (1984) demonstrated a binding capacity for natural hormones, higher for 17 β-oestradiol than for testosterone. For a long time there has been good evidence that hormonal imbalance can result in tumorigenesis in endocrine organs and their target tissues, as demonstrated experimentally by continuous stimulation of these organs with specific hormones (Gardner, 1953).

More recent data have demonstrated that continuous stimulation is not always necessary. In fact, even brief exposure of newborn mice to oestrogenic steroids leads later to a high incidence of different cancers (Dunn and Green, 1963; Kimura and Nandi, 1967; Takasugi *et al.*, 1970; Clark and McCormack, 1977).

In healthy untreated animals, sex hormone levels vary widely depending on species, sex and physiological state. For instance, in 24 h an adult male pig might produce on average 10 mg of testosterone, and a bull 40–50 mg of testosterone (Rhynes and Ewing, 1973). Production of 17β-oestradiol might vary from 28 mg/24 h in pregnant sheep (Challis *et al.*, 1971, 1974) to 0·006–0·008 mg during the oestrus cycle (Baird *et al.*, 1968). Similarly, variations in concentrations of steroid sex hormones have been found in peripheral plasma (Hunter *et al.*, 1972; Yuthasastrakosol *et al.*, 1975; Hoffmann and Karg, 1975; Hoffmann, 1983). Natural sex hormones and xenobiotic substances having hormonal action have now been used for more than two decades in controlling reproduction, in breeding programmes and as growth promoters in various domestic species. Anabolics of natural and xenobiotic origin most commonly used in animal production, generally by implant in the ear region or injection, are shown in Table 3. The studies on the hormonal treatment of farm animals have been reviewed by Van Veerden *et al.* (1981), Roche (1981) and Bouffault and Willemart (1983).

TABLE 3
Growth Promoters Exerting Hormonal Activity in Animal Production

Compounds	Oestrogenic	Androgenic	Gestogenic
Exogenous			
Natural steroids	17β-oestradiol	testosterone	progesterone
Xenobiotics			
Steroidal	oestradiol benzoate	testosterone propionate	melengestrol acetate (MGA)
	oestradiol monopalmitate	trenbolone	
		trenbolone acetate (TBA)	
Non-steroidal	diethylstilboestrol (DES)		
	hexestrol		
	dienestrol diacetate		
	zeranol		

TABLE 4
Preparation and Doses of Anabolics Used as Growth Promoters in Animal
Production

17β-Oestradiol + progesterone	20 mg + 200 mg	veal, calf
17β-Oestradiol + testosterone propionate	20 mg + 200 mg	steer, heifer, lamb
17β-Oestradiol + trenbolone acetate	20 mg + 140 mg	veal calf, steer
Hexestrol + trenbolone acetate	40 mg + 200 mg	veal, steer, lamb, swine
Trenbolone acetate	300 mg	cattle
Zeranol + trenbolone acetate	36 mg + 140 mg	veal calf, steer, heifer, lamb
Zeranol	12 mg–72 mg	veal calf, steer, heifer, lamb
DES	3 mg – 120 mg	veal calf, steer, heifer, lamb, poultry

The most relevant effects of the anabolics are to induce a considerable increase of protein deposition, often with a concomitant decrease in fat deposition, and to improve the feed conversion efficiency. Even the quality and appearance of meat appear to be improved by the treatment. Combinations of two anabolic agents are generally more effective than a single substance (Table 4). Animal weight presents an average increase of 10–25%, peaking to 47% in steers treated with combined 20 mg of oestradiol benzoate and 200 mg of progesterone (Roche, 1980). A mechanism of action of anabolic agents has been proposed by Heitzman (1975). The initial stimuli act on the hypothalamus and then, via pituitary and endocrine tissues, promote the release of steroids resulting in a stimulation of growth of non-endocrine tissues.

Endogenous hormones, present in organs and tissues, have to be considered natural constituents of foods of animal origin, scarcely affected by food processing (Hoffman and Karg, 1975). Hormone levels in tissues may vary consistently, depending on the animal's sex. In muscle tissues, for example, levels of androstenedione have been found higher than those of testosterone in female animals and calves, whereas testosterone was higher in bull muscle (Gaiani and Chiesa, 1986). Quantitative data obtained so far on steroid residues in edible tissues, after appropriate withdrawal times and discarding the implant or injection area, do not differ consistently from the levels of natural hormones (Hoffmann and Oettel, 1976; Henricks, 1981; Reid, 1981; Hoffmann, 1983; Mattioli et al., 1986).

Might the residues of steroid sex hormones in food present any risk for the consumer's health? In order to discuss this problem it might be useful to recall the hormone levels normally present in humans in relation to their different physiological states. A good review on oestrogen production in man has been published by Rubens and Vermeulen (1983). The most active oestrogen is 17β-oestradiol, then oestrone which may be transformed in tissues to 17β-oestradiol or to the less active metabolite oestriol. Concentration of oestrogens in plasma, depending on the rate of production and the metabolic clearance, is high at birth, decreases rapidly and rises again at puberty. In adult males, where oestrone is quantitatively more important, the plasma levels of oestrogens remain quite stable (6–10 mg/100 ml), showing a moderate increase during senescence. Plasma levels of oestrogen vary cyclically in women. They show a peak during pregnancy and decrease after menopause to similar or lower levels than in elderly males. Secretion of the androgen testosterone ranges from 4·4 to 6·6 mg/24 h in men; it is 0·35 mg in women, 0·100 mg in infants and decreases progressively with age.

Endogenous steroid hormones, even when secreted within the normal range, might present either hormonal or toxic side effects such as baldness, prostatic disease etc. (testosterone related), and premenstrual tension, reproductive system disorders, increased tendency to develop calculi etc. (oestrogen related). More serious are the roles played by the steroid hormones as promoters in induction of liver cancer and the more complex one in cancer of the prostate, breast and uterus. Considering the risk of steroid hormones to human subjects, Taylor (1981) concludes that low anabolic residues in agricultural products may result in little hazard to the human population, providing there is a proper control of their administration and the continuation of a search for better agents.

Similar tentative conclusions have been reached by the EEC Scientific Committee (CEC report, 1982) considering the actual amount of sex steroids consumed via food, their low oral bioavailability and the existence of liver and placental barriers.

When natural oestrogens are administered orally, an unphysiologic rise of mainly oestrone is observed, the oestradiol metabolite in the liver. Quite differently, synthetic steroidal oestrogens escape from hepatic inactivation entering unchanged into the general circulation.

Finally, it is of interest to note that some partially synthetic derivatives of natural steroids differ from the natural hormones in their biological behaviour. For example, ethynyloestradiol, with an acetylenic substituent at the 17-position, is a powerful oestrogen sufficiently resistant to metabolism in the gastrointestinal tract to be highly effective by oral administration. It has also been found that the introduction of an 11β-methoxy group increases the biological potency of steroid hormones. Both of these structural modifications result in a reduced affinity of the molecule for the serum binding proteins, and consequently an enhanced activity towards the hormonal receptors (Katzenellenbogen *et al.*, 1980). These compounds therefore, in spite of their close similarity to the natural steroids, must be regarded as wholly xenobiotic as far as their hormonal efficacy, metabolism and potentially adverse effects are concerned.

XENOBIOTICS WITH HORMONAL ACTIVITY

Many wholly synthetic compounds possess biological activity analogous to the natural hormones. Some of these compounds, particularly those exerting androgenic activity, such as trenbolone, or oestrogenic properties, such as stilbene derivatives, have been used extensively as growth promoters.

Trenbolone

Trenbolone (TBOH, *syn*-trienbolone, trienolone or 17β-hydroxytrenbolone) is a synthetic steroid with androgenic activity lower than testosterone (approximately 15%), but with greater anabolic effects. The product normally used commercially is trenbolone acetate (TBA). Chemically, trenbolone has a structure similar to testosterone except for three conjugated double bonds (Fig. 4). Information on the physical-chemical properties of trenbolone has been given by Windholtz (1976). Its administration as growth promoter is by implant at the base of the ear; the withdrawal period has been calculated as 50 days for cattle and 60 days for other animals. TBA may be implanted alone or in combination with oestradiol or with zeranol, its effect resulting in an increase in nitrogen retention, improved feed efficiency and an increase of carcass weight (Van Veerden *et al.*, 1981; Roche, 1981; Bouffault and Willemart, 1983; Roche, 1983; Foxcroft *et al.*, 1983). The meat presents no organoleptic differences from that of non-implanted animals. The metabolism of TBA has been studied in the rat, calf, heifer, cow and steer using radiometric techniques. TBA is rapidly hydrolysed to trenbolone and, together with its metabolites, excreted as glucuronides and sulphates, mostly in the bile. The predominant trenbolone metabolites identified in the extractable fractions of rat bile were a 16-OH and a 17-keto metabolite. In contrast, in cattle the major bile TBA metabolite was 17α-hydroxytrenbolone with a small amount of trenbolone and other metabolites (Pottier *et al.*, 1981).

Genotoxicity of trenbolone was examined by mutagenicity tests

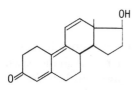

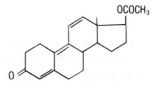

TRENBOLONE   TRENBOLONE ACETATE

FIG. 4. Structures of trenbolone and trenbolone acetate.

(Ingerowski *et al.*, 1981; Richold, 1983) and by its CBI (Barraud *et al.*, 1984). Trenbolone did not show mutagenic activity in prokaryotic systems, *in vivo* tests for bone marrow and germ cell cytogenetics. It should be noted that in the Ames salmonella/mammalian microsome assay the higher doses (2000–3000 μg/plate) displayed cytotoxic effects which prevented definite conclusions with regard to its mutagenicity. Clastogenic activity *in vitro* against human lymphocytes was negative, but tests against mouse lymphoma cells were slightly positive, to the same degree shown by testosterone and oestradiol. The CBI for trenbolone, a little higher than that found for testosterone, was shown to be dose-dependent, but not proportionally. As a function of time the CBI first increased, peaking after 24 h, then decreased indicating that the molecules fixed on DNA are probably eliminated by repair mechanisms. In Syrian hamster embryo (SHE) cells no induction of unscheduled DNA synthesis could be detected but the SHE cells were clearly transformed in their morphology by trenbolone and not by testosterone. This indicates that the transforming ability is not related to the hormonal effect (Schiffmann *et al.*, 1985).

Morphological and neoplastic transformation of SHE cells without measurable gene mutation has been reported for diethylstilboestrol (DES) (Barrett *et al.*, 1981; McLachlan *et al.*, 1982). A genetic mechanism at the chromosomal level causing neoplastic cell transformation has been proposed (Tsutsui *et al.*, 1983). It has been postulated that the capability of trenbolone to transform mammalian cells *in vitro*, possibly related to its covalently binding to protein, may indicate a carcinogenic potential of this compound difficult to detect by assays of direct DNA damage (Schiffmann *et al.*, 1985).

Studies of acute, short- and long-term toxicity have been carried out in several animal species. Trenbolone showed low acute oral toxicity. In rodents the compound caused an increased size of liver, kidney and spleen in addition to the expected changes related to the hormonal activity such as increase in ovary weight, decrease and atrophy of seminal vesicles, testis and prostate.

In long-term studies in mouse, haematological and histopathological changes were observed at the highest dose level. There was an increased incidence of nodular hyperplasia and tumours in the liver, swollen kidneys and ovarian cysts. In rat, serious histopathological changes of the reproductive apparatus and other organs have been detected, including an increased incidence of pancreatic islet cell tumours. The interpretation of the results of carcinogenicity studies in rodents is difficult because of the hormonal effect at all the dose levels employed. The increased tumour incidence at the highest dose levels is probably due to an epigenetic mechanism related to the modulating effect of the hormonal activity on tumour production (CEC report, 1982). In special studies on man, volunteers of both sexes were given i.m. 5·0 or 10·0 mg of TBA daily during 14 days. Nitrogen balance was disturbed at the low level (about 70 μg/kg) and a significant reduction of 17-ketosteroid excretion and disturbance in the menstrual cycle were observed at the higher dose level (Kruskemper et al., 1967). Determination of a no-hormonal-effect level has not yet been finalized. From available published data, residues of trenbolone in meat appear to be of the order of a few ppb (Galli et al., 1985; Hess, 1983).

Many analytical methods have been proposed in order to identify and control the trenbolone residues in biological fluids and meat (Ryan and Hoffmann, 1978). In tissues, after various purification and partition procedures, TBOH could be detected by TLC and quantitatively determined by emission spectrofluorimetry. The detection limit in meat extracts was 5 ppb. The same limit has been found using HPLC techniques (Stan and Hols, 1979). Radioimmunoassay techniques (RIA) appear to be the most adequate, detecting very low amounts of TBOH, e.g. >40 pg (Hoffmann and Oettel, 1976; Duchatel et al., 1982). Discrepancies between the total residues determined by radiotracer studies and extractable residues determined by RIA led to the conclusion that non-extractable radioactivity probably represents covalently bound residues.

It has been demonstrated that, after proteolysis, these residues become bioavailable on consumption, but probably less toxic for the consumers (Hoffmann et al., 1984; Rico and Burgat-Sacaze, 1984).

Stilbene Derivatives

Anabolic compounds derived from the stilbene structure are shown in Fig. 5. Among them, DES is certainly the compound which has been most

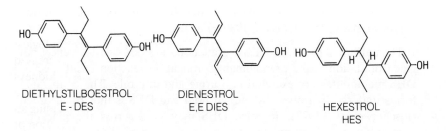

DIETHYLSTILBOESTROL   DIENESTROL
E - DES   E,E DIES   HEXESTROL
                                                                                          HES

FIG. 5. Structures of oestrogenic stilbene derivatives.

widely used either in human and veterinary medicine or as an anabolic agent. Specifications on chemical and physical properties have been reported by Windholtz (1976c). This chemical has undergone the most thorough investigation. A review on its use as an anabolic agent would be at the present time rather historical (it has been banned in many countries) if we were not considering its widespread illegal use.

When, more than 40 years ago, DES was synthesized in England (Dodds *et al.*, 1938) and its oestrogenic properties were recognized, it was used therapeutically because of its effectiveness and cheapness. Unfortunately its metabolism was not carefully studied and it was generally assumed that glucuronidation was its only metabolic pathway. Many years later the *in utero* exposure to stilbene derivatives was associated with genital tract abnormalities including adenosis, adenocarcinosis and squamous metaplasia in female human offspring. Additionally, different types of cancer have been reported in women chronically treated by DES and in men receiving DES for treatment of prostatic cancer (IARC, 1979).

Thus additional metabolic studies have been carried out and it has been suggested that electrophilic intermediates, such as the aromatic and olefinic epoxide of DES and DES semiquinone and quinone, are formed in several species and humans (Metzler *et al.*, 1980). At least four metabolic pathways are operative in DES metabolism:

Aromatic hydroxylation leading to 3'-hydroxy-DES (catechol), which is then methylated yielding 3'-methoxy-DES (Engel *et al.*, 1976)
Oxidation of the stilbenediol structure yielding Z,Z-DIES which may undergo further reactions, e.g. methoxylation, cyclization, hydroxylation
Aliphatic oxidation leading to 1-hydroxy-DES
Cleavage of the DES molecule resulting in the formation of 4'-

hydroxypropiophenone, having possibly an olefinic epoxide intermediate (Metzler et al., 1980) (Fig. 6).

The pattern of oxidative DES degradation shows species differences but glucuronidation is the predominant conjugation reaction in all species. DES metabolites are excreted into urine and into bile. The conjugated forms undergo hydrolysis by the gut flora and DES is thus re-adsorbed (Fischer et al., 1973). In mice DES may pass across the placenta, accumulating with its metabolites in the foetal genital tract (Shah and McLachlan, 1976).

DES has been tested for genotoxicity in different test systems. No mutagenicity was detected in the Ames salmonella test but the compound was active in other systems, inducing mutations in mouse lymphoma cells, sister chromatid exchanges in human fibroblasts, unscheduled DNA synthesis in activated HeLa cells and morphological and neoplastic transformation of Syrian hamster embryo fibroblasts (Glatt et al., 1979; Rudiger et al., 1979; Clive, 1977; Martin et al., 1978; McLachlan et al., 1982). This latter effect is of particular interest, being clearly not related to the oestrogenicity of the compound. Additionally, DES does not cause detectable mutations in the transformed cells at two loci always mutated by other chemical carcinogens (Barrett et al., 1981). It has been suggested that DES can transform cells to neoplastic ones without somatic mutation or exerting a mutational effect at the chromosome level.

DES binds covalently to cellular macromolecules, such as nucleic acids and proteins. In carcinogenicity studies, DES showed carcinogenic activity in several animal species, rodents, hamsters, dogs and squirrel monkeys (IARC, 1979). Apart from the genotoxicity and carcinogenic properties, other toxic effects of DES have been reported. Among them there are reports that it acts synergistically with X-rays and chemical carcinogens on mammary adenocarcinoma development in female rats (Shellabarger et al., 1976, 1980).

On the basis of the data already mentioned, international organizations have reached conclusions which may be of some interest to report:

'DES is a carcinogen when ingested by animals. Evidence in the record suggests that DES is a carcinogen when ingested by humans. There is no known no-effect level for the carcinogenic properties of DES' (Fed. Reg., 1979).

'DES is causally associated with the occurrence of cancer in humans. There is also sufficient evidence for its carcinogenicity in experimental animals' (IARC, 1979).

'Stilbene oestrogens should not be used in animal production as anabolic

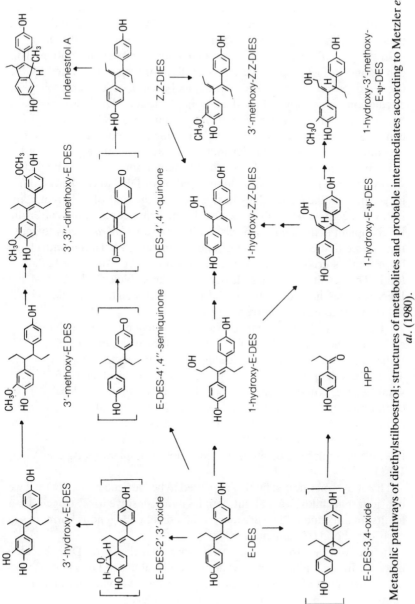

FIG. 6. Metabolic pathways of diethylstilboestrol; structures of metabolites and probable intermediates according to Metzler *et al.* (1980).

agents, because they are orally active, persistent in food, pose some environmental problems because of their low biodegradability, and because DES is a known carcinogen' (WHO working group, 1981).

In the past, DES has been used as anabolic in growth promotion. This compound in fact is effective either orally, not being inactivated by the digestive processes with prolonged life because of the enterohepatic circulation, or slowly released after implantation. DES use has been banned since 1979 in the United States and since 1981 in those EEC countries where it was still permitted. In some EEC countries, use of this substance was already forbidden many years ago, e.g. in Italy from 1961.

Early researches carried out on different hormones including DES showed that, whereas the oral administration of DES to chickens did not leave any significant residues in the meat at the end of the treatment, hormonal activity was still detectable in chicken meat 3 months after the DES implant in the animals' necks. Utilizing an *ante litteram* relay toxicity, the muscle tissue, liver and fat of poultry implanted from 3 months have been administered to ovariectomized rats every 1, 2 or 3 days for 12 days in total. The results showed a clearly dose-related biological effect of the DES residues in poultry tissues on rat uterine weight (Cubadda *et al.*, 1964*a,b*; Fratoni and Quattrucci, 1966).

Moreover, in 1980 a report on various cryptogenic breast enlargement cases in prepubertal children was carried out by paediatric hospitals. The Italian ministry of health, considering that hormones as auxinic agents in animal breeding were used to a greater extent than official information would suggest, undertook widespread controls on meat and baby foods containing veal meat. DES residues were found in veal meat and baby foods (Loizzo and Macri, 1983). The hypothesis has been made that the DES found in baby food might have arisen from processed meat containing the intramuscular depot site of the injection or implant (Karg and Vogt, 1981).

The above-mentioned finding appeared to be particularly worrying if we consider that children are about 20 times more sensitive to oestrogens than adults, mainly due to the very low production of endogenous hormones in early childhood (Hoffmann, 1981).

In many other western countries, such illegal use of DES became evident. In the United States, widespread illegal use of DES in cattle has been discovered after the total banning. Only a development of adequate routine control programmes may reduce such illegal use.

Many analytical methods for the evaluation of DES residues and/or its metabolites at ppb levels in foodstuffs have been reported; the classical method is based on the evaluation of uterus hypertrophy in immature mice after oestrogen intake (Umberger *et al.*, 1958). This method is not specific and does not allow identification of the active oestrogenic compound, which is important in view of the different biological activities of different oestrogens. Moreover, some results showed an increase of uterus weight which was linear with dose only in a limited range (Galli *et al.*, 1983). Therefore, as far as residues of DES are concerned, the results of the biological assay appear not to be quantitatively reliable. Radioimmunoassay (RIA) has been the methodological approach developed furthest and applied most widely for the detection of residues of anabolic agents in tissues, urine and faeces. RIA is a very sensitive analytical method and allows the determination of many samples at the same time (Hoffmann, 1978).

An improvement, so far as sensitivity and specificity of the gas-chromatographic quantitation is concerned, may be achieved by selective ion monitoring (SIM). By the SIM method the two synthetic oestrogens commonly used in animal breeding (DES and hexestrol) and the most potent natural oestrogen (oestradiol) were determined simultaneously. Moreover, a comparative study done by adding DES to a commercial homogenized baby food shows that SIM analysis is more reliable and sensitive than biological assay (Galli *et al.*, 1983).

OVERVIEW

The use of anabolic agents to improve beef, sheep and poultry production is increasing. It is estimated that about half of the cattle produced in the UK and more than 90% of feedlot cattle in the USA are treated with growth promoters (FAO/WHO report, 1985). These substances are not to be used in laying hens or dairy cattle but, unfortunately, they have been utilized in Europe to increase weight before slaughter of cull dairy cows still lactating. It was estimated that approximately 1·5% of the anabolic would be excreted in the milk during the first month of treatment. Another problem related to the misuse of steroid hormones and, more generally, of anabolics from all sources is that they may be injected or implanted in edible portions of the animals, resulting in large amounts of residues in food. It has been calculated that up to 30% of the activity of anabolics may remain at the implant site at normal slaughter time (FAO/WHO report, 1985).

In this panorama all the international organizations involved with food safety evaluation and legislation, e.g. FAO/WHO committees, FDA, European Scientific Committee on Food, had to deal for many years with problems related to the use of anabolics in animal breeding. Till very recently the most commonly shared opinion among them was that the use of natural hormones, and derivatives quickly yielding the parent compounds after hydrolysis, would present no harm to the consumer if appropriate technological conditions were respected. Additional information has been considered necessary before the evaluation of xenobiotics might be completed. The ethical basis for these technologies would be not to achieve a major profit but to increase availability of protein of animal origin in consideration of the impressive number of undernourished people in the world. In this respect some speculation is reasonable: is the malnutrition problem related only to food deficiencies or mainly to incorrect distribution among countries and, in the same country, among buying powers of various social groups?

Is the benefit, if any, derived from this practice so substantial as to justify the possible risk of an additional charge to the already high amounts of compounds exerting hormonal activity naturally occurring in foods? Again, how may these highly sophisticated technologies help in developing countries used to a very traditional kind of agriculture and animal breeding?

It has been calculated that the world production of milk and meat in 1975 alone might cover the minimum human demand for protein of animal origin, to which there is to be added the protein from eggs and fish (Jasiorowski and Sharly, 1975).

The distribution is presently so unbalanced as to cause the nutritionist concern about the consequences of the excess of protein intake by the population of western countries.

Consumer organizations have developed a clear, strong position against the use of anabolics. They do not accept the risk/benefit equation in this respect, considering that no real benefit for the community may result from these practices. An important expectation of consumers is the freedom to exercise a choice. This choice, in European countries, is the wish for meat from animals which are not subjected to stress, producing more slowly meat of better quality; they are prepared to pay the price (Yeomans, 1983).

With a decision welcomed by the consumers and some scientists but highly disliked by many breeders, on 20th December 1985 the EEC ministries of agriculture approved a total banning of the use of hormones starting from 1st January 1988. Probably the extra cost of maintaining for a long time thousands of kilograms of meat in the EEC stores acted in favour of this decision.

Therefore, the dilemma seems to be solved at least in Europe but still there remains the need for proper programmes to control the presence of anabolics in food of animal origin due to illegal use.

A last question mark remains on the destiny of the large quantities of hormones, mainly oestrogens, entering the environment via animal production. The fate of thousands of kilograms of these compounds in soil and water from animal excreta is still not well known. Data available on oestrogen degradation were collected in the past using analytical methodologies considered inadequate today. These compounds just disappear in the environment. We hope that there is no chance of receiving an unwanted answer to this question.

ACKNOWLEDGMENTS

The author is grateful to Dr. G. Vettorazzi (WHO) and Dr. A. Macrì (Health Institute, Rome) for providing up-to-date information and literature, and to Prof. R. Walker (Surrey University) for his encouragement and help during the preparation of the manuscript.

REFERENCES

Andrews, R. I., Thompson, B. K. and Trenholm, H. L. (1981). A national survey of mycotoxins in Canada. *J. Am. Oil Chem. Soc.*, **57**, 889–91.

Axelson, M., Kirk, D. N., Farrant, R. D., Cooley, G., Lawson, A. M. and Setchell, K. D. R. (1982). The identification of the weak oestrogen equal (7-hydroxy-3-(4'-hydroxyphenyl)chroman) in human urine. *Biochem. J.*, **201**, 353–7.

Axelson, M., Sjövall, J., Gustafsson, B. E. and Setchell, K. D. R. (1984). Soya, a dietary source of the non-steroidal oestrogen equol in man and animals. *J. Endocrinol.*, **102**, 49–56.

Baird, D. T., Goding, J. R., Ichikawa, Y. and McCracken, J. A. (1968). The secretion of steroids from the autotransplanted ovary in the ewe spontaneously and in response to systemic gonadotrophin. *J. Endocrinol.*, **42**, 283.

Barraud, B., Lugnier, A. and Dirheimer, G. (1984). Determination of the binding of trenbolone and zeranol to rat-liver DNA in vivo as compared to 17β-oestradiol and testosterone. *Food Add. Contaminants*, **1**, 147–55.

Barrett, J. C., Wong, A. and McLachlan, J. A. (1981). Diethyl-stilbestrol induces neoplastic transformation without measurable gene mutation at two loci. *Science*, **212**, 1402–4.

Bartholomew, R. N. and Ryan, D. S. (1980). Lack of mutagenicity of some phytoestrogens in the Salmonella/mammalian microsome assay. *Mutat. Res.*, **78**, 317–21.

Bennett, G. A. and Shotwell, O. L. (1979). Zearalenone in cereal grains. *J. Am. Oil Chem. Soc.*, **56**, 812–19.

Berger, T., Esbenshade, K. L., Diekman, M. A., Hoagland, T. and Tuite, J. (1981). Influence of prepubertal consumption of zearalenone on sexual development of boars. *J. Anim. Sci.*, **53**, 1559–64.

Betina, V. (1984). Zearalenone and brefeldin A. In: *Mycotoxins: Production, Isolation, Separation and Purification*, V. Betina (Ed.), Elsevier, Amsterdam, pp. 237–57.

Blaney, B. J., Moore, C. J. and Tyler, A. L. (1984). Cytotoxins and fungal damage in maize harvested during 1982 in far north Queensland. *Austral. J. Agric. Res.*, **35**, 463–71.

Bouffault, J. C. and Willemart, J. P. (1983). Anabolic activity of trenbolone acetate alone or in association with estrogens. In: *Proc. OIE Symp. Anabolics in Animal Production*, ISBN 92-9044-118-6, pp. 155–79.

Bradbury, R. B. and White, D. E. (1954). Estrogens and related substances in plants. *Vit. Horm.*, **12**, 207–33.

Brookes, P. and Lawley, P. D. (1964). Evidence for the binding of polynuclear aromatic hydrocarbons to the nucleic acids of mouse skin: relation between carcinogenic power of hydrocarbons and their binding to DNA. *Nature*, **202**, 781–4.

Brown, R. G. (1973). Ausscheidungsstudie über Zeranol. *Tierärzl. Umschau*, 179–85.

Brown, R. G. (1983). Zeranol implants. In: *Proc. OIE Symp. Anabolics in Animal Production*, ISBN 92-9044-118-6, pp. 181–92.

Carter, M. W., Matrone, G. and Smart, W. W. G., Jr. (1955). Effect of genistin on reproduction of the mouse. *J. Nutr.*, **55**, 639–45.

Challis, J. R. G., Harrison, F. A. and Heap, R. B. (1971). Uterine production of estrogens and progesterone at parturition in the sheep. *J. Reprod. Fertil.*, **25**, 306.

Challis, J. R. G., Harrison, F. A. and Heap, R. B. (1974). The extraction of estrogen and the rate of secretion of estrone and 17β-estradiol by the uterus in the pregnant sheep. *J. Endocrinol.*, **61**, 277.

Chang, K., Kurtz, H. J. and Mirocha, C. J. (1979). The effect of the mycotoxin zearalenone on swine reproduction. *Am. J. Vet. Res.*, **40**, 1260–7.

Christensen, C. M., Mirocha, C. J., Nelson, G. H. and Quast, J. F. (1972). Effect on young swine of consumption of rations containing corn invaded by Fusarium roseum. *Appl. Microbiol.*, **23**, 202.

Clark, J. H. and McCormack, S. A. (1977). Clomid or Nafoxidine administered to neonatal rats causes reproductive tract abnormalities. *Science*, **197**, 164–5.

Clark, J. H., Watson, C., Upchurch, S., McCormack, S. A., Padykula, H., Markaverich, B. and Hardin, J. W. (1980). Estrogen action in normal and abnormal cell growth. In: *Estrogens in the Environment*, J. A. McLachlan (Ed.), Elsevier/North Holland.

Clive, D. (1977). A linear relationship between tumorigenic potency in vivo and mutagenic potency at the heterozygous thymidine kinase ($TK^{+/-}$) locus of L5178y mouse lymphoma cells coupled with mammalian metabolism. In: *Progress in Genetic Toxicology*, D. Scott, B. A. Bridges and F. H. Sobelo (Eds), Elsevier/North Holland, Amsterdam, pp. 241–7.

Comm. Europ. Commun. (1982). Report of the Scientific Working Group on

Anabolic Agents in Animal Production. VI/2924.

Cubadda, R., Fabriani, G., Fratoni, A. and Quattrucci, E. (1964a). Effetti dell'azione protratta del dietilstibestrolo su polli. *Quad. Nutr.*, **24**, 1–28.

Cubadda, R., Fabriani, G., Fratoni, A. and Quattrucci, E. (1964b). Ricerche dei residui ormonali nelle carni di pollo trattati con estrogeni, *Quad. Nutr.*, **24**, 187–201.

Davis, G. J., McLachlan, J. A. and Lucier, G. W. (1977). Fetotoxicity and teratogenicity of zearanol in mice. *Toxicol. Appl. Pharmacol.*, **41**, 138–9.

Dixon, S. N. (1980). Radioimmunoassay of the anabolic agent zeranol. I. Preparation and properties of a specific antibody zeranol. *J. Vet. Pharm. Therap.*, **3**, 177–81.

Dixon, S. N. and Heitzman, R. J. (1981). Residues of anabolic agents in beef, cattle and sheep. In: *Anabolic Agents in Beef and Veal Production*, CEC Workshop, ISBN-0-905442-54-7, pp. 58–9.

Dodds, E. C., Golberg, L., Lawson, W. and Robinson, R. (1938). Estrogenic activity of certain synthetic compounds. *Nature*, **141**, 247–8.

Duchatel, J. P., Evrard, P. and Magbruin-Rogister, G. (1982). Dosage radioimmunologique de trenbolone dans le plasma et les muscles de jeunes taureaux implantes au moyen d'un melange d'acetate de trenbolone et de 17β-oestradiol (Torelor). *Ann. Med. Vet.*, **126**, 147–56.

Duffy, M. J. and Duffy, G. J. (1978). Estradiol receptors in human liver. *J. Ster. Biochem.*, **9**, 233–5.

Dunn, T. B. and Green, A. W. (1963). Cyst of the epididymus, cancer of the cervix, granular cell myoblastoma and other lesions after estrogen injection in newborn mice. *J. Nat. Cancer Inst.*, **31**, 425.

Eisenfeld, A. J., Aten, R. F. and Dickson, R. B. (1980). Estrogen receptor in the mammalian liver. In: *Estrogens in the Environment*, J. A. McLachlan (Ed.), Elsevier/North Holland.

Elakovich, S. D. and Hampton, J. M. (1984). Analysis of coumestrol, a phytoestrogen, in alfalfa tablets sold for human consumption. *J. Agric. Food Chem.*, **32**, 173–5.

Eldridge, A. C. and Kwolek, W. F. (1983). Soybean isoflavones: effect of environment and vaiety on composition. *J. Agric. Food Chem.*, **31**, 394–6.

Engel, L. L., Weidenfeld, J. and Merriam, G. R. (1976). Metabolism of diethylstilbestrol by rat liver: a preliminary report. *J. Toxicol. Environ. Health*, Suppl. 1, 37–44.

Eppley, R. M., Stoloff, L., Trucksess, M. W. and Chung, C. W. (1974). Survey of corn for Fusarium toxins. *J. Assoc. Off. Anal. Chem.*, **57**, 632–5.

FAO/WHO Report (1985). *Expert Consultation on Residues of Veterinary Drugs in Foods*, FAO Food Nutr. Paper, 32.

Farnsworth, N. R., Bingel, A. S., Cordell, G. A., Crane, F. A. and Fong, H. H. S. (1975). Potential value of plants as sources of new antifertility agents, II. *J. Pharm. Sci.*, **64**, 717–54.

Federal Register (1979). **44**, 85, 54900.

Fischer, L. J., Kent, T. H. and Weissinger, J. L. (1973). Absorption of diethylstilbestrol and its glucuronide conjugate from the intestines of five- and twenty-five-day-old rats. *J. Pharmacol. Exp. Ther.*, **185**, 163–70.

Foxcroft, G. R., Cameron, D. M. and Bouffault, J. C. (1983). Preliminary study of the hormonal no-effect level of 17β-trenbolone acetate in the mature male pig. *Proc. OIE Symp. Anabolics in Animal Production*, ISBN 92-9044-118-6, pp. 347–51.

Fratoni, A. and Quattrucci, E. (1966). Studio comparativo sull'accrescimento, l'utilizzazione della dieta e la composizione delle carni in polli trattati con diversi ormoni. *Quad. Nutr.*, **26**, 1–25.

Gaiani, R. and Chiesa, F. (1986). Physiological levels of androstenedione and testosterone in some edible tissue from calves, bulls and heifers. *Meat Science*, **17**, 177–85.

Galli, C. L., Marinovich, M., Sautebin, L., Galli, G. and Paoletti, R. (1983). Selected ion monitoring, a method of choice of the determination of estrogen residues in food. *Tox. Lett.*, **155**, 193–8.

Galli, C. L., Macri, A. and Quattrucci, E. (1985). Growth promoters: residues in food. In: *Food Toxicology: Real or Imaginary Problems?*, G. G. Gibson and R. Walker (Eds), Taylor and Francis, London, pp. 289–300.

Gardner, W. U. (1953). Hormonal aspects of experimental tumorigenesis. *Adv. Cancer Res.*, **1**, 173.

Gilbert, J. (1984). The detection and analysis of Fusarium mycotoxins. In: *The Applied Mycology of Fusarium*, M. O. Moss and J. E. Smith (Eds), Cambridge University Press, pp. 188–93.

Glatt, H. R., Metzler, M. and Oesch, F. (1979). Diethylstilbestrol and 11 derivatives. A mutagenicity study with Salmonella typhimurium. *Mutat. Res.*, **67**, 113–21.

Greenhalgh, R., Gilbert, J., King, R. R., Blackwell, B. A., Startin, J. R. and Shephard, M. J. (1986). Synthesis, characterization and occurrence in bread and cereal products of an isomer of 4-deoxymivalenol (vomitoxin). *J. Agric. Food Chem.*, **32**, 1416–20.

Hagler, W. M., Jr., Tyczkowska, K. and Hamilton, P. B. (1984). Simultaneous occurrence of deoxynivalenol, zearalenone and aflatoxin in 1982 scabby wheat from the midwestern United States. *Appl. Environ. Microbiol.*, **47**, 151–4.

Heitzman, R. J. (1975). The effectiveness of anabolic agents in increasing rate of growth in farm animals. In: *Environmental Quality and Safety*, Suppl. Vol. IV, *Anabolic Agents in Animal Production*, F. C. Lu and J. Rendel (Eds), Georg Thieme Verlag, Stuttgart, pp. 89–98.

Henricks, D. M. (1981). In: *International Symposium on Steroids in Animal Production*, H. Jasiorowski (Ed.), Ars Polonaruch, Warsaw, pp. 161–70.

Hess, D. L. (1983). Determination of the hormonal no-effect level of 17β-trenbolone and Altrenogest in the macaque. *Proc. OIE Symp. Anabolics in Animal Production*, ISBN 92-9044-118-6, pp. 359–78.

Hidy, P. H., Baldwin, R. S., Greasham, R. L., Keith, C. L. and McMullen, J. R. (1977). Zearalenone and some derivatives: production and biological activities. *Adv. Appl. Microbiol.*, **22**, 59–82.

Hoffmann, B. (1978). Use of radioimmunoassay (RIA) for monitoring hormonal residues in edible animal products. *J. Assoc. Off. Anal. Chem.*, **61**, 1263.

Hoffmann, B. (1981). Levels of endogenous anabolic sex hormones in farm animals. In: *Anabolic Agents in Beef and Veal Production*, Proc. CEC Workshop, Brussels, pp. 96–112.

Hoffmann, B. (1983). Naturally occurring hormones in animal foods: testosterone.

In: *Handbook of Naturally Occurring Food Toxicants*, M. Rechcigl, Jr. (Ed.), CRC Press, Boca Raton, Florida, pp. 287–94.

Hoffmann, B. and Karg, H. (1975). Metabolic fate of anabolic agents in treated animals and residue levels in their meat, Proc. FAO/WHO Symp. Anabolic Agents in Animal Production. In: *Environmental Quality and Safety*, Suppl. Vol. V, F. C. Lu and J. Rendell (Eds), Georg Thieme Verlag, Stuttgart, pp. 181–91.

Hoffmann, B. and Oettel, G. (1976). Radioimmunoassay for free and conjugated trenbolone and for trenbolone acetate in bovine tissue and plasma samples. *Steroids*, **27**, 509–23.

Hoffmann, B., Schopper, D. and Karg, H. (1984). Investigations on the occurrence of non-extractable residues of trenbolone acetate in cattle tissues in respect to their bioavailability and immunological reactivity. *Food Add. Contaminants*, **3**, 252–9.

Horning, E. C., Thenot, J. P. and Helton, E. D. (1978). Toxic agents resulting from the oxidative metabolism of steroid hormones and drugs. *J. Toxicol. Environ. Health*, **4**, 341.

Hunter, P. H. F., Hall, J. P., Cook, B. and Taylor, P. D. (1972). Oestrogens and progesterone in porcine peripheral plasma before and after induced ovulation. *J. Reprod. Fertil.*, **31**, 499.

IARC (1979). *Evaluation of the Carcinogenic Risk of Chemicals to Humans*, Monograph 21, pp. 173–231.

Ingerowski, G. H., Scheutwinkel-Reich, M. and Stan, H. J. (1981). Mutagenicity studies on veterinary anabolic drugs with the Salmonella/microsome test. *Mutat. Res.*, **91**, 93–8.

Janski, A. M. (1983). Development of a sensitive method for extraction and assay of zeranol residues in animal tissues and the use of the method in a multiple implant study in cattle. *Proc. OIE Symp. Anabolics in Animal Production*, ISBN 92-9044-118-6, pp. 443–56.

Jasiorowski, H. A. and El Sharly, K. (1975). World production of animal protein and the need for a new approach. *FAO/WHO Symp. on Use of Anabolic Agents in Animal Production and its Public Health Aspects*, FAO, Rome.

Karg, H. and Vogt, K. (1981). Residues of diethylstilbestrol (DES) in veal calves. In: *Anabolic Agents in Beef and Veal Production*, CEC Workshop, Brussels, pp. 70–83.

Katzenellenbogen, J. A., Katzenellenbogen, B. S., Tatee, T., Robertson, D. W. and Landvatter, S. W. (1980). The chemistry of estrogens and antiestrogens: relationships between structure, receptor binding and biological activity. In: *Estrogens in the Environment*, J. A. McLachlan (Ed.), Elsevier/North Holland.

Kiang, D. T., Kennedy, B. J., Pathre, S. V. and Miroka, C. J. (1978). Binding characteristics of zeralenone analogs to oestrogen receptors. *Cancer Res.*, **38**, 3611–5.

Kimura, T. and Nandi, S. (1967). Nature of induced persistent vaginal carnification in mice IV. Changes in the vaginal epithelium of old mice treated neonatally with estradiol or testosterone. *J. Nat. Cancer Inst.*, **39**, 75–93.

Kroes, R. and Huis in't Veld, L. G. (1975). Methods for controlling the application of anabolics in farm animals. In: *Anabolic Agents in Animal Production*, FAO/WHO Symposium (March 1975), pp. 192–202.

Kruskemper, H. L., Morgner, K. D. and Noell, G. (1967). Klinische pharmakologie von trienolonen, eine Gruppe neuartiger anabol wirksamer Oestran-Derivate, *Arzneim. Forsch.*, **17**, 449–54.

Kumagai, S., and Shimizu, T. (1982). Neonatal exposure to zearalenone causes persistent anovulatory estrus in the rat. *Arch. Toxicol.*, **50**, 279–86.

Kurtz, H. J., Nairn, M. E., Nelson, G. H., Christensen, C. M. and Mirocha, C. J. (1969). Changes in the genital tracts of swine fed estrogenic mycotoxin. *Am. J. Vet. Res.*, **30**, 551.

Lee, U. S., Jang, H. S., Tanaka, T., Hasegawa, A., Oh, Y. J. and Ueno, Y. (1985). The coexistence of the Fusarium mycotoxins nivalenol, deoxynivalenol and zearalenone in Korean cereal harvested in 1983. *Food Add. Contaminants*, **3**, 185–92.

Lee, Y. J., Notides, C. A., Tsay, Y. and Kende, A. S. (1977). Coumestrol, NBD-norhexestrol and dansyl-norhexestrol, fluorescent probes of oestrogen-binding proteins. *Biochemistry*, **16**, 2896–910.

Loizzo, A. and Macri, A. (1983). Toxicology of estrogens in babyfood: multiposal predictive toxicometrics of DES. In: *Application of Behavioural Pharmacology in Toxicology*, G. Zbinden *et al.* (Eds), Raven Press, New York, pp. 315–8.

Loizzo, A., Gatti, G. L., Macri, A. and Moretti, G. (1984). The case of brands of babyfood containing estrogen treated veal meat in Italy: methodological and toxicological aspects, *Ann. Int. Symp. Sanita*.

Lovelace, C. E. A. and Nyathi, C. B. (1977). Estimation of the fungal toxins zearalenone and aflatoxin contaminating opaque beer in Zambia. *J. Sci. Food Agric.*, **28**, 288–92.

Lutz, W. K. (1979). In vivo covalent binding of organic chemicals to DNA as a quantitative indicator in the process of chemical carcinogenesis. *Mutat. Res.*, **65**, 289–356.

Marasas, W. F. O., Van Rensburg, S. J. and Mirocha, C. J. (1979). Incidence of Fusarium species and the mycotoxins deoxynivalenol and zearalenone in corn produced in oesophageal cancer areas in Transkei. *J. Agric. Food Chem.*, **27**, 1108–12.

Martin, P. M. D. and Keen, P. (1978). The occurrence of zearalenone in raw and fermented products from Swaziland and Lesotho. *Sabrouaudia*, **16**, 15–22.

Martin, C. N., McDermid, A. C. and Garner, R. C. (1978). Testing of known carcinogens and noncarcinogens for their ability to induce unscheduled DNA synthesis in HeLa cells. *Cancer Res.*, **38**, 2621–7.

Mattioli, M., Galeati, G., Gaiani, R. and Chiesa, F. (1986). Detection of oestrogen residues in meat by radioreceptor assay. *Meat Science*, **16**, 79–89.

McLachlan, J. A., Wong, A., Degen, G. H. and Barret, J. C. (1982). Morphological and neoplastic transformation of Syrian hamster embryo fibroblasts by diethylstilboestrol and analogs. *Cancer Res.*, **42**, 3040–5.

McNutt, S. H., Purwin, P. and Murray, C. (1928). Vulvovaginitis in swine. *J. Am. Vet. Med. Assoc.*, **73**, 484–92.

Medina, M. B. and Sherman, J. T. (1986). High performance liquid chromatographic separation of anabolic oestrogens and ultraviolet detection of 17β-oestradiol, zeranol, diethylstilboestrol or zearalenone in avian muscle tissues extracts. *Food Add. Contaminants*, **3**, 263–72.

Mercier-Bodard, C., Renoir, J. M. and Baulieu, E. E. (1979). Further characterization and immunological studies of human sex steroid plasma binding protein. *J. Ster. Biochem.*, **11**, 253–9.

Metzler, M., Gottschlich, R. and McLachlan, J. A. (1980). Oxidative metabolism of stilbene oestrogens. In: *Estrogens in the Environment*, J. A. McLachlan (Ed.), Elsevier, Amsterdam, pp. 293–303.

Micco, C., Grossi, M., Onori, R., Chirico, M. and Brera, C. (1986). Aflatossina B$_1$, ocratossina A e zearalenone in mais nazionale: monitoraggio della produzio ne relativa agli anni 1982, 1983 e 1984. *Riv. Soc. Ital. Sci. Alim.*, **15**, 113–6.

Migdalof, B. H., Dugger, H. A., Heider, J. G. and Coombs, R. A. (1983). Biotransformation of zeranol. I. Disposition and metabolism in the female rat, rabbit, dog, monkey and man. *Xenobiotica*, **13**, 209–21.

Miller, J. K., Hacking, A. and Gross, V. J. (1973). Stillbirths, neonatal mortality and small litters in pigs associated with the ingestion of Fusarium toxin by pregnant sows. *Vet. Res.*, **93**, 555.

Mirocha, C. J. and Christensen, G. M. (1974). Oestrogenic mycotoxins synthesised by Fusarium. In: *Mycotoxins*, I. F. H. Purchase (Ed.), Elsevier, New York, pp. 129–48.

Moss, M. O. and Smith, J. E. (Eds) (1984). *The Applied Mycology of Fusarium*, Cambridge University Press, Cambridge.

Nottle, M. C. and Beck, A. B. (1974). Urinary sediments in sheep feeding on oestrogenic clover. 3. The identification of 4-O-methyl equol as a major component of some sediments. *Austral. J. Agric. Res.*, **25**, 509–14.

Osborne, B. G. (1982). Mycotoxins and the cereals industry: a review. *J. Food Technol.*, **17**, 1–9.

Pottier, J., Cousty, C., Heitzman, R. J. and Reynolds, I. P. (1981). Differences in the biotransformation of a 17β-hydroxylated steroid, trenbolone acetate, in rat and cow. *Xenobiotica*, **11**, 489–500.

Powell-Jones, W., Raeford, S. and Lucier, G.W. (1981). Binding properties of zearalenone mycotoxins to hepatic oestrogen receptors. *Mol. Pharmacol.*, **20**, 35–42.

Price, K. R. and Fenwick, G.R. (1985). Naturally occurring oestrogens in foods: a review. *Food Add. Contaminants*, **2**, 73–106.

Reid, J. F. S. (1981). Significance of natural oestrogen-implanted beef to human health. In: *The Use, Residues and Toxicology of Growth Promoters*, ISBN-0-905442-44-X, p. 24.

Rhynes, W. E. and Ewing, L. L. (1973). Testicular endocrine function in Hereford bulls exposed to high ambient temperature. *Endocrinology*, **92**, 509.

Richold, M. (1983). An evaluation of the mutagenicity of anabolic hormones with particular reference to trenbolone. *Proc. OIE Symp. Anabolics in Animal Production*, ISBN 92-9044-118-6, pp. 297–306.

Rico, A. G. and Burgat-Sacaze, V. (1984). Toxicological significance of covalently-bound residues. *Food Add. Contaminants*, **2**, 157–61.

Rico, A. G., Burgat-Sacaze, V., Braun, J. P. and Bernard, P. (1981). Metabolism of endogenous and exogenous anabolic agents in cattle. In: *Anabolic Agents in Beef and Veal Production*, Proc. EEC Workshop, Brussels, pp. 45–56.

Roche, J. F. (1980). The use of growth promoters in beef cattle. In: *The Use, Residues and Toxicology of Growth Promoters*, Proc. An Foras Taluntais Conference, Dublin, pp. 1–12.

Roche, J. F. (1981). Effect of repeated implantation with zeranol on daily gain, carcass weight, and residues in tissue of steers. *Am. Soc. Anim. Sci.*, 73rd, Meeting, Abstract N. 161.

Roche, J. F. (1983). The use of natural steroids, hormones and xenobiotics. *Proc. OIE Symp. Anabolics in Animal Production*, ISBN 92-9044-118-6, pp. 119–27.

Roe, F. J. C. (1983). Results of long-term rodent studies with special reference to cancer risks and hormonal no-effect levels. *Proc. OIE Symp. Anabolics in Animal Production*, ISBN 92-9044-118-6, pp. 339–46.

Rubens, R. and Vermeulen, A. (1983). Oestrogen production in man. *Proc. OIE Symp. Anabolics in Animal Production*, ISBN 92-9044-118-6, pp. 141–55.

Rudiger, H. W., Haenisch, F., Metzler, M., Oesch, F. and Glatt, H. R. (1979). Metabolites of diethylstilbestrol induce sister chromatid exchange in human cultured fibroblasts. *Nature*, **281**, 392–4.

Ryan, J. J. and Hoffman, B. (1978). Trenbolone acetate: experiences with bound residues in cattle tissues, *J. Assoc. Off. Anal. Chem.*, **61**. 1274–9.

Schiffmann, D., Metzler, M., Neudecker, T. and Henschler, D. (1985). Morphological transformation of Syrian hamster embryo fibroblasts by the anabolic agent trenbolone. *J. Cancer Res. Clin. Oncol.*, **109**, 18.

Schoental, R. (1979). The role of Fusarium mycotoxins in the aetiology of tumours of the digestive tract and of certain other organs in man and animals. *Front. Gastr. Res.*, **4**, 17–24.

Scott, P. M., Panalaks, T., Kanhere, S. and Miles, W. F. (1978). Determination of zearalenone in cornflakes and other corn-based foods by thin-layer chromatography, high pressure liquid chromatography and gas-liquid chromatography-high resolution mass spectrometry, *J. Assoc. Off. Anal. Chem.*, **61**, 593–600.

Seo, A. and Morr, C. V. (1984). Improved high performance liquid chromatographic analysis of phenolic acid and isoflavonoids from soybean protein products. *J. Agric. Food Chem.*, **32**, 530–33.

Setchell, K. D. R., Borriello, S. P., Hulme, P., Kirk, D. N. and Axelson, M. (1984). Non-steroidal estrogens of dietary origin: possible roles in hormone dependent disease. *Am. J. Clin. Nutr.*, **40**, 569–78.

Shah, H. C. and McLachlan, J. A. (1976). The fate of diethystilbestrol in the pregnant mouse. *J. Pharmacol. Exp. Ther.*, **197**, 687–96.

Sharp, G. D. and Dyer, I. A. (1972). Zearalenol metabolism in steers. *J. Anim. Sci.*, **34**, 176–9.

Shellabarger, C. J., Stone, J. P. and Holtzman, S. (1976). Synergism between neutron radiation and diethylstilbestrol in the production of mammary adenocarcinomas in the rat. *Cancer Res.*, **36**, 1019–22.

Shellabarger, C. J., McKnight, B., Stone, J. P. and Holtzman, S. (1980). Interaction of dimethylbenzanthracene and diethylstilbestrol on mammary adenocarcinoma formation in female ACI rats. *Cancer Res.*, **40**, 1808–11.

Shutt, D. A. (1967). Interaction of genistein with oestradiol in the reproductive tract of the ovariectomized mouse. *J. Endocrinol.*, **37**, 231.

Shutt, D. A. (1976). The effect of plant oestrogens on animal reproduction. *Endeavour*, **35**, 110–13.

Shutt, D. A. and Braden, A. W. H. (1968). The significance of equol in relation to the oestrogenic responses in sheep ingesting clover with a high formonetin content. *Austral. J. Agric. Res.*, **19**, 545–53.

Stan, H. J. and Hols, F. W. (1979). Nachweis von Trenbolon- und Testosteron-

Rückständen in Fleisch durch Hockdruckflüssigkeitschromatographie. *Z. Lebensm. Unters. Forsch.*, **169**, 266–70.

Stob, M. (1973). Estrogens in foods. In: *Toxicants Occurring Naturally in Foods*, Nat. Acad. Sci., Committee of Food Protection Nat. Res. Conc., Washington, DC.

Stob, M. (1983). Naturally occurring food toxicants: estrogens. In: *Handbook of Naturally Occurring Food Toxicants*, M. Rechcigl, Jr. (Ed.), CRC Press, Boca Raton, Florida, pp. 81–100.

Stob, M., Baldwin, R. S., Tuite, J., Andrews, F. N. and Gillette, K. G. (1962). Isolation of an anabolic uterotrophic compound from corn infected with Gibberella zeae. *Nature*, **196**, 1318.

Stoloff, L. and Dalrymple, B. (1977). Aflatoxin and zearalenone occurrence in dry-milled corn products. *J. Assoc. Off. Anal. Chem.*, **60**, 579–82.

Stoloff, L., Henry, S. and Francis, O. J. Jr (1976). Survey for aflatoxins and zearalenone in 1973 crop corn stored on farms and in country elevators. *J. Assoc. Off. Anal. Chem.*, **59**, 118–21.

Takasugi, N., Kimura, T. and Mori, T. (1970). Irreversible changes in mouse vaginal epithelium induced by early post-natal treatment with steroid hormones. In: *The Post-Natal Development of Phenotype*, Butterworths, London.

Tanaka, T., Hasegawa, A., Matsuki, Y., Ishii, K. and Ueno, Y. (1985a).Improved methodology for the simultaneous detection of the trichothecene mycotoxins deoxynivalenol and nivalenol in cereals. *Food Add. Contaminants*, **2**, 125–37.

Tanaka, T., Hasegawa, A., Matsuki, Y. and Ueno, Y. (1985b). A survey of the occurrence of nivalenol, deoxynivalenol and zearalenone in foodstuffs and health foods in Japan. *Food Add. Contaminants*, **2**, 259–65.

Taylor, W. (1981). Toxicology and carcinogenicity of anabolic agents in human subjects. In: *Anabolic Agents in Beef and Veal Production*, Proc. CEC Workshop, Brussels, pp. 27–44.

Tsutsui, T., Maizumi, H., McLachlan, J. A. and Barrett, J. C. (1983). Aneuploidy induction and cell transformation by diethylstilbestrol: a possible chromosomal mechanism in carcinogenesis. *Cancer Res.*, **43**, 3814–21.

Ueno, Y. and Kubota, K. (1976). DNA-attacking ability of carcinogenic mycotoxins in recombination-deficient mutant cells of Bacillus subtilis. *Cancer Res.*, **36**, 445–51.

Umberger, E. J., Gass, G. H. and Curtis, J. M. (1958). Design of biological assay method for the detection and estimation of estrogenic residues in the edible tissues of domestic animals treated with estrogens, *Endocrinology*, **63**, 806–15.

Urry, W. H., Wejrmeister, H. L., Hodge, E. B. and Hity, P. H. (1966). The structure of zearalenone. *Tetrahedron Lett.*, No. 27, 3109.

Van Veerden, E. J., Berende, P. L. M. and Huisman, J. (1981). Application of endogenous and exogenous anabolic agents in veal calves. In: *Anabolic Agents in Beef and Veal Production*, Proc. CEC Workshop, ISBN 0-905443-54-7, pp. 1–26.

Verdeal, R. and Ryan, D. S. (1979). Naturally occurring oestrogens in plant foodstuffs: a review. *J. Food Protect.*, **42**, 577–83.

Verdeal, K., Brown, R. R., Richardson, T. and Ryan, D. S. (1980). Affinity of phytoestrogens for the oestradiol-binding proteins and effect of coumestrol on the growth of 7,12-dimethylbenz(a)anthracene-induced rat mammary tumours.

J. Nat. Cancer Inst., **64**, 285–90.

Walz, E. (1931). Isoflavone and saponin glycosides in soya hispida. *Liebigs Ann.*, **489**, 118.

Wehner, F. C., Marasas, W. F. O. and Thiel, P. G. (1978). Lack of mutagenicity to *Salmonella typhimurium* of some Fusarium mycotoxins. *Appl. Environ. Microbiol.*, **35**, 659–62.

WHO Working Group Report (1981). *Health Aspects of Residues of Anabolics in meat*, Bilthoven.

Windholtz, M. (Ed.) (1976*a,b,c*). *The Merck Index*, 9th edn, Merck & Co., Rahway, New York: *a*, 9781; *b*, 9271; *c*, 3113.

Yeomans, L. (1983). Food safety standard regulations of anabolic drugs: the consumer viewpoint. *Proc. OIE Symp. Anabolics in Animal Production*, ISBN 92-9004-118-6, pp. 545–51.

Yuthasastrakosol, P., Palmer, W. M. and Howland, B. E. (1975). Luteinizing hormone, oestrogen and progesterone levels in peripheral serum of anoestrus and cyclic ewes as determined by radioimmunoassay. *J. Reprod. Fertil.*, **43**, 57.

Chapter 6

MYCOTOXINS

Yoshio Ueno

Department of Toxicology and Microbial Chemistry, Science University of Tokyo, Japan

139

INTRODUCTION

Fungi produce many secondary metabolites, and some of these organic compounds such as antibiotics, organic solvents and other fermentation products are useful for human life. However, several metabolites are toxic to human and animal health. An association of toxic fungal metabolites, so-called mycotoxins, with human and animal health has been made since biblical times when ergotism was suspected to be a toxicosis resulting from the ingestion of such mycotoxins. A notable finding has been the neuro-toxin mycotoxin citreoviridin from *Penicillium citreoviride* Biourge. During the last three centuries, in rice-eating countries including Japan, an acute type of cardiac beriberi (Shoshin-kakke in Japanese) has been prevalent, with characteristic symptoms such as convulsion, vomiting, ascending paralysis, and respiratory arrest. In 1891, Dr. Sakaki, a Japanese physician, suspected that rice grains infested with fungi were responsible for the development of the acute cardiac beriberi. The experi-ments of Sakaki, Uraguchi and Hirata demonstrated that an alcohol extract and its toxic principle 'citreoviridin' induced symptoms in animals which are similar to cardiac beriberi in humans. This is the first experi-mental toxicology on toxic fungal metabolites, as reviewed by Uraguchi (1969, 1971) and the present author (Ueno, 1974, 1983*a*).

This fungi–rice–mycotoxicosis hypothesis led many Japanese scientists to discover several hepatotoxic mycotoxins such as luteoskyrin from *Penicillium islandicum* Sopp and nephrotoxic mycotoxins such as citrinin from *P. citrinum* Thom, which were isolated from imported and domestic rice grains (Saito *et al.*, 1971). The hypothesis was expanded to a fungi–barley–mycotoxicosis relationship, and a number of surveys have demonstrated a scabby wheat and barley (Akakabi in Japanese) associated intoxication in man and farm animals, characterized by vomiting, diarrhea, hemorrhage and dermal inflammation, that originated from several tricho-thecene mycotoxins from *Fusarium* and other fungi (Tatsuno *et al.*, 1968; Ueno, 1977, 1980, 1983*b*).

In 1960, a massive illness of turkeys (turkey-X disease) had developed in England and a toxic metabolite, aflatoxin B_1 (AFB$_1$), was isolated from the suspected fungus *Aspergillus flavus*. Since this mycotoxin significantly contaminated groundnuts, corn and other commodities in tropical and subtropical countries, and possessed a potent hepatocarcinogenicity in experimental animals, AFB$_1$ was suspected to be one cause of human liver cancer (Goldblatt, 1969). Actually, AFB$_1$ was frequently detected from foods in the high risk area. However, recent epidemiology has revealed a close relationship with hepatitis B virus. The significance of AFB_1 in food is under re-evaluation with respect to human liver cancer.

In Yugoslavia, Bulgaria, and other Balkan countries, an endemic nephropathy developed sporadically in humans and swine, and a nephrotoxic mycotoxin, ochratoxin A (OT-A), was isolated from the metabolites of *Aspergillus ochraceus* and identified as a causal agent. Chemical epidemiology has demonstrated a close relationship between the contamination of this mycotoxin in foods and the incidence of endemic Balkan nephropathy (Krogh, 1977). This endemic Balkan nephropathy is also associated with the incidence of tumors of the urinary system in the endemic area. Kanisawa and Suzuki (1978), Japanese pathologists, have demonstrated the liver and renal carcinogenicity of OT-A in mice. In this respect, this mycotoxin is grouped with the carcinogenic mycotoxins.

During the last 20 years, more than a hundred mycotoxins have been isolated from the metabolites of toxigenic fungi, and their chemical and toxicological characters elucidated. However, only certain members, such as the trichothecenes, ochratoxins and aflatoxins, are considered to be the toxicants in foods in relation to human exposure.

In this chapter, the author has aimed to summarize recent concepts of the mycotoxins, with special reference to their contamination in foods and human diseases.

TRICHOTHECENES

The trichothecenes are a family of closely related sesquiterpenoids produced by several plant pathogenic fungi. In the early stages of trichothecene problems, the first compound, trichothecin, was isolated from a culture of *Trichothecium roseum* as an antifungal agent, and subsequent studies identified verrucarins A to J and roridins A to E from *Myrothecium verrucaria* and *M. roridum*, respectively, as antifungal metabolites.

During the course of a survey of gibberellin production, a potent phytotoxic metabolite, diacetoxyscirpenol, was detected from cultures of *F. scirpi*. In 1967, all the spiroepoxy-containing sesquiterpenoids, formerly called scirpenes, were renamed trichothecenes, and now more than 80 compounds are listed as trichothecenes. The structures and fungal origin of the major trichothecenes are shown in Fig. 1 and Table 1.

Alimentary toxic aleukia (ATA), or septic angina, has been a well-documented food-borne toxicosis in man and farm animals in the Soviet

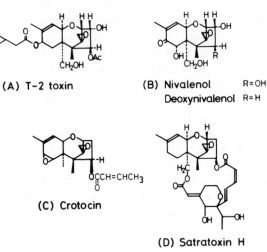

(A) T-2 toxin

(B) Nivalenol   R=OH
    Deoxynivalenol R=H

(C) Crotocin

(D) Satratoxin H

FIG. 1. Major trichothecenes.

TABLE 1
Major Trichothecene-producing Fungi

Group	Fungi	Major trichothecenes
A	*Fusarium sporotrichioides*	T-2 toxin, HT-2 toxin, neosolaniol, diacetoxyscirpenol
	F. semitectum	diacetoxyscirpenol
	F. equiseti	diacetoxyscirpenol
B	*F. graminearum*	nivalenol, deoxynivalenol
	F. culmolum	deoxynivalenol
C	*Cephalosporium crotocinigenum*	crotocin
D	*Myrothecium roridum*	roridin A, D, E
	M. verrucaris	verrucarin A, B
	Stachybotrys atra	satratoxin F, G, H

Union since the 19th century. The typical symptoms of the disease are fever, necrosis, leukopenia, hemorrhage, exhaustion of bone marrow and death. *F. sporotrichioides* and other toxigenic fungi were detected in overwintered millet and other cereals (Forgacs and Carll, 1962), and this was followed by discovery of T-2 toxin and other related trichothecenes as metabolites of this fungus (Ueno *et al.*, 1972). T-2 toxin was also found to be causative agent of moldy corn toxicosis in cows in the United States. This trichothecene and its deacylated compound, HT-2 toxin, were isolated from cultures of *F. tricinctum*, one of the causative fungi in moldy corn (Bamburg and Strong, 1971).

Other important trichothecenes are deoxynivalenol (DON) and nivalenol (NIV) of *F. graminearum* (*Gibberella zeae* in sexual stage). In Japan, China, Canada, the United States and other countries, scabby wheat and barley intoxication sporadically developed when low temperature and high humidity continued in the harvest season of crops. This intoxication is characterized by vomiting, diarrhea, hemorrhage of intestines, and malfunction of the hematopoietic system. Tatsuno *et al.* (1968) isolated NIV from cultures of *F. nivale* Fn 2B (presumably a variety of *F. graminearum*). Yoshizawa and Morooka (1973) and Vesonder *et al.* (1973) isolated DON (vomitoxin) from the suspected barley and corn.

In Hungary and other parts of central Europe, a massive illness of horses and other farm animals was found to be caused by toxic components of straw infected with *Stachybotrys atra*, and this intoxication was named stachybotryotoxicosis. Dermal inflammation and necrosis, hemorrhagic changes in intestines and muscles followed by death were characteristic symptoms (Forgacs and Carll, 1962). Eppley and Bailey (1973) isolated the toxic trichothecenes satratoxin H and others from cultures of this fungus. Chemically, these satratoxins possess a macrocyclic linkage similar to the verrucarins and roridins (Fig. 1). Evidence of human satratoxicosis is not often reported (Hintikka, 1977); however, satratoxins and the related macrocyclic trichothecenes have been detected from house dust in the United States, in a case where severe dermal inflammation was observed in the family (Croft *et al.*, 1986). Possible contamination by these satratoxins in food remains to be solved in the future.

As summarized above, various derivatives of the trichothecenes were detected from the metabolites of *Fusarium*, *Trichoderma*, *Trichothecium*, *Stachybotrys* and other fungi; among these fungi, the most important species is *F. graminearum* which selectively invades our important crops such as wheat, barley, corn and others, and produces NIV and DON in the fields. Therefore, current research on the trichothecenes problem in food is focusing on the heavy contamination of these trichothecenes in cereal grains. As will be discussed later, the safety evaluation of NIV and DON and their carry-over to various kinds of food from contaminated cereals is very important in food toxicology.

Mycology

The major trichothecene-producing fungi are listed in Table 1. To date, many trichothecene-producing fungi have been found under natural circumstances, particularly in plant pathogenic strains and food and feed contaminants. For example, *Stachybotrys atra* is selectively parasitic on straw and other cellulose-rich materials.

From the viewpoint of food hygiene, the most important producers are the fungi of *Fusarium* spp. The taxonomy of *Fusarium* spp. is confusing and has not been agreed upon by mycologists (Ueno, 1980). Booth (1971) reported a new taxonomic system for *Fusarium* in which he established 12 sections containing 51 species and varieties, and Marasas *et al.* (1984) summarized the toxigenic *Fusarium* species.

Fusarium sporotrichioides produces T-2 toxin, HT-2 toxin and other related trichothecenes in cultures (Ueno and Ishii, 1985), and is widely detected in cereals, but its plant pathogenicity is not so far specific. *F. graminearum* produces NIV, DON and their esters such as 4-acetyl-NIV (fusarenon-X) (Ueno *et al.*, 1969) and 3- and 15-acetyl-DON (Yoshizawa and Morooka, 1973). The plant pathogenicity of this fungus is selective, particularly for wheat, barley and other crops, and trichothecene production on these cereals is closely matched to their harvest period. Therefore, upon parasiting these cereals, the fungus produces toxins when environmental factors such as temperature and humidity are favorable for toxin production.

Our taxonomical approaches on '*F. graminearum*' have revealed two chemotypes: one is the nivalenol producer (NIV type) and the other is the deoxynivalenol producer (DON type) (Fig.2), and there are some regional differences in their distribution (Ichinoe *et al.*, 1983). Under laboratory conditions, the former type produces NIV, 4-acetyl-NIV and 4,15-diacetyl-NIV, and the latter produces DON, 3-acetyl-DON and 15-acetyl-

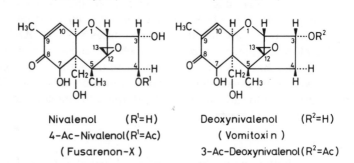

FIG. 2. Two chemotypes of *Fusarium graminearum* (*Gibberella zeae*).

DON. However, during storage of harvested cereals these acetyl esters of trichothecenes are hydrolyzed into the parent NIV and DON, and therefore NIV and DON remain as the contaminants in cereal grains.

During the course of screening for anti-tumor agents from natural sources, the macrocyclic trichothecenes, named baccharins and baccharinols, were isolated from a tropical plant, *Baccharis megapotamica* (Jarvis, 1984). This is the first report which suggested a plant origin for trichothecene compounds. However, later surveys have demonstrated that the macrocyclic trichothecenes produced by soil fungi such as *M. verrucaria* and *roridum* spp. are accumulated by plant tissues. This indicates an ecological association between fungi and plants.

Chemistry
At present, more than 80 kinds of trichothecene derivatives have been isolated from the metabolites of *Fusarium* spp. and others; in addition, several interesting trichothecenes were detected in the biotransformed products catalyzed by animal and microbial systems.

In the early stage of the trichothecene problem, the present author classified these trichothecenes into four groups according to their chemical properties and the producing fungi (Ueno *et al.*, 1973). The first (type A) is represented by T-2 toxin, HT-2 toxin, diacetoxyscirpenol and others. The second (type B) has a carbonyl function at C-8 and is represented by NIV and DON. The third is characterized by a second epoxide at C-7,8 or C-9,10 (type C), and the last (type D) includes those containing a macrocyclic ring between C-4 and C-5 with two ester linkages. Currently, the author has added two groups: the fifth (type E) is represented by the macrocyclic trichothecenes in which the macrocyclic ring is opened; the sixth group (type F) is represented by verrucarin K, in which the 12,13-epoxide function is changed to a vinyl linkage, and thereby the oxygen atom in the epoxide ring is removed. These compounds are presumed to be intermediates produced during the biosynthesis of macrocyclic trichothecenes.

A de-epoxidized metabolite was also detected when DON was incubated with dermal flora under anaerobic conditions (Fig. 3). Therefore the type F trichothecenes, characterized by a vinyl bond at C-12, are presumed to be intermediates formed during the biosynthetic and bio-degradative reactions of the trichothecenes.

The fundamental skeleton of trichothecene mycotoxins is named 'trichothecane'. The majority of trichothecanes possess a double bond at C-9,10 and an epoxide ring at C-12,13, and therefore they are termed '12,13-

epoxy-trichothecenes'. The epoxide ring is extremely stable to nucleo-philic attack. Heating under acid conditions causes an intramolecular rearrangement of the trichothecene skeleton to the apo-trichothecene ring system. Heating of DON has been shown to result in iso-DON (Greenhalgh *et al.*, 1984) (Fig. 4), and this demonstrates that the iso-DON may remain in food when cereal flours contaminated with DON are baked for food processing.

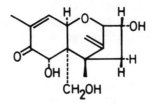

FIG. 3. Structure of de-epoxydeoxynivalenol (DOM-1).

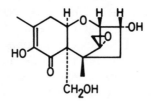

FIG. 4. Structure of iso-deoxynivalenol (iso-DON).

All the trichothecenes possessing an ester group are hydroxylated to the corresponding parent alchohols upon treatment with bases. For example, T-2 toxin changes to T-2 tetraol via HT-2 toxin and T-2 triol. 4-Acetyl-NIV and 3-acetyl-DON are changed to NIV and DON, respectively. The macrocyclic trichothecenes such as verrucarins and satratoxins give rise to verrucarol.

T-2 toxin and the macrocyclic trichothecenes, which possess ester and macrocyclic linkages, are highly soluble in organic solvents such as ether, acetone, ethyl acetate and chloroform. However, the highly hydroxylated NIV and DON are sparingly soluble in these solvents but soluble in water. Such a wide difference in solubility in organic solvents may give rise to difficulty during chemical analysis for the presence of trichothecenes in food and other biological materials.

Toxicological Properties

After the finding that trichothecene mycotoxins were associated with human and animal toxicosis, many experiments have been performed in order to elucidate their biological and toxicological features, as summarized by the author (Ueno, 1980, 1983b, 1984a, 1985b).

LD_{50} values of the representative trichothecenes are listed in Table 2. The oral LD_{50} of T-2 toxin is 10·5 mg/kg in mice, 3·05 mg/kg in guinea pigs, 5·2 mg/kg in rats, and 6·1 mg/kg in trout. An interesting finding is the high toxicity of T-2 toxin when administered subcutaneously. The LD_{50} values (mg/kg) of T-2 toxin using different administration routes are 2·1 (s.c.), 4·2 (i.v.), 5·2 (i.p.) and 10·5 (p.o.) in mice. These data are unexceptional in toxicology, and it is presumed that T-2 toxin administered subcutaneously may be rapidly distributed to the target organs (Ueno, 1984a).

The i.p. LD_{50} values in mice of NIV and DON, which are significantly detected in cereals as food contaminants, as will be discussed later, are 4·1 and 70 mg/kg, respectively. Most animals administered with a lethal dose

TABLE 2
LD_{50} Values of the Major Trichothecenes (Ueno, 1985b)

Trichothecenes	Animals	Routes	LD_{50} (mg/kg)
T-2 toxin	mouse	i.p.	5·2
	rat	p.o.	5·2
	swine	i.v.	1·21
Diacetoxyscirpenol	mouse	i.p.	23·0
	rat	p.o.	7·3
	rabbit	i.v.	1·0
	swine	i.v.	0·37
Nivalenol	mouse	i.p.	4·1
Fusarenon-X	mouse	p.o.	4·5
	rat	p.o.	4·4
Deoxynivalenol	mouse	p.o.	46
Crotocin	mouse	p.o.	1 000
Roridin A	mouse	i.p.	1·0
Verrucarin A	mouse	i.p.	1·5
	rat	i.v.	0·87
	rabbit	i.v.	0·54
Verrucarin B	mouse	i.v.	7·0
Verrucarin J	mouse	i.p.	0·5
Satratoxin H	mouse	i.p.	5·69
Satratoxin G	mouse	i.p.	1·29

of trichothecenes died 1–2 days after the administration, and diarrhea and hemorrhagic changes in intestines were the major symptoms.

Vomiting is one of the most significant symptoms of trichothecene toxicosis in man and animals. The i.v. injection of 4-acetyl-NIV (fusarenon-X) to dogs has been shown to induce emesis and vomiting 5–15 min after injection, and this effect was antagonized by the prior administration of metoclopramide or chloropromazine. Such data indicate an involvement of the chemoreceptor trigger zone (CTZ) in trichothecene-induced vomiting.

Diarrhea is also one of the important symptoms of trichothecene toxicosis. Currently, the author's group have investigated the pharmacological mechanism of trichothecene-induced diarrhea, and have estimated the intestinal volume by employing entero-pooling assays. In rats injected with fusarenon-X, the intestinal water volume increased in a time- and dose-dependent manner, and the maximum plateau was observed about 6 h after i.p. injection of 1·5 mg/kg of fusarenon-X. Prior treatment of rats with hydrocortisone markedly reduced the fusarenon-X-induced increment of intestinal water volume. No protective effect was observed with indomethacin, and other pharmacological reagents (Muto, Ishii and Ueno, unpublished data). The lethal toxicity of trichothecenes to mice was also prevented by the pretreatment of animals with steroidal anti-inflammatory agents such as prednisolone and naloxone, whereas no protective effect was observed with non-steroidal anti-inflammatory agents that inhibit the biosynthesis of prostaglandins, serotonin and histamine (Ryu et al., 1987). It is well known that steroidal anti-inflammatory agents possess various pharmacological activity, including the regulation of lipocortin release from the hypothalamus. Lipocortin gives rise to various physiological activities involving the control of biogenesis of prostaglandins and leukotrienes. The preventive action of steroidal anti-inflammatory agents on the lethal toxicity and diarrhea suggests an involvement of the lipocortin system in trichothecene toxicosis.

Russian people exposed to moldy millets and other crops have developed severe hematological disorders (Forgacs and Carll, 1962). Since this ATA was presumed to be caused by an intake of trichothecenes, the author has investigated the hematological changes in mice, rats and cats (Ueno, 1984a). In cats, an increment of circulating white blood cells occurred after intake of T-2 toxin, and its marked decrease was observed after repeated intakes of the toxin. Similarly leukocytosis and leukopenia were also demonstrated in mice and rats. Leukocytosis is induced by the release of white blood cells from lymph nodes by a kind of shock stimulation, and the leukopenia is induced by the malfunction of hematopoietic tissues. Pathological observations, characterized by severe lesions of bone marrow, thymus and spleen, confirmed the toxicological nature of trichothecenes.

One of the main features of acute and subacute toxicities of trichothecenes is the depletion of lymphoid tissues, as mentioned above. This characteristic of trichothecene mycotoxins indicates that they are potent modifiers of immune responses. In mice and other animals, delayed type hypersensitivity (DTH), antibody formation, and other immunological responses are markedly affected by the trichothecenes, and therefore the trichothecene mycotoxins are classified as immunodepressors (Obara *et al.*, 1984). Contamination of trichothecenes in food may give rise to serious problems in food toxicology.

Analytical Methods

Thin-layer chromatography (TLC) has always been a convenient method for detecting mycotoxins because of its simplicity and low cost. The trichothecenes present on the plates are detected by spraying with H_2SO_4, *p*-anisaldehyde and other reagents. The treatment of trichothecenes such as NIV and DON with $AlCl_3$ followed by heating gives a blue fluorescence under UV light, and this method is applied in chemical surveys of DON in foods (Trucksess *et al.*, 1984).

Gas–liquid chromatography (GC) is widely used for the survey of trichothecenes in feeds, foods and food products. Formation of derivatives of these trichothecenes is important before analysis (Scott, 1982).

Confirmation of the trichothecenes can be accomplished by combined GC and mass spectrometry (MS) with a selected ion monitoring system. Extraction and subsequent clean-up procedures are critical for good resolution of the toxins (Rosen and Rosen, 1984). Tanaka *et al.* (1985*b*) have developed an improved method for simultaneous detection of NIV and DON in cereals. Firstly, the cereals were extracted with a mixture of acetonitrile and water $(3:1)$; after defatting with n-hexane, the aqueous phase was cleaned up by a two-step column with Florisil and Sep-Pak, followed by GC-MS analysis. The trimethylsilyl (TMS) derivatives of NIV and DON were monitored by fragment ions of m/z 512, 422, 407 and 325 (DON) and m/z 510, 379, 349 and 323 (NIV).

Negative ion (NI) MS of DON under resonance electron capture conditions has been developed, and this NI technique applied to the identification of DON in grains and foods by using on-column injection capillary GC (Brumley *et al.*, 1985).

Radioimmunoassay (RIA) and enzyme-linked immunosorbent assay (ELISA) are recently used techniques for detecting environmental toxicants (Chu *et al.*, 1979; Peters *et al.*, 1982). Recently, the author's group have developed a sensitive ELISA for T-2 toxin by employing monoclonal antibodies. The minimum detectable amount of T-2 toxin by this assay is 25 pg (Ohtani *et al.*, 1985).

Trichothecenes in Cereals and Foods

Of over 80 kinds of trichothecene compounds, only limited numbers arc detected in cereals and foods. The major naturally occurring toxins are T-2 toxin, diacetoxyscirpenol, DON, NIV and satratoxins.

In Canada, the United States, South Africa and England, DON is the sole trichothecene present in corn, wheat, barley and other cereals. In Canada, Scott (1984a) demonstrated that the Canadian grains were contaminated with DON and that the average levels showed geographical difference between eastern and western Canada. In Ontario soft winter wheat, the average of DON (ppm) was 0·06 (1979 crop year), 0·42 (1980), 0·22 (1981) and 0·74 (1982); in Quebec hard spring wheat it was 0·93 (1980), 3·03 (1981) and 0·33 (1982), and in Western hard wheat 0·02–0·03 (1981–2). Corn, corn flour, rye flour and wheat flour were also found to be contaminated with DON. Significant contamination of DON in cereals has also been observed in the United States (Eppley *et al.*, 1984), England (Gilbert *et al.*, 1983b) and South Africa (Marasas *et al.*, 1977).

In contrast, both NIV and DON are detected in barley and wheat produced in Japan. Yoshizawa (1983) reported that 153 out of 205 samples examined, were positive for NIV and DON, and their contents were 0·07–22·9 and 0·06–49·6 ppm, respectively (Table 3).

By adopting a new methodology proposed by Tanaka *et al.* (1985b), we have surveyed extensively the contamination of NIV and DON in cereals sampled from various countries, and the data revealed that these two trichothecenes were detected from wheat, barley, malt barley, corn and others collected from Korea (Lee *et al.*, 1985), China (Ueno *et al.*, 1986a,b) and England (Tanaka *et al.*, 1986). More than 80% of the total samples were contaminated with both NIV and DON. Furthermore these tricho-thecenes were detected in health foods such as pressed barley, popcorn and Job's tears (Tanaka *et al.*, 1985a). Job's tears (Hatomugi in Japanese) is the seed of *Coix lacryma-jobi* L. var. *ma-yuen* Stapt (family Gramineae), and in Japan and other Asian countries this seed is widely consumed as herb medicine and health food. Chemical analysis revealed a heavy contamina-tion with NIV. Another important finding is the presence of DON in popcorn imported from the United States.

TABLE 3
Natural Occurrence of Nivalenol and Deoxynivalenol in Cereals and Foods

Country	Cereals and foods	Nivalenol [mg/kg (positive/total samples)]	Deoxynivalenol	References
Canada	corn		0·02–0·62 (105)	Scott (1984a)
	corn meal		0·11 (35)	Scott (1984a)
	corn flour		0·18 (27)	Scott (1984a)
	wheat		0·03–0·74 (939)	Scott (1984a)
	cookies		0·08 (35)	Scott (1984a)
	crackers		0·27 (20)	Scott (1984a)
	baby cereals		0·043 (30)	Scott (1984a)
England	feed barley		0·01–0·1 (21/43)	Gilbert et al. (1983a)
	malt barley		0·01–0·1 (13/42)	Gilbert et al. (1983a)
W. Germany	cereals	0·04–0·2 (11/42)	0·03–2·0 (16/42)	Blaas et al. (1984)
Japan	barley/wheat	0·07–22·0 (153/205)	0·06–49·6 (153/305)	Yoshizawa (1983)
	wheat flour	24 (12/36)	38 (26/36)	Tanaka et al. (1985b)
	barley flour	28 (6/6)	23 (3/6)	Tanaka et al. (1985b)
	polished pressed barley	68 (13/14)	18 (10/14)	Tanaka et al. (1985b)
	popcorn (USA)	0 (0/7)	84 (7/7)	Tanaka et al. (1985b)
	Job's tears	140 (11/14)	274 (2/14)	Tanaka et al. (1985b)
Korea	barley	546 (28/28)	118 (26/28)	Lee et al. (1985)
	malt	243 (4/4)	1 596 (4/4)	Lee et al. (1985)
S. Africa	corn		1·3–7·4	Marasas et al. (1977)
USA	corn		0·5–10 (24/52)	Vesonder et al. (1978)
	total feeds		0·1–41·0 (274/342)	Côté et al. (1984)
	feeds (corn)		0·1–22·0 (134)	Côté et al. (1984)

TABLE 4

World-wide Occurrence of *Fusarium* Mycotoxins Nivalenol (NIV), Deoxynivalenol (DON) and Zearalenone (ZEN) in Cereals and Foods

Countries and districts	Crop year	Cereals and foods	NIV	DON	ZEN	References
			Means (ng/g) in positives (positives/samples)[a]			
Argentine	1983	wheat	0 (0/20)	15 (3/20)	10 (20/20)	Unpublished
		barley	25 (15/20)	237 (18/20)	5 (13/20)	
		corn	0 (2/20)	111 (2/20)	6 (15/20)	
Austria	1983	wheat	25 (3/4)	360 (3/4)	ND (0/4)	Ueno et al. (1985c)
Bulgaria	1983	wheat	32 (1/2)	211 (1/2)	ND (0/2)	Ueno et al. (1985c)
Canada	1984	wheat	23 (4/10)	1 257 (4/10)	9 (9/10)	Unpublished
China						
Taiwan	1984	wheat	74 (6/12)	562 (9/12)	16 (9/12)	Ueno et al. (1986)
	1985	barley	634 (4/4)	83 (4/4)	19 (2/2)	
	1985	wheat	22 (4/10)	245 (3/10)	ND (0/10)	
Beijing	1984	wheat	6 644 (1/5)	1 710 (1/5)	ND (0/5)	Unpublished
Xi-an	1984	wheat	162 (3/4)	4 284 (4/4)	78 (4/4)	Unpublished
Shanghai	1985	wheat flour	ND (0/7)	129 (7/7)	4 (5/7)	Unpublished
England	1984	wheat	101 (17/31)	31 (20/31)	1 (4/31)	Ueno et al. (1986)
France	1984	wheat	42 (2/2)	86 (1/2)	ND (0/2)	Ueno et al. (1985c)
W. Germany						
Bavaria	1984	wheat	0 (0/6)	712 (2/6)	5 (1/6)	Unpublished
	1984	barley	0 (0/10)	190 (2/10)	16 (2/10)	
	1984	oats	1 464 (1/8)	60 (3/8)	49 (3/8)	
Münster	1984	rye	12 (4/22)	406 (4/22)	5 (3/22)	
	1984	rye flour	3 (2/12)	174 (2/12)	0 (0/12)	

TABLE 4 — contd.

Countries and districts	Crop year	Cereals and foods	NIV	DON	ZEN	References
			Means (ng/g) in positives (positives/samples)[a]			
Hungary	1984	wheat	4 (1/2)	671 (2/2)	ND (0/2)	Ueno et al. (1985c)
Italy	1984	barley	23 (1/5)	195 (2/5)	56 (1/5)	Unpublished
Japan	1983	barley	708 (5/5)	249 (5/5)	9 (3/3)	Tanaka et al. (1985a)
Hokkaido	1984	scabby wheat	205 (7/18)	3 812 (18/18)	189 (18/18)	Tanaka et al. (1985c)
Korea	1984	barley	489 (31/31)	124 (31/31)	24 (29/31)	Lee et al. (1986)
Nepal	1984	corn	892 (6/9)	541 (3/9)	819 (5/9)	Unpublished
Poland	1984	wheat	41 (43/48)	95 (13/48)	76 (1/48)	Ueno et al. (1985c)
	1984	barley	78 (3/6)	390 (1/6)	ND (0/6)	
Scotland	1984	barley	391 (3/8)	42 (5/8)	10 (8/8)	Tanaka et al. (1985d)
USSR	1984	oats	1 100 (1/1)	31 (1/1)	ND (0/1)	Ueno et al. (1986)
Yemen	1983	sorghum	91 (1/6)	ND (0/6)	ND (0/6)	Unpublished
	1984	barley	13 (2/3)	19 (2/3)	43 (3/3)	

[a]Detection limits: 2 ng/g for NIV and DON; 1 ng/g for ZEN. ND = not detected.

The rapid and sensitive methods for simultaneous detection of *Fusarium* mycotoxins proposed by us (Tanaka *et al.*, 1985*b,d*) were adopted for the survey on natural occurrences of NIV, DON and ZEN in cereals and foods sampled from more than 20 countries and districts. The data obtained are summarized in Table 4. The results reveal the co-contamination of cereals with NIV and DON, along with ZEN.

Carry-over of the Trichothecenes
Current approaches have revealed that DON and NIV are significant contaminants in cereals such as wheat, barley, corn, rye and others, and therefore the transmission of these toxins in cereals into foods is a serious problem in safety evaluation of foods.

The milling of corn and wheat has little palliative effect, and DON has been found to be distributed throughout the milled products (Gilbert *et al.*, 1983*a*; Scott *et al.*, 1984; Hart and Braselton, 1983). Young *et al.* (1984) also investigated the fate of DON during wheat processing. In this study, milling of Ontario soft winter wheat naturally contaminated with DON at 0·45 mg/kg was cleaned and milled in an industrial pilot plant. After milling, fractions containing both DON and ergosterol were found, with increased levels in the outer kernel (e.g. bran) portions and decreased levels in the inner flour portions. A positive correlation between DON and ergosterol levels indicated that the level of DON production was releated to the incidences of fungal growth, and that some parts of DON in cereals are transmitted into finished flour.

Further researches revealed that the trichothecene contaminants in cereal flour are carried over into foodstuffs such as bread, snack foods and cakes. In another study, the baking process of wheat flour was also found not to diminish the content of DON in breads (El-Banna *et al.*, 1983). Scott (1984*b*) has reviewed the fate of trichothecenes and other mycotoxins in food processing.

The above-mentioned evidence reveals that cereal grains such as wheat, barley, corn, rye and others are significantly contaminated with NIV and DON, the major toxins of *F. graminearum*, at a high frequency, and that they are transmitted into finished foodstuffs and health foods. Their incidences and levels are significantly higher than those of aflatoxin B_1, a potent hepatocarcinogen of *Aspergillus flavus*. In this respect, we have to pay more attention to their contamination in foodstuffs especially with reference to their long-term toxicity.

Regulation

Following the observations that Canadian grains are significantly contaminated with DON, and that this mycotoxin is carried over to finished cereal flours and foodstuffs, a guideline for DON in soft wheat was proposed in 1983, as shown in Table 5 (Scott, 1984a).

TABLE 5
Guidelines for Deoxynivalenol in Soft Wheat, 1983 (Scott, 1984a)

Unclean soft wheat	≤2·0 ppm
except	
Unclean soft wheat for infant foods	≤1·0 ppm
Unclean soft wheat for bran manufacture	≤2·0 ppm
Imported non-staple foods	≤1·2 ppm (on flour or bran basis)

This guideline was set by the Canadian health protection branch. After toxicological studies on DON, the tentative tolerable daily DON intake for adults was set at 3 μg/kg body weight, and the maximum DON level of 2·0 ppm in raw unclean soft wheat is expected to be reduced to approximately 1·2 ppm in the flour portion of finished foods.

At present, no guideline or regulation for the trichothecenes is officially proposed in other countries.

OCHRATOXINS

During a survey of toxic secondary fungal metabolites, ochratoxin A (OT-A) and related isocoumarin derivatives were isolated from *Aspergillus ochraceus*, and their toxicity characterized (van der Merwe *et al.*, 1965). OT-A contains a 7-carboxy-5-chloro-8-hydroxy-3,4-dihydro-3R-methyl-substituted isocoumarin linked through the carboxy group to L-β-phenylalanine (Fig. 5). This compound is the most toxic OT among the related metabolites, and frequently detected in cereals, foods and animal tissues.

OT-A has been shown to be a probable cause of nephropathy in humans (Balkan endemic nephropathy) and in pigs (Danish porcine nephropathy). After demonstration of its renal and hepatic carcinogenicity in mice, contamination by OT-A is considered one of the serious problems in food toxicology.

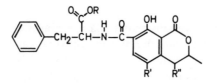

R=H, R'=Cl, R'=H   : OA
R=R'=R''=H   : OB
R=Et, R'=Cl, R'=H   : OC (OA ethyl ester)
R=Me,R'=Cl, R'=H   : OA methyl ester
R=Et, R'=R'=H   : OB ethyl ester
R=Me,R'=R'=H   :: OB methyl ester
R=H, R'=Cl, R'=OH   : 4-OH,OA

FIG. 5. Ochratoxins.

Krogh (1977), Steyn (1984) and the present author (1985*b*) have reviewed the chemistry, toxicology and biological activity of OT-A.

Ochratoxin-producing Fungi

OT-A was first isolated from *A. ochraceus* K-804, a strain isolated from sorghum grain. *A. sulphureus*, *A. sclerotiorum*, *A. alliaceus*, *A. melleus*, *A. ostianus* and *A. petrakii* are listed as producers of OT-A. Besides the *Aspergillus* group, several *Penicillium* species, e.g. *P. viridicatum*, *P. palitans*, *P. commune*, *P. purpurescens*, *P. verruculosum*, *P. variabile* and *P. cyclopium*, have been identified as producers of OT (van Walbeek *et al.*, 1969). Among these OT producers, *A. ochraceus* and *P. viridicatum* are the most important fungi as regards OT-A contamination.

Chemistry

OT is a colorless crystalline compound. Upon crystallization from benzene, it contains 1 mol of benzene. It is highly soluble in polar organic solvents, very slightly soluble in water and disssolves in aqueous sodium hydrogen carbonate.

OT-B, a less toxic metabolite, lacks the C-5 chlorine, and the methyl and ethyl esters of both OT-A and OT-B have been isolated as minor metabolites of the culture of *A. ochraceus*. The toxicity of the esters of OT-A is similar to that of OT-A, whereas those of OT-B are not toxic.

Hutchison *et al.* (1971) isolated 4-hydroxy-OT-A from *P. viridicatum*, and the same compound was identified from the metabolites of OT-A in animals administered with OT-A.

Mellein and 4-hydroxymellein, which are structurally related to the dihydroisocoumarin moiety of OT-A, have been isolated from *A. ochraceus* and other strains.

Toxicological and Biological Actions

The LD_{50} values (p.o., mg/kg) of OT-A are 28 (male rats), 20 (female rats), 3·90 (neonatal rats), 9·1 (male guinea pigs) and 8·1 (female guinea pigs). The i.p. LD_{50} to rainbow trout is 5·53 mg/kg (Steyn, 1984).

OT-A is very toxic to chick embryos, as shown by the LD_{50} value which is less than 0·01 μg for 6-day-old eggs injected via the air cell, whereas for unincubated eggs it was about 0·05 μg/egg via injection into the yolk sac (Choudhury *et al.*, 1971).

OT-A is a potent teratogen in rats, hamsters and mice, and has been shown to produce severe craniofacial abnormalities (Brown *et al.*, 1976). Still *et al.* (1971) have presented data demonstrating a relationship between OT-A contamination in feeds and bovine abortion.

The initial toxicological effect of OT-A is displayed on the nephron, and the proximal tubule is the primary target site. Changes of renal function in OT-A administered swine, for example, are characterized by damage to proximal tubular function, indicated by a decrease of the ratio Tm_{PAM}/C_{IN}, the ability to concentrate urine, and by an increased urinary excretion of glucose (Krogh, 1977).

Biochemical approaches have revealed that OT-A inhibits renal gluco-neogenesis through the depression of renal phosphoenolpyruvate carboxykinase (Meisner and Selenik, 1979; Meisner *et al.*, 1983). Recently, the author has demonstrated that, in isolated nephron segments of rats, OT-A induces the release of alanine aminopeptidase and leucine aminopeptidase which is specifically localized in the proximal tubule, and that this release is inhibited by probenecid, a selective inhibitor of the anion transport system. Therefore it is presumed that OT-A interferes specifically with the anion transport mechanism which is localized on the surface of the brush border facing vesicles, thus leading to the release of membrane-bound enzymes (Endou *et al.*, 1984).

Other evidence of toxicity is the inhibitory effect that OT-A has on protein synthesis and OT-A has been shown to cause inhibition of protein synthesis both in bacteria and in mammalian cells (Creppy *et al.*, 1983*b*,*c*). This inhibition is competitive and its acting site is phenylalanyl-tRNA synthetase. Since OT-A is composed of L-phenylalanine and the isocoumarin moiety, the synthetase enzyme recognizes the L-phenyl-alanine moiety of OT-A. The reduction of OT-A toxicity both *in vitro* and *in vivo* by phenylalanine gives support to the above biochemical evidence (Creppy *et al.*, 1980, 1984; Röschenthaler *et al.*, 1984; Moroi *et al.*, 1985).

Genotoxicity tests with *Rec*-assay in *Bacillus subtilis* (Ueno and Kubota, 1976) and Ames assay in *Salmonella typhimurium* (Ueno *et al.*, 1978) have revealed no mutagenic activity of OT-A. Long-term feeding experiments in mice, however, have demonstrated tumorigenic changes in liver and kidneys (Kanisawa and Suzuki, 1978). In these studies male ddY mice were fed diets containing 40 ppm of OT-A for 50 weeks, and pathological observation revealed hepatic cell tumors and hyperplastic nodules and adenoma in the kidneys.

Several mammalian enzyme systems biotransform OT-A into isocoumarin and hydroxylated metabolites in both *in vivo* and *in vitro* systems. Galtier *et al.* (1979) have reported the half-life of the toxin to be about 55 h after either oral or intravenous administration in rats, and that approximately 56% of the toxin was excreted via urine and feces, both as the free metabolite and hydrolyzed as ochratoxin α during 120 h following dosing. Experiments with [^{14}C]OT-A indicated that the toxin was distributed in serum (90% of dose), liver (4·5%) and kidney (4·4%) 30 min after i.p. injection (Chang and Chu, 1977). Storen *et al.* (1982) have also reported the presence of ochratoxin α and 4-hydroxy-OT-A in rat urine. Previously this group had demonstrated that, when incubating OT-A with hepatic microsomes, this 4-hydroxy-OT-A was detected in the metabolites (Størmer and Pedersen, 1980; Størmer *et al.*, 1981) (Fig. 6). As for the toxicity of OT-A metabolites, Creppy *et al.* (1983*a*) have reported that 4

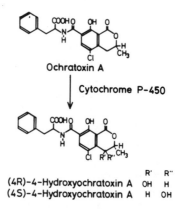

FIG. 6. Cytochrome P-450 dependent hydroxylation of ochratoxin A.

(*R*)-hydroxy-OT-A was toxic similarly as the parent OT-A, whereas ochratoxin α was inactive.

Detailed experiments with microsomes and purified cytochrome P-450 systems in the author's laboratory have revealed the following sequence of events (Ueno, 1985a). In hepatic microsomes of untreated rats, 4(*R*)-hydroxy-OT-A is the major metabolite, and pretreatment of rats with PCB or 3-methylcholanthrene accelerated this hydroxylation reaction in the microsomal system. In a reconstituted cytochrome P-450 system, cyto-chrome P-450 II-a (CO differential maximal spectrum at 448 nm and a high-spin form) prepared from PCB-treated rat livers catalyzed this hydroxylation, whereas the formation of 4(*S*)-4-hydroxy-OT-A was observed with various isozymes of cytochrome P-450 type. Therefore the author came to the conclusion that the cytochrome P-450 II-a (one of P-448 type) catalyzes the stereospecific hydroxylation of OT-A, and plays an important role in the metabolism of OT-A, in a manner similar to that of hydroxylation of aflatoxin B_1 into aflatoxin M_1 (Ueno *et al.*, 1985) and emodin into 2-hydroxyemodin (Tanaka *et al.*, 1987).

The biotransformation of OT-A has also been observed with a ruminant system. When OT-A was incubated with the content of stomachs of cows, OT-A was detoxicated into ochratoxin α and phenylalanine, and 4 nmol of OT-A was degraded by 1·5 g of rumen content in 4 h. Assuming that the same reaction velocity is obtained in the living cow and that the stomach content has a retention time of 48 h, every kilogram of content will degrade 30 μmol or 12 mg of OT-A. This suggests that a cow should be able to degrade OT-A in feed contaminated up to the level of 12 mg/kg (Hult *et al.*, 1976).

Analysis of Ochratoxin A in Foods

Several quantitative and semi-quantitative methods for the determination of low levels of OT-A in various commodities and biological samples have been developed, as reviewed by Krogh (1977) and Steyn (1984). The procedures include TLC (Nesheim *et al.*, 1973), mini-column techniques (Hald and Krogh, 1975), HPLC (Howell and Tayler, 1981) and enzyme-linked immunosorbent assay (ELISA) (Pestka *et al.*, 1981b).

Patterson and Roberts (1979) applied two-dimensional TLC for analysis of OT-A in feedstuffs. Several confirmative techniques have been intro-duced for the TLC assays. A generally used method is the viewing of the plates under UV light (366 nm), when OT-A appears as a green fluorescent spot and OT-B as a blue-green spot. The fluorescence of the OTs changes to a purple-blue fluorescence upon exposure to ammonia fumes or on spraying with aqueous sodium hydrogen carbonate. OT-A is also confirmed by formation of the fluorescent methyl and ethyl esters. Upon heating the plates in boron trifluoride–methanol for 10 min, OT-A changes to its methyl ester (Scott *et al.*, 1972*a*).

Numerous HPLC methods have been introduced for detection of OT-A in foodstuffs. Phillips *et al.* (1983) introduced a new HPLC method for determination of OT-A as *O*-methyl, methyl ester derivatives. OT-A was derivatized to an *O*-methyl, methyl ester (Me$_2$) with diazomethane and then determined by HPLC. This novel method is applicable for the determination of OT-A in animal tissues and analysis of the biological fate of OT-A.

A simple and rapid radioimmunoassay (RIA) of OT-A has been developed for OT-A in barley (Rousseau *et al.*, 1985). In this method, a highly radioactive [^{14}C]OT-A was synthesized; the detection limit is 2 ng per assay. As for ELISA of OT-A, the author's laboratory have developed a sensitive ELISA with a monoclonal antibody for OT-A; the detection limit is 5 pg per assay (Chiba *et al.*, 1985).

Natural Occurrence and Human and Animal Health
After the finding of ochratoxins among the fungal metabolites, the first evidence that OT-A was a contaminant in corn was reported by Shotwell *et al.* (1969*c*) in the United States, and it was followed by Scott *et al.* (1970) who detected OT-A in Canadian wheat. Table 6 shows the frequency and level of OT-A contamination in agricultural commodities. These data indicate the world-wide distribution of OT-A in groundnuts, corn, wheat, barley, sorghum and animal feeds. In general, the level of OT-A in animal feeds is much higher than that found in cereals.

Case reports on the acute poisoning by ingestion of OT-A have not been frequently reported, except the reports of lethal effects in poultry, rabbits and dogs in Bari, Italy (Visconti and Bottalico, 1983). This toxicosis appeared as acute gastroenteritis, causing the death of several farm animals and dogs, and HPLC analysis of causative moldy bread revealed the presence of 80 mg of OT-A and 9·6 mg of OT-B per kg of dry bread, which was colonized by *A. ochraceus*.

OT-A is also an important toxicant of chicks and hens. Several literature reports have cited outbreaks of disease in chickens in association with the contamination of feedstuffs with OT-A up to 2 ppm.

In 1928 a peculiar renal damage was discovered in pigs from Denmark who had been fed moldy cereal feeds. The renal damage included degeneration of the proximal tubules, interstitial fibrosis and hyalinization

TABLE 6
Natural Occurrence of Ochratoxin A in Agricultural Commodities

Commodity	Country	No. of samples	Contamination (%)	Ochratoxin A (μg/kg)	References
Corn	USA			110–150	Shotwell et al. (1969c)
Wheat (red spring)	Canada	4	100	20–100	Scott et al. (1970)
Corn	India	21		30–50	Rao et al. (1979)
Wheat	India	24	8	30–50	Rao et al. (1979)
Sorghum	India	24	12·5	50–70	Rao et al. (1979)
Grund nut	India	18	11	50–200	Rao et al. (1979)
Wheat (red winter)	USA	291	1	25–35	Shotwell et al. (1976)
Wheat (red spring)	USA	286	2·8	15–115	Shotwell et al. (1976)
Animal feeds and tissues	Canada	496	1·1	50–200	Prior (1981)
Coffee beans	USA	267	7·1	22–360	Levi et al. (1974)
Moldy bread	Italy	1		80 000	Visconti et al. (1983)
Porcine kidney	Poland	122	50	≥1	Golinski et al. (1985)
Porcine serum	Poland	388	38	1–450	Golinski et al. (1985)
Porcine serum	Sweden	279	16	≥2	Hult et al. (1980)
Nuts	Germany	150	5	0·2–8·6 (ng)	Kiermeier (1985)
Beans	Bulgaria	24	16·7	25–27	Petkova-Bocharova and
Corns	Bulgaria	22	27·3	25–35	Castegnaro (1985)

of the glomeruli. This disease is endemic in Denmark, with an incidence rate of 0·6–65·9 per 10 000 pigs in 1971 (Krogh, 1977). A close association between the rate of endemic swine nephropathy and the level of OT-A has been reported in Denmark, Sweden, Norway, Hungary, Finland and other countries.

Another important problem is the transmission of OT-A in feedstuffs to edible tissues. According to a current report of Buchmann and Hald (1985), condemnation rates (%) due to OT-A residue in porcine kidney (over 25 ppb) were 25 in 1980, 11 in 1981, 10 in 1982, 20 in 1983 and 11 in 1984. In 1983, 3% of a total of 7639 kidneys contained more than 150 μg/kg and 29% more than 25 μg/kg of OT-A.

Golinski et al. (1985) reported spontaneous occurrence of OT-A residues in porcine kidneys and serum samples in Poland. During the period April 1983 to July 1984, 214 700 swine were processed in a slaughterhouse in Poznan, Poland, and 122 (0·057%) carcasses exhibited microscopic kidney damage typical for porcine nephropathy, among which 52 were positive with OT-A (over 1 ng/g). Of 388 serum samples, 148 exhibited OT-A residue from 1 to 520 ng/ml, and the average concentration in the serum samples for the whole period was 7·6 ng/ml. The above findings indicate the contamination of blood and kidneys of swine with OT-A in Denmark, Sweden and other European countries.

Balkan endemic nephropathy is a fatal chronic disease affecting inhabitants of rural areas of Yugoslavia, Rumania and Bulgaria. This is characterized by contracted kidneys, with tubular degeneration, interstitial fibrosis, and hyalinization of glomeruli (Krogh, 1977). Because of the similarity between porcine endemic nephropathy and Balkan endemic nephropathy, OT-A was presumed to be a common causative agent. Further evidence for human exposure in these areas has been provided by the evidence of OT-A in the blood of 9·8–13·5% of the inhabitants, compared to 3·6% in the controls (Krogh, 1983).

Long-term feeding experiments have shown that OT-A is a renal and hepatic carcinogen in mice (Kanisawa and Suzuki, 1978). It is the first experiment which has demonstrated the carcinogenic potential of OT-A in experimental animals. According to Ceovic et al. (1976) and Chernozemky et al. (1977), Balkan endemic nephropathy is strongly associated with a very high incidence of tumors of the urinary system. Hult et al. (1982) detected OT-A in the blood of people living in areas of endemic nephropathy in Yugoslavia, and Petkova-Bocharova and Castegnaro (1985) demonstrated that the OT-A contents in beans and corns in the endemic area were 2–3 times higher than those in a control area in Bulgaria. These data may provide some support for the hypothesis that OT-A is an etiological factor both in Balkan endemic nephropathy and in tumors of the urinary system.

AFLATOXINS

Aflatoxin (AF) is well known as a potent hepatocarcinogen in experimental animals, and its contamination of foods gives rise to serious problems in human and animal health. Although *Aspergillus flavus* is associated with most food and feed contaminants with AF, only a few strains of *A. flavus* actually produce this toxic metabolite.

The majority of the more than 2000 publications about AF which have appeared during the past 20 years reflect an interest in mycotoxins, and more specifically in AF problems. This interest was primarily induced by the outbreak of turkey X disease in England in 1960 (Sargent *et al.*, 1961). Subsequent surveys demonstrated that the toxic manifestations were caused by ingestion of certain mold-contaminated feeds containing imported Brazilian peanut meal, and the toxins showed a characteristic fluorescence pattern on TLC plates. This physical property greatly facilitated their isolation and characterization, culminating in the determination of the molecular formulas of four components designated as AF B_1, B_2, G_1 and G_2 (Asao *et al.*, 1965). Additional AF compounds such as AFM_1 and AFM_2 were isolated from the milk of cows feeding on AF-contaminated fodder (Allcroft and Carnaghan, 1963).

After the finding that toxic peanut meal and the isolated AFs developed liver cell carcinoma in experimental animals, extensive surveys on the contamination of AFs in feeds and foodstuffs and its significance on human liver cancer have been carried out, with concomitant development of chemical detection methods, as reviewed in the literature (Goldblatt, 1969; Wyllie and Morehouse, 1977; Stoloff, 1977; Wogan, 1977; Egan *et al.*, 1982: Newberne, 1984; Hsieh and Ruebner, 1984; Ueno, 1985*b*).

In this section, the aim is to focus attention on the AF problem, with particular regard to contamination, modern analytical methods, toxicology, metabolism and the evaluation of its role in human liver cancer.

Chemistry
The term aflatoxins normally refers to the group of bisfuranoisocoumarin metabolites isolated from the *A. flavus* group of fungi. Aflatoxins fluoresce strongly in UV light (*ca.* 365 nm); B_1 and B_2 produce a blue whereas G_1 and

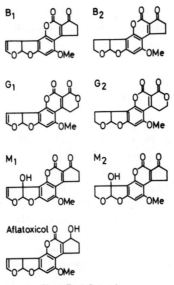

FIG. 7. Aflatoxins.

G_2 produce a green fluorescence, and this physical property makes a convenient marker for detection and monitoring of AFs in foods and biological materials. A number of chemically close derivatives, namely aflatoxicol, AFM_1 and parasiticol are also produced by the *A. flavus* group. The major AF derivatives are shown in Fig. 7.

AFB_1 ($C_{17}H_{12}O_6$) possesses the following spectral characteristics: $[\alpha]_D^{CHCl_3}$ $-558°$; λ_{max}^{EtOH} 223, 265 and 632 nm (ϵ 25 600, 13 400 and 21 800, respectively); $\nu_{max}^{CHCl_3}$ 1760 (intense), 1684 (weak), 1632, 1598 and 1562 cm^{-1}.

Lactating animals, on ingestion of AFB_1, secrete a metabolite in their milk, and this toxin, AFM_1, has been isolated and characterized. The infrared and UV spectra of AFB_1 and AFM_1 are similar; however, an extra band at 3425 cm^{-1} has been detected in the infrared spectrum of AFM_1, which suggests the presence of a hydroxy group.

An additional milk toxin, named AFM_2, has been isolated from crude extracts of fungal cultures. It is a dihydro-AFM_1. Two 2-hydroxy derivatives of AFB_2 and G_2 have been designated AFB_{2A} and AFG_{2A}, with AFB_{2A} identical to AFB_1 hemiacetal. They were isolated from cultures of *A. flavus* and formed by acid-catalyzed addition of water. Since these derivatives are not toxic, the formation of such derivatives is important as evidence of a detoxication reaction.

As mentioned above, the chemical decontamination of AFB_1 is very important for the safety evaluation of feeds and foodstuffs. In this regard, several chemical reactions of AF derivatives have been reported. AFs in the dry state are heat stable up to their melting point (269°C). In the presence of moisture, however, the destruction of AFs takes place at elevated temperatures. The opening of the lactone ring followed by decarboxylation is presumed in this reaction.

The hydrolysis of the lactone ring is also observed in alkaline solution, and an ammoniation process has now been introduced for chemical decomposition of AFB_1 in cereals and cottonseed meal. However, current research (Fremy and Quillardet, 1985) has revealed the interesting finding that the milk of lactating cows fed ammoniated and autoclaved groundnut

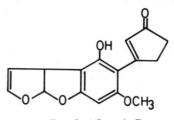

FIG. 8. Aflatoxin D_1.

meal contained an unusually high level of AFM_1 as expected from the detoxication process. AFD_1, the major product of ammoniated AFB_1 (Fig. 8), is 130-fold less mutagenic than AFB_1 in the Ames test (Schroeder *et al.*, 1985).

Many oxidizing agents such as sodium hypochlorite, potassium permanganate, hydrogen peroxide and sodium perborate react with AF and change its structure.

Reduction of AFB_1 by hydrogen gives tetrahydrodeoxy-AF, and reduction with sodium borohydride yields AF RB_1 and RB_2. These compounds arise as a result of opening the lactone ring followed by reduction of the acid group and keto group in the cyclopentenone ring.

The details of chemical and biological modifications of AFs have been reviewed by Goldblatt and Dollear (1977) and Jones (1977a).

Chemical Analysis

As summarized by Stoloff (1982), many chemical and biological methods for the detection and quantification of AFB_1 and related compounds have been proposed during the past 20 years. The early observations of Sargent *et al.* (1961), concerning the chemical properties of toxic components in suspected groundnut meal, form the basic technology for the separation and detection procedures, an extraction of AFs with chloroform and detection of their fluorescence under UV exposure.

The analysis of AFs involves separation/extraction of the mycotoxins, clean-up procedures and quantification. In some cases, a confirmation process is included.

As for the extraction process, in almost all the proposed methods the following solvent systems are now used: methanol–water (55:45 v/v), acetone–water (85:15), acetonitrile–water (9:1), chloroform–water (50% of dry substrate) and methylene dichloride–water (50% of dry substrate).

The clean-up process is very important for determination of AFs and other environmental toxins in foods. In most cases, lipids are the major components which interfere with the subsequent steps of quantification, and the procedures for lipid removal depend on the solvents employed for extraction of AFs. Extracts with hydrophilic organic solvents (methanol, acetone, acetonitrile) are defatted by hexane or isooctane. Adsorbent columns are often introduced for the removal of interfering materials; silica gel, alumina, Florisil and other adsorbents are offered in several official methods. In several cases, with extracts from plant origins, pigments cause a disturbance of the analysis, and lead acetate, zinc acetate and cupric carbonate are used to overcome this problem.

For the quantification of AFs in cleaned-up samples, TLC and HPLC are often used in several official methods. Since TLC is simple, economic and easy to handle, this is a powerful separation and detection tool, and this technique is incorporated in methods used by a number of European and other countries for regulatory purposes (Schuller *et al.*, 1970). Two-dimensional TLC has also been introduced for determination of AFs in meat, milk and eggs (Trucksess and Stoloff, 1979).

HPLC is now employed for the determination of AFs in foods and biological fluids. Pons (1976) was the first to propose HPLC for resolution of AFs. The AFs were completely resolved as sharp peaks in the order B_1–B_2–G_1–G_2 on a small-particle porous silica gel column in 7–13 min by a water-saturated chloroform–cyclohexane–acetonitrile elution solvent (25:7·5:1·0), with detection by ultraviolet absorption at 360 nm.

The relative fluorescence intensities of AFs in solution are different, and this makes a problem for HPLC–fluorometric detection. Normal phase columns packed with microparticulate silica gel (e.g. μPorasil, Zorbak SIL, LiChrosorb Si 60) are employed, and reverse-phase columns are packed with microparticulate silica gel, but the active hydroxyl sites are bound through a silyl group to an organic radical, mostly octadecyl (e.g. μBondapak C_{18}, Spherisorb ODS).

Currently, HPLC methodology is employed for the detection of AFB_1 and related toxins in cottonseed products (Pons and Franz, 1977), AFM_1 in milk and dairy products (Chambon *et al.*, 1983), AFB_1 and AFG_1 in human urine (Anukarahanonta, 1983), and others. Fremy and Quillardet (1985) applied this HPLC technique for analysis of 'carry-over' of AFB_1 into milk of cows fed ammoniated rations. The Association of Official Analytical Chemists (1981) has proposed an official HPLC method for AFs.

Modern technology has led to the introduction of mass spectrometry (MS). Because AFs are found in low concentrations and are not amenable to gas chromatography, several steps are necessary to prepare samples sufficiently pure for identification by MS. Field desorption (FD) MS has been used to screen extracts for AFs (Sphon *et al.*, 1977), but FD has not found widespread application because it is a difficult technique to use.

Electron impact (EI) MS with low-resolution full scan and high-resolution selected ion monitoring (HRSIM) modes was introduced for identification of AFs (Haddon *et al.*, 1977). This method detects AFs in samples at the 10–100 ppb level after extraction and TLC clean-up. Negative ion chemical ionization (NICI) obtained from resonance capture conditions in the CI source has also been proposed for confirmation of AFB_1 and AFM_1 in foods at levels as low as 10 ppb. This NICI-MS technique also requires extraction, silica gel column chromatography, two-dimensional TLC and a second extraction from the gel (Brumley *et al.*, 1981).

With the aim to reduce the many clean-up steps, a quadruple MS/MS technique has recently been introduced for the identification and confirmation of AFs. Since chemical noise is the major problem in MS analysis, the technique of tandem MS or MS/MS has generated considerable interest as a method to help overcome the chemical noise problem in the chemical analysis. Essentially, MS/MS uses one mass filter to select the compound of interest from the matrix. These selected ions then undergo collisionally activated dissociation (CAD) to yield characteristic products which are separated by the second mass filter (Plattner *et al.*, 1984). This MS/MS with NICI is applicable for confirmation of AFs in materials without the preparative TLC clean-up step, and the detection limit is 10 ppb. This technique has been applied for detection of aflatoxin D in ammoniated corn (Grove *et al.*, 1984).

Immunochemical Analysis

In a search for simpler and more specific methods, several immuno-chemical methods with polyclonal and monoclonal antibodies have been developed for determination of mycotoxins including AFs. Chu (1984) reviewed the modern concept of the immunoassay of mycotoxins, and Garner *et al.* (1985) summarized the data on monitoring AFs and their metabolites in human body fluids.

The development of an immunoassay includes at least four categories: conjugation of mycotoxins to protein for immunization; formation of antibodies against mycotoxins; characterization of their specificity; and application of specific antibodies for survey determination.

Generally, most mycotoxins are small organic molecules, and it is essential to conjugate the mycotoxins to carrier proteins. A water-soluble carbodiimide or mixed anhydride method is generally used for the con-jucation process. AFB_1 contains a carbonyl group, which is conjugated to protein after the formation of a carboxymethyl oxime (CMO) derivative. In this method a CMO group is generally introduced at the carbonyl position in the cyclopentenone ring of AFB_1 and AFM_1 (Chu and Ueno, 1977) and AFB_{2a} and AFQ_1 are converted to hemiglutarate and hemi-succinate, respectively, and then conjugated to the protein.

The antibodies produced by use of AF conjugated through the cyclo-pentenone portion generally recognize the dihydrofuran moiety of AF, and those produced by the conjugate through the dihydrofuran moiety, e.g. AFB_{2a}, recognize the cyclopentenone portion of the mycotoxin.

The technology for immunoassay can be briefly divided into either radioimmunoassay (RIA) or enzyme-linked immunosorbent assay (ELISA). The RIA requires highly labeled AFs, and the specific activity of the radioactive ligand plays an essential role in the sensitivity of RIA. Furthermore, the sensitivity of RIA is increased by a simple clean-up procedure after extraction of samples to be tested. The detection limit of AFB_1 is 5·8 ppb in corn, peanut and wheat (El-Nakib *et al.*, 1981) and that of AFM_1 in milk is 5 ppb (Pestka *et al.*, 1980, 1981a).

In general, the sensitivity of ELISA for mycotoxins is about 10–100 times more than RIA when pure mycotoxins are used (Chu, 1984), and this method does not use radioactive substances. The latter point is a great advantage in practice. Actually, 10–25 ppt levels of AFM are detectable with ELISA when the samples are cleaned up with C_{18} reverse phase Sep-pak cartridge prior to assay (Hu *et al.*, 1983).

These immunochemical methods are expected to cover the monitoring of AF exposure in human life; as reviewed by Garner *et al.* (1985), the field application of immunoassays for AFB_1, AFM_1 and DNA-binding form(s) of AF metabolites will promote understanding of the causative agents in human liver cancer.

Occurrence in Foods

After the finding that AF was a potent hepatocarcinogen, numerous surveys have been carried out during the past 20 years. However, as pointed out by Jones (1981), some caution is required in evaluating information on the natural occurrence of the AFs. It had been demonstrated on the laboratory scale that the *A. flavus* group can grow and produce AFs on cereals. It does not mean that AF production will in fact occur under natural conditions. Fungal growth or mold contamination is not necessarily an indication of AF production on the specified commodity. Furthermore, many reports on the natural occurrence of AF indicate the presence of fluorescent spots on TLC plates without a confirmation test being performed.

Among foods and foodstuffs, peanut and peanut products, which are widely grown and utilized for food and feedstuffs in the tropical and subtropical countries, would seem to be significantly contaminated with AF and therefore play an important role in AF risk evaluation. As reviewed by Jones (1977b), the contamination of peanuts and their products with AF has been reported in the United States, Africa, Asian countries and India, as well as in other countries. AF has also been found in other kinds of edible nuts, including almonds, hazelnuts and pistachio nuts, although the levels have been relatively low.

Table 7 summarizes various information on AF contamination in cereals and cereal products. *Aspergillus flavus* is able to infect several kinds of cereals, in particular corn, and produces AF prior to harvest. The levels and frequency of AF contamination are significantly high, and corn heavily contaminated with AFB_1 may induce acute-type hepatitis in man.

AFB_1 and related mycotoxins are often detected in cereals such as corn, barley, wheat, sorghum, oats, millet, rice, beans and other local edible grains and foods. Although their contents are low relative to the levels found in peanuts and corn, these commodities are important as dietary foods in the whole world.

Dairy products are sometimes contaminated with AFB_1 and AFM_1. Consumption of AFB_1-contaminated feeds by lactating animals results in the extraction of metabolites such as AFM_1. The relative amount of AFM_1 excreted is related to the amount of AFB_1 in the feed, and about $0 \cdot 1\%$ of AFB_1 ingested is excreted into milk as AFM_1. Kiermeier and Mashaley

TABLE 7
Natural Occurrence of Aflatoxins in Cereals and Cereal Products

Products	Country	Aflatoxins (μg/kg)	Remarks	References
Corn	USA	3–27	2·7% positive	Shotwell et al. (1969b)
Yellow corn	USA	4–308	34·6% positive	Shotwell et al. (1973)
Corn	USA	10 000	associated with AF toxicoses in chickens	Smith and Hamilton (1970)
White corn (feed grade)	Nigeria	100–1 000	100% positive	Oyeniran (1973)
Corn	Nepal	8·8–37·5 B_1	51% positive	Karki et al. (1979)
Corn	China	89·5	36% (<30 μg/kg)	Liu (1985)
Corn	Philippines	400	35% positive	Campbell and Salamat (1971)
Corn	Thailand	93 B_1		Shank et al. (1972)
Corn	Japan	131–340 B_1	commercial samples	Saito et al. (1984)
Corn	India	6 250–15 600	acute hepatitis	Krishnamachari et al. (1975)
Corn	Kenya	3 200–12 000	acute hepatitis	Ngindu et al. (1982)
Corn	Philippines	45·9	84% positive	Bulatao-Jayme et al. (1982)
Wheat	USA	2–19	0·4% positive	Shotwell et al. (1969a)
Wheat	France	0·25–180	47% positive	Lafont and Lafont (1970)
Wheat flour	France	0·25–150	28% positive	Lafont and Lafont (1970)
Spaghetti	Canada	13	isolated sample	van Walbeek et al. (1968)
Sorghum	Uganda	1–1 000	37·7% positive	Alpert et al. (1971)
Sorghum	France	0·25–100	25% positive	Lafont and Lafont (1970)
Oats	Sweden	2 600		Pettersson et al. (1978)
Oats	France	0·25–100	42% positive	Lafont and Lafont (1970)
Barley	France	0·25–10	7% positive	Lafont and Lafont (1970)
Millet	Uganda	1–100	16·4% positive	Alpert et al. (1971)

TABLE 7 —contd.

Products	Country	Aflatoxins ($\mu g/kg$)	Remarks	References
Millet	Thailand	248		Shank et al. (1972)
Millet	Nigeria	1·4		Emerole et al. (1982)
Rye	France	0·25–100		Lafont and Lafont (1970)
Rice	Philippines	16		Campbell and Saramat (1971)
Rice	Thailand	98	2% positive	Shank et al. (1972)
Rice and rice products	Philippines	30	38% positive	Bulatao-Jayme et al. (1982)
Boiled rice	Philippines	0·6	20% positive	Bulatao-Jayme et al. (1982)
Rough rice	Brazil	400		Jones (1957)
Raw rice	Nepal	5–10		Karki et al. (1979)
Rice		40		Emerole et al. (1982)
Garri (Manihot flour)	Nigeria	1 600		Emerole et al. (1982)
Red pepper	Nigeria	700		Emerole et al. (1982)
Yam flour	Nigeria	400		Emerole et al. (1982)
Beans	Japan	B_1 1·3–26·9	1·8% positive	Saito et al. (1979)
		B_2 0·4– 6·9	1·8% positive	Saito et al. (1979)
Cassava	Philippines	467·5	100% positive	Bulatao-Jayme et al. (1982)
Yam	Philippines	88·8	39% positive	Bulatao-Jayme et al. (1982)
Sweet potato	Philippines	60·6	84% positive	Bulatao-Jayme et al. (1982)
Cocoa		50·6	70% positive	Bulatao-Jayme et al. (1982)
Pistachio nut	Japan	2·0–800 B_1		Saito et al. (1979)
		0·4–180 B_2		
		0·6–51·4 G_1		
		0·2–16·3 G_2		
		1·8–39·3 M_1		

(1977) reported that AFM_1 was detected in 8 dried milk products out of 166 samples in the range $0 \cdot 7$–$2 \cdot 0$ $\mu g/kg$, which corresponds to $0 \cdot 08$–$0 \cdot 26$ $\mu g/$ liter.

Meat and meat products are also contaminated with AF when farm animals are fed with AF-contaminated rations. Furthermore, many meat products such as 'country style' hams and certain sausages, are traditionally mold-ripened. As suggested by Leistner (1984), undesirable *Penicillium* and other fungi grow quite frequently on meat products, especially on fermented sausages (salami) and raw hams. Natural inoculation has been the basis for the traditional methods, but now there is a trend to control the ripening process using selected starter non-toxic strains.

Currently, the survey of AF contamination is expanding to traditional foods and commodities, and these data show a world-wide distribution of AF, particularly in Africa and Asia. As shown in Table 5, in the Philippines rice and rice products were contaminated with 30 ppb AFB_1 in 38% positive samples, and cassava and cassava products, one of the major dietary foods, contained $467 \cdot 5$ ppb AFB_1 (average of 142 samples) (Bulatao-Jayme *et al.*, 1982).

AF has also been shown to occur in spices, including cayenne pepper, Indian chilli powder, dried chilli peppers, black pepper, capsicum peppers and nutmeg (Jones, 1977*b*), and Kiermeier (1985) has summarized the data on AFB_1 contents in 15 550 samples during 1980–3.

Acute Hepatitis and Aflatoxins

Though epidemiological studies have suggested that AF may be responsible for human diseases, there are few reports so far which directly correlate AF and human diseases, particularly acute toxicosis.

In two adjacent states (Gujarat and Rajasthan) in India, a food-borne toxicosis started during late October 1974 in rural areas where the staple food was corn. In October 1974 there were unseasonal rains which drenched the standing corn crop, and a total of 397 patients were affected and 106 died (Krishnamachari *et al.*, 1975). Clinical features were characterized by jaundice, vomiting, anorexia, and followed by ascites, which appeared rapidly within a period of 2–3 weeks. The liver was enlarged and tender in only a few cases. Death was usually sudden, and in most cases was preceded by massive gastrointestinal bleeding. Twice as many males as females were affected. Liver histopathology revealed extensive bile duct proliferation with periductal fibrosis.

During the outbreak and for several weeks afterwards, a large number of dogs developed ascites and icterus, and died within 2–3 weeks of the onset.

Affected corn grains obtained from afflicted households showed the presence of A. *flavus*, and chemical analysis revealed the presence of AF in the range 6·25–15·6 ppm. Since an adult consumes about 350 g of corn daily, the patients would have ingested 2–6 mg of AF daily for several weeks. These findings indicated that the hepatitis was due to the uptake of AFB_1. The follow-up of clinical signs including cirrhosis and hepatic cancer is continuing on about 250 survivors by the National Institute of Nutrition, Hyderabad.

Another outbreak of acute hepatitis caused by AF poisoning was observed in Kenya. Between March 28 and June 3, 1983, 20 patients (8 women and 12 men aged from 2½ to 45 years) were admitted to Makueni, Makindu or Machakos hospitals with jaundice. The early symptoms were abdominal discomfort, anorexia, general malaise, and low-grade fever. Of 20 patients, 8 improved with return of appetite, clearing of jaundice, and were discharged from hospitals within 6–20 days. Hepatic failure developed in the remaining 12 patients and they died between 1 and 12 days after admission. Massive ascites and gastrointestinal hemorrhage were observed (Ngindu *et al.*, 1982).

Histopathologically the liver of patients showed evidence of toxic hepatitis—marked centrolobular necrosis with minimal inflammatory reaction. There was only slight fatty infiltration and no proliferation of bile ducts. Elevation of serum transaminases was observed, while attempts to isolate viruses were negative. Three of 29 sera were positive for hepatitis B surface antigen (HBsAg). TLC analysis revealed the presence of 3200 and 12 000 ppb of AFB_1 in corn from the homes where there had been acute illness and death (Table 5), while corn from the unaffected homes had a maximum of 500 ppb of AFB_1. The liver samples, which came from 2 of the children of the family in which 6 died, contained 39 and 89 ppb of AFB_1.

This acute hepatitis observed in Kenya was presumed to be caused by the ingestion of corn contaminated with 3–12 ppm levels of AFB_1.

Primary Liver Cancer, Aflatoxin and Hepatitis B Virus

Despite increasing incidence of human primary hepatocellular carcinoma (PHC) in the world, it is still controversial whether PHC is caused by hepatic viruses or by mycotoxins. Before the discussion of PHC, it is necessary to clarify the histological classification of tumors of the liver, biliary tract and pancreas. WHO (1978) divided primary liver cancer (i.e. malignant epithelial neoplasia arising from the liver) into six categories: (1) hepatocellular carcinoma (liver cell carcinoma), an intrahepatic malignant tumor composed of cells resembling hepatocytes; (2) cholangiocarcinoma (intrahepatic bile duct carcinoma), an intrahepatic malignant tumor composed of cells resembling those of biliary epithelium; (3) bile duct cysto-adenocarcinoma, a malignant cystic tumor lined by mucus-secreting epithelium with papillary infoldings; (4) combined hepatocellular and cholangiocarcinoma, a tumor containing unequivocal elements of both hepatocellular and cholangiocarcinoma; (5) hepatoblastoma, a malignant tumor composed of cells resembling primitive hepatic parenchymal cells, with or without mesenchymal elements; (6) undifferentiated carcinoma, a malignant epithelial tumor which is so poorly differentiated that it cannot be placed in any of the above categories.

In the following sub-sections the cause of human primary liver cancer will be discussed in relation to aflatoxin intake and hepatic viruses.

Primary Liver Cancer Rate and Aflatoxin Intake
The interpretation of mortality and incidence of primary liver cancer (PLC) has been analyzed in detail (Linsell, 1984; International Union against Cancer, 1982). The geographical distribution can be presented by arbitrary classification into three groups: age-adjusted incidence rates higher than 20 per 100 000 males (south and west Africa, China, south Asia, Hong Kong, Singapore, etc.), intermediate rates of 5–20 per 100 000 (Nigeria, Brazil, Switzerland, Spain, Poland, New Zealand, etc.), and low incidence rates less than 5 per 100 000 (United States, Israel, etc.)

High rates are found in southern and western Africa, and in rural southern Africa PLC presents at a relatively young age with a peak incidence in the third, fourth and fifth decades. The youngest patients are Mocambican Shangaans, who have a mean age of 33·4 years and of whom 50% are less than 30 years of age. In almost all parts of the world, PLC occurs predominantly in men. In sub-Saharan Africa and in the Far East, male preponderance is more striking, with ratios as high as 8:1.

The relationship between PLC rates and AF intake in a high-incidence area in South Africa was reported by van Rensburg *et al.* (1974, 1975). In the Inhambane district of Mozambique, the cancer rates for 1964–8 and 1969–71 were 35·5 and 25·4 per 100 000 per year, and the randomly sampled 880 meals were positive for AF with an average of 7·8 μg/kg wet food (9·3% positive), and a mean daily per capita consumption of 224·4 ng/kg body weight (15 μg/adult/day). The pooling of these data with similar investigations in lower incidence areas revealed a positive correlation between the intake of AF and the liver cancer rate.

Retrospective evaluation of data from Kenya, Thailand and Mozambique has shown that the liver cancer rates were 4·2, 6·0 and 25·4 per 100 000, respectively, and the daily intakes of AFB_1 were estimated as 10·0, 45·0 and 222·4 ng/kg body weight, respectively (Munro, 1976; Enwonwu, 1984). These data also indicated the positive relationship between the primary liver cancer rates and the exposure to AFB_1.

Liu (1985) reported epidemiological data on cancer rates and AFB_1 levels in foods in China. In two districts of high incidence of liver cancer, namely Fusui district of Guiangxi and Qidong district of Jiangsu, the mortalities from liver cancer were 58·6 and 49·0 per 100 000, respectively, but for the whole of China it was 9·6 per 100 000. Fusui Institute of Liver Cancer analyzed about 2000 food samples collected in Fusui, and AFB_1 was positively identified in 51·4% of corn and 62·9% of wheat in 1980. The average content of AFB_1 was 89·0 ppb in corn samples. Significant contamination of AFB_1 in corn was also indicated by feed-borne intoxication of pigs in the high liver cancer district of Guiangxi in 1974. In six parts of Guiangxi, 'yellow-fat disease', characterized by a yellow color of fat and by liver damage, developed in 10 145 pigs during July to October, and the mortality of affected young pigs reached 48·83%. Guiangxi Institute of Veterinary Science clarified that the yellow fat disease was caused by moldy corn contaminated with AFB_1, and 74·1% of 172 feed samples based on corn were positive for AFB_1, with values above 500 ppb (Liu, 1985).

Bulatao-Jayme et al. (1982) reported on the PLC risk from aflatoxin exposure in the Philippines. In this study, only confirmed PLC hospital cases were used. Among 90 PLC cases (74 males and 16 females), the peak age was between 35 and 44 years, within which 26·7% of the cases were found, and the mean ages of the cases were 47 years for the males and 36 years for the females. Ninety controls, individually matched with the cases as to age and sex, were patients from the surgical and medical wards, who showed normal livers after liver function tests.

Chemical analysis of 3510 samples from over 100 food items revealed that cassava and cassava products and peanut butter were positive for AFB_1 in almost all the samples tested, with 467·5 and 143·6 ppb respectively (Table 5), followed by yam and yam products (88·8 ppb), sweet potato and sweet potato products (60·6 ppb), cocoa and cocoa products (50·6 ppb) and peanuts and peanut products (49·1 ppb). Of the total AF load, 51·2% came from cassava, 20·3% from corn, 6·8% from peanuts and 5·8% from sweet potato. The statistical analysis indicated that the mean AF load per day of the PLC cases was 4·4-fold higher than the control. Another factor was found to be the intake of alcohol, which had a synergistic and statistically significant effect on the development of PLC.

These three reports in southern Africa, China and the Philippines indicate a positive relationship between primary liver cancer rates and levels of AFB_1 intake. Current attempts to establish the relationship have been made by the introduction of modern technology for detection of AFB_1 and its metabolites in human biological materials. Urine and serum samples from humans have been subjected to HPLC, RIA, ELISA and HPLC-RIA analysis for detection of AFB_1, AFM_1 and other metabolites. Data have indicated their presence in urine samples in Gambia (Martin *et al.* 1985), Quidong in China (Sun and Chu, 1984), the Philippines (Campbell *et al.*, 1974), the United States (Yang *et al.*, 1980; Siraj *et al.*, 1981; Wray and Hayes, 1980) and Japan (Tsuboi *et al.*, 1984). Lampiugh and Hendrickse (1983) detected 4900 pg/g AFB_1 and 8500 pg/g aflatoxicol in the livers of African children, and Autrup *et al.* (1983) and Groopman *et al.* (1985) detected a putative adduct, 2,3-dihydro-2-(7'-guanyl)-3-hydroxy-AFB_1, in human urine.

These data present evidence for exposure of humans to AF, but at the moment there are not sufficient samples to evaluate these data in connection with the incidence of PLC. However, Chinese scientists have also demonstrated (using poly- and mono-clonal antibodies against AFM_1 and other AF derivatives for immunoconcentration) that 100 ng of AFM_1 could be present in 24-h urine in high-risk areas, while only below 2 ng of AFM_1 was present in low-risk areas of PLC (Sun and Chu, 1984; Sun *et al.*, 1983).

An opposite hypothesis, namely that AF is not involved in the incidence of PLC, was recently proposed by Stoloff (1983). PLC mortality ratios, computed from death certificate records compiled by the National Center for Health Statistics, for the periods 1968–71 and 1973–6 were sorted according to race, sex and region. Comparative studies on rural white males from the south-east and the north and west regions with regard to mortality ratios and dietary exposure to AF revealed that the expected average daily ingestion of AFB_1 was 13–197 ng/kg body weight for the south-east and 0·2–0·3 ng/kg body weight for the north and west. However, the age-adjusted excess PLC in the south-east population was only 10% at all ages and 6% for the 30–49 age group compared to that calculated in the north and west populations. The remaining major portion of the PLC mortality in the south-east was presumed to be due to many unidentified causes, leaving in doubt the validity of any attribution of the excess PLC mortality to AF exposure. A large excess over average United States PLC mortality was observed in Orientals resident in the United States and for urban black males, and the study came to the conclusion that the high incidence of PLC in Orientals was related to the presence of hepatitis B virus markers in the serum.

Primary Liver Cancer and Hepatitis B Virus

As is well known, hepatitis B virus (HBV) seems to be closely related to PLC as a causative agent for the following reasons.

(a) There is a close geographical correlation of incidence between PLC and HBV. In Africa (Kew, 1981; Kew *et al.*, 1983) and Asia, the carrier rate of hepatitis B surface antigen (HBsAg) is 10–12%, and the annual mortality due to PLC is 20–150 per 100 000 population per year, with at least 80% of PLC patients carrying HBsAg. In Quidong district, a high-incidence area of PLC in China, the incidence rate of PLC and the mortality during 1972–81 are 50·31 and 48·37/10^5/year, respectively, and this PLC incidence rate increased to 234/10^5/year in HBV carriers and decreased to 13·5/10^5/year in non-carriers (Sun and Chu, 1984).

(b) Biopsy and autopsy specimens of the liver of chronic hepatitis and cirrhosis in the course of HBV infection have revealed several characteristic lesions of liver parenchymal cells. In these lesions, small basophilic cells were characteristic, showing aggregation of mitochondria in perinuclear regions and proliferation of rough endoplasmic reticulum (Itakura, 1982–3).

(c) Cell lines derived from a PLC patient in S. Africa were shown to excrete a large amount of HBsAg (Macnab *et al.*, 1976), and integrated HBV DNA in a human liver cell has been detected in continuous cell lines expressing HBsAG from HBV carriers with PLC. Injection of tumor cell lines containing HBV DNA into nude mice produced nodules of PLC (Shouval *et al.*, 1981). Immunopathological studies have revealed the presence of HBsAG in the cytoplasm or hepatitis B core antigen (HBcAG) in the nucleus of liver parenchymal cells in HBV infection.

(d) Experimental infection with human HBV has been successful only in chimpanzees and a few other mammals. Typical hepatic cirrhosis or PLC in these animals caused by HBV has not yet been obtained.

(e) Viral hepatitis type B in woodchuck (*Marmota monax*) and that in Pekin ducks (*Anas domesticus*) have been identified as animal models of hepatitis. These viruses can induce cirrhosis and PLC in their respective hosts (Snyder *et al.*, 1982; Sun and Wang, 1983). Tiollais *et al.* (1985) has reviewed the HBV problem.

This accumulated information has demonstrated positive and strong evidence for HBV as a cause of human liver cancer. Besides HBV, some viral-like particles, non-A and non-B have been identified both in PLC patients and in chimpanzees. Detailed studies are in progress, and currently the surface antigen for non-B hepatitis virus is being applied for clinical diagnosis of PLC (Seto and Gerety, 1985).

As mentioned above, epidemiological, pathological and immunochemical evidence suggests that HBV plays the most important role in the induction of PLC. It was recently concluded (World Health Organization, 1985) that HBV is second only to tobacco (cigarette smoking) products among the known human carcinogens. However, in order to confirm the etiological role of HBV in PLC, it must be shown that HBV is truly oncogenic by both transformation of cells in cultures and induction of PLC in animal experiments. The problem is that usually there is no histologically identifiable human-type chronic hepatitis or hepatic (macronodular, postnecrotic) cirrhosis in those experiments.

As for AFB_1, its potent mutagenicity and carcinogenicity are well known in experimental models, and the epidemiological surveys also support the hypothesis that AFB_1 is the most suspected cause for incidence of PLC, as mentioned above. However, direct evidence for AFB_1 as the causative agent of human PLC must be presented.

At present, several approaches are being carried out in order to cover this great gap between the two hypotheses of AFB_1 and HBV origins in PLC. The binding of AFB_1 to various high molecular weight DNAs from human normal liver and cancer cell lines, Alexander primary liver carcinoma (PLC) and Mahlavu hepatocellular carcinoma (hHC) has been tested by Yang et al. (1985). In this study preferential binding was observed with the hepatocellular carcinoma DNA at two subgenomic, Hind III restricted DNA fragments, and such preferential binding was not observed with normal liver DNA.

From this evidence that AFB_1 preferentially attacks a 3·1 kb Hind III restriction fragment of Mahlavu hHC DNA, in which a Nar I restriction endonuclease site reading GCCGGC is located, and because the Nar I restriction endonuclease recognition sequence has been considered to be the reading sequence for the 12th amino acid (GGC = glycine) of the n-ras oncogene, AFB_1 is presumed to possess a high affinity with the second G in a tetranucleotide of CGGC. The modified G is unable to pair with C but rather mis-pair with A, thus resulting in a (GC to AT) transversion-type mutation, as observed previously in bladder carcinoma.

Such an approach indicates that AFB_1 may possess the ability to mutate preferentially the DNA sequence of tumorigenic DNA, and the modification of a specific site of DNA could be expected to activate the protooncogene integrated in the host cells. If such activation of integrated HBV takes place in the hepatic cells, it is highly possible to speculate that AFB_1 may act as a co-carcinogen in PLC.

Another approach was taken in the author's laboratory using rats and cultured cells. In the hepatocarcinoma in rats induced by AFB_1 feeding, both c-myc and c-Ha-ras proto-oncogenes were overexpressed (Tashiro et $al.$, 1986a). Such expression was also observed in Kagura-1, the established cell line from AFB_1 induced hepatocarcinoma (Tashiro et $al.$, 1986b). These evidences are expected to give a key to the analysis of the carcinogenic process induced by AFB_1.

It is well established that carcinogenesis and cellular differentiation are closely regulated by glucocorticoids. In order to solve the association between AFB_1 induced gene expression and glucocorticoids, the effect of AFB_1 on the enzyme induction was analyzed with Reuber hepatoma cells, which possess many liver-specific enzymes. Tyrosine aminotransferase (TAT) and others are induced by hydrocortisone, and this induction was inhibited by a small amount of AFB_1. Detailed analysis on glucocorticoid receptors revealed that AFB_1 caused an impairment of the enzyme system which regulates glucocorticoid-receptor levels in the cells (Tashiro et $al.$, 1986c).

AFB_1 is capable of inducing endogenous murine retrovirus in AKR mouse embryo fibroblasts, and inhibition of DNA methylation by AFB_1 and other chemical carcinogens is involved in this process (Rascati and McNeely, 1983). Experiments with Alexander hepatocellular carcinoma cells and HBcAG transfected human cells have also shown that HBcAG expression is partly controlled by methylation (Miller and Robinson, 1983).

Such approaches are expected to present direct evidence for the contribution of AFB_1 and other environmental carcinogens in the etiology of PLC in geographic areas contaminated with these potent carcinogens.

Dietary Factors Influencing the Hepatocarcinogenicity of Aflatoxins

Among numerous fungal metabolites, AFB_1 is the most potent hepatocarcinogen in experimental animals. Detailed evaluation has shown that AFB_1 is carcinogenic in mice, rats, fish, ducks, marmosets, tree shrews and monkeys, by several routes of administration (Wogan, 1977) as summarized in Table 8. Rats are frequently used as an experimental model for AFB_1 carcinogenicity; among several strains, male Fischer rats are the most susceptible, and the liver cancer frequency is dose-dependent in a range of 1–100 μg/kg feed. Oral administration of AFB_1 in a dose of 25 μg/kg body weight 5 days a week for 8 weeks causes a high incidence of liver cancer 42 weeks later. The tumors are more readily produced in males and in the young, and mice are rather resistant to AFB_1.

Biochemical and toxicological approaches to the potent carcinogenicity of AFB_1 have revealed that AFB_1 is metabolized by microsomal and

TABLE 8

Carcinogenicity of Aflatoxin B_1 (Wogan, 1977)

Species	Dose	Duration of observation	Tumor frequency	
Duck	30 μg/kg in diet	14 months	8/11	(72%)
Trout	8 μg/kg in diet	1 year	27/65	(40%)
Tree shrew	24–66 mg total	3 years	9/12	(75%)
Marmoset	5·0 mg total	2 years	2/3	(65%)
Monkey	100–800 mg total	over 2 years	3/42	(7%)
Rat	100 μg/kg in diet	58–88 weeks	28/28	(100%)
Mouse	150 μg/kg in diet	80 weeks	0/60	(0%)

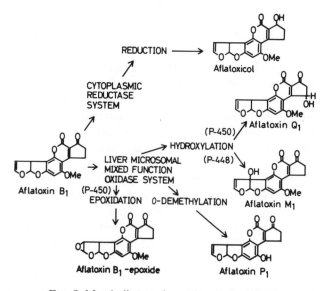

FIG. 9. Metabolic transformation of aflatoxin B_1.

nuclear mixed function monooxygenase systems into an 'active form' (AFB_1 epoxide) which binds with macromolecules such as DNA, RNA and protein. The hydroxylation and demethylation of AFB_1 produce AFM_1 and AFP_1, respectively, and cytosol enzymes catalyze the reduction of AFB_1 to aflatoxicol, as shown in Fig. 9 (Hsieh, 1981; Ueno 1985b). Among these metabolic processes, the epoxidation reaction is considered to be an 'activation reaction', and hydroxylation as well as demethylation are 'detoxication reactions'. Furthermore, water-soluble glucuronides and sulfate conjugates of AFB_1, which are not mutagenic in the Ames test, are excreted into urine of the monkey, rat and mouse (Wei et al., 1985). These activation and detoxication processes of AFB_1 are mediated by the microsomal, nuclear and cytosolic enzyme systems and the cofactors in target cells, and these metabolic potentials are greatly influenced by dietary components and xenobiotics.

An investigation by Novi (1981) demonstrated the regression of AFB_1-induced hepatocellular carcinomas by reduced glutathione (GSH) in rats, and an AFB_1-GSH conjugate was identified as the major biliary metabolite in rats (Degen and Neumann, 1981). In vitro experiments clarified that, among several isozymes of GSH transferases, 1-1 and 1-2 isozymes catalyzed the conjugation of AFB_1 with GSH (Coles et al., 1985).

Resistance to the acute toxicity of AFB_1 has been correlated with the formation of AFB_1-GSH conjugate in rat, mouse and other species (O'Brien et al., 1983).

It has been well established that microsomal and nuclear monooxygenase systems play an important role in the activation of many carcinogens including AFB_1 and polycyclic hydrocarbons, and that the cytochrome P-450 system is regulated by internal and external drug-metabolizing inducers, as evaluated by in vivo carcinogenicity tests and in vitro systems such as the Ames/microsomes test and the DNA-binding assay.

Wattenberg and Lam (1981) reported on the anticarcinogenic properties of β-naphthoflavone (βNF) and vegetables of the cabbage family Cruciferae. These properties have been attributed to the presence of flavones and indoles, which are capable of inducing aryl hydrocarbon hydroxylase. Actually, both cabbage and cauliflower have been shown to depress the toxicity and carcinogenicity of AFB_1 (Boyd et al., 1982). Experiments with rainbow trout have revealed a 50% reduction in AFB_1– DNA binding (Witham et al., 1982) and an 80% reduction in the incidence of hepatomas after βNF treatment (Nixon et al., 1984). A similar experiment showed that 100% incidence of liver cancer was observed in male Fischer rats treated with AFB_1 at a dose of 25 μg × 5/week for 8 weeks after 42 weeks, while a 75% reduction of liver cancer rates was observed in rats fed 0·015% βNF in the diet. A single i.p. injection of βNF in doses of 20 and 150 mg/kg has been shown to result in an increment of AFM_1 excretion 3- and 4-fold higher than the control (Gurtoo et al., 1985). These results are in accord with the suggestion that the induction of cytochrome P-450, which preferentially leads to the formation of AFM_1, may be associated with the inhibition of AFB_1 hepatocarcinogenicity.

Several antioxidants, notably 2(3)-t-butyl-4-hydroxyanisole (BHA) and 3,5-di-t-butyl-4-hydroxytoluene (BHT), are added to foods, cosmetics, drugs and animal feeds to prevent oxygen-induced lipid peroxidation. In some cases, these antioxidants can interact with other environmental compounds to protect against some toxicities. As reviewed by Wattenberg (1985), treatment with the antioxidant food additive BHT inhibits the neoplastic effect of many structurally different chemical carcinogens in rodent tissues. As far as AFB_1 is concerned, treatment with BHT in vivo has induced protection against AFB_1-induced cytotoxicity and covalent binding in primary cultures of rat hepatocytes (Salocks et al., 1981), and another antioxidant, ethoxyquin (EQ), was shown to inhibit the hepato-carcinogenic effect of AFB_1 in rats (Cabral and Neal, 1983).

Detailed experiments have demonstrated that pretreatment of rats with BHT enhances the total *in vitro* metabolism of AFB_1 by the hepatic fraction toward the formation of AFM_1 and decreases the mutagenicity of AFB_1 in the Ames/S-9 test (Fukuyama and Hsieh, 1984). In rats fed diets containing antioxidants such as BHT, BHA, EQ or oltipraz [5-(2-pyrizinyl)-4-methyl-1,2-dithiol-3-thione], the formation of the AFB_1 metabolite–DNA adduct, mainly 8,9-dihydro-8-(N^7-guanyl)-9-hydroxy-AFB_1 (Fig. 10), was substantially reduced in the livers and kidneys. Concordantly, the specific activities of hepatic enzymes such as epoxide hydrase and glucuronyl and glutathione transferases, which are important for the detoxification process of AFB_1 and others, were significantly elevated by all antioxidants (Kensler *et al.*, 1985).

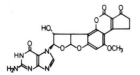

8,9-Dihydro-8-(N^7-guanyl)-
9-hydroxy-aflatoxin B_1
(AFB_1-Gua)

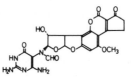

8,9-Dihydro-8-(N^5-formyl-
2',5',6'-triamino-4'-oxo-
N^5-pyrimidyl)-9-hydroxy-
aflatoxin B_1
(AFB_1-triamino-Py)

FIG. 10. Major DNA adducts of aflatoxin B_1.

Dithiothiones are present in cruciferous vegetables such as cabbage, which reduced AFB_1-induced carcinogenesis, as mentioned above (Boyd *et al.*, 1982), and oltipraz is known to protect against CCl_4 hepatotoxicity, as observed with AFB_1. Such approaches are very interesting, and their chemoprotective actions have to be evaluated with special regard to their anticarcinogenic activity.

Another view on AFB_1 metabolism is the promotion of its genotoxicity by environmental toxicants and related reagents. It has been demonstrated that cytochrome P-450s are composed from multi-isozymes, and more than a dozen isozymes of cytochrome P-450s have been fractionated from polychlor biphenyl (PCB)-induced rat microsomes. From their profile on column chromatography and spectral characters, they are subdivided into two groups: type I (maximal CO differential spectra at 450 nm) and type II (at 448 nm). As mentioned earlier, the reconstituted cytochrome system has proven that cytochrome P-450 I-a exhibited a high affinity for the activation (DNA binding) of AFB_1, while cytochrome P-450 II-a possessed a high activity for the formation of AFM_1 (Ueno *et al.*, 1983,1985). This means that various cytochrome P-450 isozymes recognize the structure of AFB_1 and are able to catalyze the epoxidation, hydroxylation and demethylation steps. Such region-selective modification of AFB_1 has also been clarified by estimating a fluorescence energy transfer of the complexes (AFB_1-cytochrome P-450s) (Omata and Ueno, 1985). Another factor which has a great influence on the activation of AFB_1 is cytochrome b_5 (Ueno *et al.*, 1983, 1985).

These basic approaches to the mechanism of AFB_1 activation suggest that the activation of AFB_1 into DNA-binding form(s) and direct-acting mutagen(s) may be mediated by selected cytochrome P-450 among numerous isozymes, and male-type cytochrome P-450 and cytochrome b_5 may initiate the male predominance of PLC.

Furthermore, PLC is greatly influenced by nutritional factors such as dietary fat, vitamins, trace elements and dietary contaminants (N-nitroso compounds, organochlorine pesticides, etc.) (Newberne, 1984).

Multifactoral Etiology of Primary Liver Cancer

As already mentioned, HBV and AFB_1 are considered to be the major etiological causes of liver cell cancer in the areas of prevalence. However, it is still hypothetical as to how these etiologically important agents associate with each other. Harris and Sun (1984) and Sun and Chu (1984) have presented the hypothesis that AFB_1 plays the role of a complete carcinogen and HBV mainly acts as an important promoter. This is consistent with the evidence that PLC only occurs in a small percentage of chronic carriers, most of whom have chronic hepatitis with persistent hepatic hyperplasia. The increase of liver cell turnover in the hyperplastic process followed by hepatic injury, which may be caused by HBV and/or AFB_1 and accelerated by immuno-response modifiers, makes the hepatic cells more sensitive to the carcinogenic effect of AFB_1.

Figure 11 presents a hypothetical schema for the development of PLC. The activation process of AFB_1 mediated by the cytochrome P-450 system is regulated genetically and by dietary factors, and the reactive AFB_1 (AFB_1 epoxide) attacks some promoter/regulation locus of HBV integrated into the host DNA, which leads to the expression of the proto-oncogenic property of HBV. Impairments of the immuno surveillance system by AFB_1 and other mycotoxins such as trichothecenes (see Trichothecenes section), and tumor-promoting agents in dietary foods, may cause the acceleration of tumorigenicity of the hepatic cells.

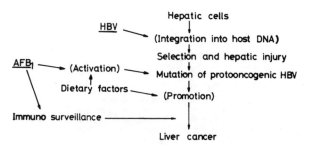

FIG. 11. Multifactoral etiology of primary liver cancer.

Regulation

To protect the public health from hazardous toxicants, food laws in many countries prohibit the sale of any kinds of foods that contain chemicals that may cause injury to humans. Particularly, as far as carcinogenic compounds are concerned, no tolerance level is permitted. Since AFB_1 and related metabolites are one of the potent carcinogens, and there are many possibilities for contamination in food and dairy products (Table 5), many countries have proposed the establishment of tolerance levels in the respective commodities. The details of the limits and regulations on AFB_1, AFM_1 and other related compounds are summarized by Schuller *et al.* (1982, 1983).

OTHER MYCOTOXINS

Sterigmatocystin

Sterigmatocystin (ST) is produced by fungi such as *Aspergillus versicolor*, *A. sydowi*, *A. nidulans*, *Bipolaris* spp., *Chaetomiun* spp. and *Emericella* spp. ST is characterized by a bisdihydrofuran ring fused to a substituted anthraquinone, and the terminal double bond of ST which is important for its mutagenic and carcinogenic activity is similar to AFB_1 (Fig. 12). Terao (1983) has summarized the toxicological and carcinogenic properties of ST.

After the finding that ST was a contaminant in brown rice stored in warehouses under natural conditions (Manabe and Tsuruta, 1975), several reports have cited the presence of ST in cereals and green coffee beans. The Food and Drug Administration of the United States did not detect ST in an analysis of more than 500 samples during 1974–5 (Stoloff, 1976).

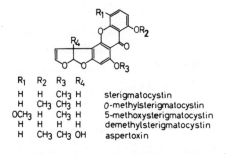

R_1	R_2	R_3	R_4	
H	H	CH₃	H	sterigmatocystin
H	CH₃	CH₃	H	O-methylsterigmatocystin
OCH₃	H	CH₃	H	5-methoxysterigmatocystin
H	H	H	H	demethylsterigmatocystin
H	CH₃	CH₃	OH	aspertoxin

FIG. 12. Sterigmatocystin and related compounds.

Vesonder and Horn (1985) detected 7·75 μg/g of ST in dairy cattle feed associated with acute clinical symptoms of bloody diarrhea and death. It is difficult to evaluate the ST contamination in relation to human disease, although ST possesses potent mutagenic potential both to *Salmonella* (Ueno *et al.*, 1978) and to mammalian cells (Noda *et al.*, 1981).

Patulin and Citrinin

Patulin (Fig. 13) is produced by *Penicillium expansum*, which is pathogenic to apples. After the finding that patulin causes tumors in rats when given by subcutaneous injection, and is mutagenic in bacterial systems (Ueno and Kubota, 1976), the possibility that patulin could occur in foods made from fungal contamination has caused some concern.

The first report on the natural occurrence of patulin in apple juice revealed its presence at the 1 ppm level in commercial samples in Canada (Scott *et al.*, 1972*b*). Kiermeier (1985) has summarized the analytical data from more than 67 reports during 1980–3; out of 356 samples analyzed, 16 apple juice and related products were found to be contaminated with more than 50 ng/kg of patulin.

The established tolerance level of patulin is zero in all foods in Belgium,

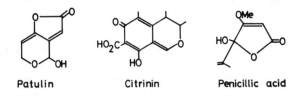

Patulin   Citrinin   Penicillic acid

FIG. 13. Toxic lactones.

and 50 ng/g in apple juice in Norway, Sweden and Switzerland (Schuller *et al.*, 1982, 1983).

Citrinin (Fig. 13) is also one of the toxic lactones produced by several species of fungi. The most important fungus is *Penicillium citrinum*, which was reported as one of the causative fungi of 'yellow rice toxicosis' in Japan (Saito *et al.*, 1971). Citrinin is nephrotoxic, in a similar fashion to OTA (see Ochratoxins section), and has been detected in wheat (Scott *et al.*, 1972*a*), corn flour (Takahashi *et al.*, 1982) and barley (Hald *et al.*, 1983). Long-term feeding experiments have revealed that citrinin alone is not tumorigenic in rats,.but that it synergistically increases the renal tumor induced by a nephrotoxic chemical, N-(3,5-dichlorophenyl)succinimide (DDPS) (Shinohara *et al.*, 1976).

Zearalenone

Zearalenone (ZEN) is a uterotropic mycotoxin produced by *Fusarium graminearum* (*Gibberella zeae* in sexual stage), which often invades barley, wheat, corn and other cereals (see Trichothecenes section) (Fig. 14). Feeds contaminated with significant levels of ZEN induce hyperestrogenism in farm animals. Current surveys in our laboratory have revealed significant contamination of ZEN in barley, wheat and other cereals harvested in Japan, Korea and other countries (Tanaka *et al.*, 1985*a,c,d*; Lee *et al.*, 1985), and this mycotoxin co-exists with NIV and DON, which are also produced by the same fungus *F. graminearum*.

ZEN exhibits uterotropic activity in a similar manner to β-estradiol. Firstly, ZEN binds with the cytosolic estrogen receptor of uterine tissue, followed by translocation to a nuclear receptor and induction of mRNA synthesis (Kawabata *et al.*, 1982). Metabolic studies on ZEN have shown

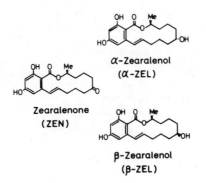

α-Zearalenol
(α-ZEL)

Zearalenone
(ZEN)

β-Zearalenol
(β-ZEL)

FIG. 14. Zearalenone and its metabolites.

that the hepatic ZEN-reductase(s) catalyzes the transformation of ZEN into α- and β-zearalenol (Fig. 14), and the estrogenic activity of α-zearalenol is much higher than the parent ZEN (Ueno and Tashiro, 1981).

Possible transmission of ZEN residues in cereals into foodstuffs and the transformation into more active metabolite(s) are of great concern in evaluating health hazards. Furthermore, agricultural industries are applying this phytoestrogen ZEN as a growth promoter to farm animals. The residues of ZEN and its metabolite in dairy products and edible tissues have to be investigated.

Viomellein

As described in the Ochratoxins section, OTA, a nephrotoxic and naturally occurring mycotoxin, is produced by several fungi such as *Penicillium viridicatum* and *Aspergillus ochraceus*. These fungi are also known as producers of xanthomegnin and viomellein (Fig. 15). Mice fed these mycotoxins for 10 days develop identical lesions, predominantly in the liver, including necrotizing cholangitis, focal hepatic necrosis and hyperplasia of the biliary epithelium, with only minor changes in the kidneys (Carlton *et al.*, 1976). Hald *et al.* (1983) have surveyed these mycotoxins in a barley batch which was associated with field cases of mycotoxic porcine nephropathy. The data revealed the presence of 1 mg/kg of viomellein, along with 1·9 mg/kg of OTA and 0·8 mg/kg of citrinin. These findings indicate the natural co-occurrence of these nephrotoxic and hepatotoxic mycotoxins in barley. Systematic surveys on the natural

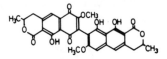

Viomellein

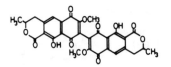

Xanthomegnin

FIG. 15. Viomellein and xanthomegnin.

occurrence of these mycotoxins in foods are required for their evaluation in food toxicology.

Emodin and Related Anthraquinones

As mentioned in the Introduction, hepatotoxic and hepatocarcinogenic mycotoxins such as luteoskyrin and rugulosin (Fig. 16) have been isolated from *Penicillium islandicum* and other fungi which significantly invade imported rice, and these findings led to a proposed rice–fungi–mycotoxins hypothesis in connection with the high incidence rate of PLC in Asia, as reviewed by Saito *et al.* (1971).

However, no extensive surveys of these anthraquinoid mycotoxins have been carried out on imported and domestic rice during the last 20 years,

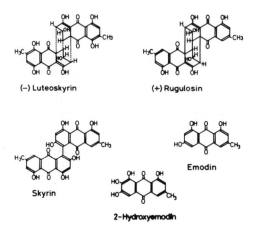

FIG. 16. Anthraquinoid mycotoxins.

and there are no data which indicate the natural occurrence of these mycotoxins, although the author has proposed a sensitive and rapid method for TLC analysis of luteoskyrin in rice (Ueno, 1982).

Particularly, after the finding of AFB_1 and its association with the PLC problem, no detailed studies are reported on these and other mycotoxins, except for biochemical and pathological investigations.

Recently, the author focused attention on emodin (Fig. 16), one of the fungal metabolites and also a constituent of rhubarb, an oriental medicine. This anthraquinone is produced by several *Penicillium* species (Ueno, 1984*b*), and chemically composed of versicolorin A, in which emodin is fused with a bisfuranoid ring. In rhubarb, this compound and related anthraquinones such as chrysophanol and aloe-emodin compose about 1–2% of the total weight.

In the Ames/microsome test, emodin is mutagenic to TA 1537, and is transformed into several hydroxylated metabolites, among which 2-hydroxyemodin (1,2,3,8-tetrahydroxy-6-methylanthraquinone) (Fig. 16) is a direct-acting mutagen (Masuda and Ueno, 1984; Masuda et al., 1985; Tanaka et al., 1987). These findings reveal that emodin, an anthraquinoid metabolite of fungi and plants, is a potent mutagen in the Ames test. Free radicals derived from 2-hydroxyemodin attack DNA, which leads to mutation in bacterial cells (Kodama et al., 1987). Further study is required for the evaluation of the toxicity of emodin and related anthraquinones, which are present in several medicinal plants.

REFERENCES

Allcroft, R. and Carnaghan, R. B. A. (1963). Groundnut toxicity: an examination for toxin in human food products from animals fed toxic groundnut. *Vet. Rec.*, **75**, 259–63.

Alpert, M. E., Hutt, M. S. R., Wogan, G. N. and Davidson, C. S. (1971). Association between aflatoxin content of food and hepatoma frequency in Uganda. *Cancer*, **28**, 253–60.

Anukarahanonta, T. (1983). High performance liquid chromatography of aflatoxins in human urine. *J. Chromatog.*, **276**, 387–93.

Asao, T., Büchi, G., Abdel-kader, M. M., Chang, S. B., Wick, E. L. and Wogan, G. N. (1965). Structures of aflatoxin B_1 and G_1. *J. Am. Chem. Soc.*, **87**, 882–6.

Association of Official Analytical Chemists (1981). *Official Methods of Analysis*, Ch. 26, Natural Poisons, AOAC, Arlington, Virginia.

Autrup, H., Bradley, A., Shamsuddin, A. K. M., Wakhisi, J. and Wasunna, A. (1983). Detection of putative adduct with fluorescence characteristics identical to 2,3-dihydro-2-(7'→guanyl)-3-hydroxyaflatoxin B_1 in human urine collected in Murang's district, Kenya. *Carcinogenesis*, **4**, 1193–5.

Bamburg, J. R. and Strong, F. M. (1971). 12,13-Epoxytrichothecenes. In: *Microbial Toxins*, Vol. 7, Algal and Fungal Toxins, S. Kadis and A. S. J. Ciegler (Eds), Academic Press, New York, pp. 207–92.

Blaas, W., Kellert, M., Steinmeyer, S., Tiebach, R. and Weber, R. (1984). Untersuchung von Cerealien auf Deoxynivalenol und Nivalenol im unteren μg/kg Bereich. *Z. Lebensm. Unters. Forsch.*, **179**, 104–8.

Booth, C. (1971). *The Genus Fusarium*, Commonwealth Mycological Institute, Kew, London.

Boyd, J. N., Babish, J. G. and Stoewsand, G. S. (1982). Modification by beet and cabbage diets of aflatoxin B_1-induced rat plasma α-fetoprotein elevation, hepatic tumorigenesis and mutagenicity of urine. *Food Chem. Toxicol.*, **20**, 47–52.

Brown, M. N., Szczech, G. M. and Purmalis, B. P. (1976). Teratogenic and toxic effects of ochratoxin A in rats. *Toxicol. Appl. Pharmacol.*, **37**, 331–8.

Brumley, W. C., Nesheim, S., Trucksess, M. W., Trucksess, E. W., Dreifuss, P. A., Roach, J. A. G., Andrzejewski, D., Eppley, R. M., Pohland, A. E., Thorpe, C. W. and Sphon, J. A. (1981). Negative ion chemical ionization mass spectrometry of aflatoxins and related mycotoxins. *Anal. Chem.*, **53**, 2003–6.

Brumley, W. C., Trucksess, M. W., Adler, S. H., Cohen, C. K., White, K. D. and Sphon, J. A. (1985). Negative ion chemical ionization mass spectrometry of deoxynivalenol (DON): application to identification of DON in grains and snack foods after quantitation/isolation by thin layer chromatography. *J. Agric. Food Chem.*, **33**, 326–30.

Buchmann, N. B. and Hald, B. (1985). Analysis, occurrence and control of ochratoxin A residues in Danish pig kidneys. *Food Add. Contam.*, **2**, 193–9.

Bulatao-Jayme, J., Almero, E. M., Castro, M. C. A., Jardeleza, M. T. R. and Salamat, L. S. (1982). A case-control dietary study of primary liver cancer risk from aflatoxin exposure. *Int. Epidemiol.*, **11**, 112–9.

Cabral, J. R. P. and Neal, G. E. (1983). The inhibitory effects of ethoxyquin on the carcinogenic action of aflatoxin B_1 in rats. *Cancer Lett.*, **19**, 125–32.

Campbell, T. C. and Salamat, L. (1971). Aflatoxin ingestion and excretion by humans. In: *Symposium on Mycotoxins in Human Health*, I. F. H. Purchase (Ed.), Elsevier, Amsterdam, pp. 271–80.

Campbell, T. C., Sinnhuber, R. C., Lee, D. J., Wales, J. H. and Salamat, L. (1974). Hepatocarcinogenic material in urine specimens from humans consuming aflatoxin. *J. Nat. Cancer Inst.*, **52**, 1647–9.

Carlton, W. W., Stack, M. E. and Eppley, R. M. (1976). Hepatic alterations produced in mice by xanthomegnin and viomellein, metabolites of *Penicillium viridicatum*. *Toxicol. Appl. Pharmacol.*, **38**, 455–9.

Ceovic, S., Crims, P. and Mitar, T. (1976). The incidence of tumors of the urinary organs in the region of endemic nephropathy and in control region. *Lijecnicki Vjesnik*, **98**, 301–4.

Chambon, P., Dano, S. D., Chambon, R. and Geahchan, A. (1983). Rapid determination of aflatoxin M_1 in milk and dairy products by high performance liquid chromatography. *J. Chromatog.*, **259**, 372–4.

Chang, F. C. and Chu, F. S. (1977). The fate of ochratoxin A in rats. *Food Cosmet. Toxicol.*, **15**, 199–204.

Chernozemsky, I. N., Stoyanov, I. S., Petkova-Bocharova, T., Nicolov, I. G., Draganov, I. V., Stoichev, I. I., Tanchev, Y., Naidenov, D. and Kalcheva, N. (1977). Geographic correlation between the occurrence of endemic nephropathy and urinary tumors in Vratza district, Bulgaria. *Int. J. Cancer*, **19**, 1–11.

Chiba, J., Kajii, H., Kawamura, M., Ohi, K., Morooka, N. and Ueno, Y. (1985). Production for monoclonal antibodies reactive with ochratoxin A: enzyme-linked immunosorbent assay for detection of ochratoxin A. *Proc. Jap. Assoc. Mycotoxicol.*, **21**, 289 (in Japanese).

Choudhury, H., Carlson, C. W. and Semeniuk, G. (1971). Ochratoxin toxicity in hens. *Poultry Sci.*, **50**, 1855–9.

Chu, F. S. (1984). Immunochemical studies on mycotoxins. In: *Toxigenic Fungi: Their Toxins and Health Hazard*, H. Kurata and Y. Ueno (Eds), Elsevier, Amsterdam, pp. 234–44.

Chu, F. S. and Ueno, I. (1977). Production of antibody against aflatoxin B_1. *Appl. Environ. Microbiol.*, **33**, 1125–8.

Chu, F. S., Grossman, S., Wei, D. R. and Mirocha, C. J. (1979). Production of antibody against T-2 toxin. *Appl. Environ. Microbiol.*, **37**, 104–8.

Coles, B., Meyer, D. J., Ketterer, B., Stanton, C. A. and Garner, R. C. (1985). Studies on the detoxication of microsomally activated aflatoxin B_1 by glutathione and glutathione transferases *in vitro*. *Carcinogenesis*, **6**, 693–7.

Côté, L. M., Reynolds, J. D., Vesonder, R. F., Buck, W. B., Swanson, S. P., Coffey, R. T. and Brown, D. C. (1984). Survey of vomitoxin-contaminated feed grains in midwestern United States and associated health problems in swine. *J. Am. Vet. Med. Assoc.*, **184**, 189–92.

Creppy, E. E., Schlegel, M., Röschenthaler, R. and Dirheimer, G. (1980). Phenylalanine prevents acute poisoning by ochratoxin A in mice. *Toxicol. Lett.*, **6**, 77–80.

Creppy, E. E., Størmer, F. C., Röschenthaler, R. and Dirheimer, G. (1983*a*). Effects of two metabolites of ochratoxin A, (4R)-4-hydroxyochratoxin A and ochratoxin α, on immune response in mice. *Infec. Immun.*, **39**, 1015–8.

Creppy, E. E., Størmer, F. C., Kern, D., Röschenthaler, R. and Dirheimer, G. (1983*b*). Effects of ochratoxin A metabolites on yeast phenylalanyl-tRNA synthetase and on the growth and *in vivo* protein synthesis of hepatoma cells. *Chem. Biol. Interact.*, **47**, 239–47.

Creppy, E. E., Nern, D., Steyn, P. S., Vleggaar, R., Röschenthaler, R. and Dirheimer, G. (1983*c*). Comparative study of the effect of ochratoxin A analogues on yeast aminoacyl-tRNA synthetases and on the growth and protein synthesis of hepatoma cells. *Toxicol. Lett.*, **19**, 217–24.

Creppy, E. E., Röschenthaler, R. and Dirheimer, G. (1984). Inhibition of protein synthesis in mice by ochratoxin A and its prevention by phenylalanine. *Food Chem. Toxicol.*, **22**, 883–6.

Croft, W. A., Jarvis, B. B. and Yatamara, C. S. (1986). Airborne outbreak of trichothecene toxicosis. *Atmos. Environ.*, **20**, 549–52.

Degen, G. H. and Neumann, H. G. (1981). Differences in aflatoxin B_1 susceptibility of rat and mouse are correlated with the capability *in vitro* to inactivate aflatoxin B_1 epoxide. *Carcinogenesis*, **12**, 299–306.

Egan, H., Stoloff, L., Castegnaro, M., Scott, P., O'Neil, I. K. and Bartsch, H. (1982). *Environmental Carcinogens: Selected Methods of Analysis*, IARC Scientific Publications, No. 44, IARC, Lyon.

El-Banna, A. A., Lau, P.-Y. and Scott, P. M. (1983). Fate of mycotoxins during processing of foodstuffs. II. Deoxynivalenol (vomitoxin) during making of Egyptian bread. *J. Food Protection*, **46**, 484–6.

El-Nakib, O., Pestka, J. J. and Chu, F. S. (1981). Analysis of aflatoxin B_1 in corn, wheat and peanut butter by an enzyme-linked immunosorbent assay and a solid-phase radioimmunoassay. *J. Assoc. Off. Anal. Chem.*, **64**, 1077–82.

Emerole, G. O., Uwaifo, A. O., Thabrew, M. I. and Bababunmi, E. A. (1982). The presence of aflatoxin and some polycyclic aromatic hydrocarbons in human foods. *Cancer Lett.*, **15**, 123–9.

Endou, H., Obara, T. and Ueno, Y. (1984). Use of isolated nephron segments and isolated renal cells for the evaluation of nephrotoxicity. *Second Int. Symp. Nephrotoxicity* (Univ. Surrey, Guildford, England), August 9, pp. 535–8.

Enwonwu, C. O. (1984). The role of dietary aflatoxin in the genesis of hepatocellular cancer in developing countries. *Lancet*, October 27, 956–7.

Eppley, R. M. and Bailey, W. J. (1973). 12,13-Epoxy-delta-trichothecenes as the probable mycotoxins responsible for stachybotryotoxicosis. *Science*, **181**, 758–60.

Eppley, R. M., Trucksess, M. W., Nesheim, S., Thrope, C. W., Wood, G. E. and Pohland, A. E. (1984). Deoxynivalenol in winter wheat; thin layer chromatographic method and survey. *J. Assoc. Off. Anal. Chem.*, **67**, 43–5.

Forgacs, E. E. and Carll, W. T. (1962). Mycotoxicoses. *Adv. Vet. Sci.*, **7**, 273–382.

Fremy, J. M. and Quillardet, P. (1985). The carry-over of aflatoxin into milk of cows fed ammoniated rations: use of an HPLC method and a genotoxicity test for determining milk safety. *Food Add. Contam.*, **2**, 201–7.

Fukuyama, M. Y. and Hsieh, D. P. H. (1984). The effects of butylated hydroxytoluene on the *in vitro* metabolism, DNA-binding and mutagenicity of aflatoxin-B_1 in the rat. *Food Chem. Toxicol.*, **22**(5), 355–60.

Galtier, P., Boneu, B., Charpenteau, J. L. and Bodin, G. (1979). Physiopathology of haemorrhagic syndrome related to ochratoxin A intoxication in rats. *Food Cosmet. Toxicol.*, **17**, 49–53.

Garner, C., Ryder, R. and Montesano, R. (1985). Monitoring of aflatoxins in human body fluids and an application to field studies. *Cancer Res.*, **45**, 922–8.

Gilbert, J., Shepherd, M. J. and Howell, M. V. (1983a). Studies on the fate of trichothecene mycotoxins during food processing. In: *Proc. Eur. Food Chem. II* (Rome/Italy), March 15–18, pp. 253–62.

Gilbert, J., Shepherd, M. J. and Startin, J. R. (1983b). A survey of the occurrence of the trichothecene mycotoxin deoxynivalenol (vomitoxin) in UK grown and in imported maize by combined gas chromatography–mass spectrometry. *J. Sci. Food Agric.*, **34**, 86–92.

Goldblatt, L. A. (Ed.) (1969). Aflatoxin: scientific background, control, and implications. In: *Food Science and Technology*, Academic Press, New York.

Goldblatt, L. A. and Dollear, F. G. (1977). Detoxication of contaminated crops. In: *Mycotoxins in Human and Animal Health*, J. V. Rodricks, C. W. Hesseltine and M. A. Mehlman (Eds), Pathotox Publ., Park Forest South, Illinois, pp. 139–50.

Golinski, P., Hult, K., Grabarkiewicz-Szczesna, J., Chelkowski, J. and Szebiotko, K. (1985). Spontaneous occurrence of ochratoxin A residues in porcine kidney and serum samples in Poland. *Appl. Environ. Microbiol.*, **49**, 1014–5.

Greenhalgh, R., Gilbert, J., King, R. R., Blackwell, B. A., Startin, J. R. and Shepherd, M. J. (1984). Synthesis, characterization and occurrence in bread and cereal products of an isomer of 4-deoxynivalenol (vomitoxin), *J. Agric. Food Chem.*, **32**, 1416–20.

Groopman, J. D., Donahue, P. R., Zhu, J., Chen, J. and Wogan, G. L. (1985). Aflatoxin metabolism in humans: detection of metabolites and nucleic acid adducts in urine by affinity chromatography. *Proc. Nat. Acad. Sci.*, **82**, 6492–6.

Grove, M. D., Plattner, R. D. and Peterson, R. E. (1984). Detection of aflatoxin D in ammoniated corn by mass spectrometry–mass spectrometry. *Appl. Environ. Microbiol.*, **48**, 887–9.

Gurtoo, H. L., Koser, P. L., Bansal, S. K., Fox, H. W., Sharma, S. D., Mulhern, A. I. and Pavelic, Z. P. (1985). Inhibition of aflatoxin B_1 hepatocarcinogenesis in rats by β-naphthoflavone. *Carcinogenesis*, **6**(5), 657–78.

Haddon, W. F., Masri, M. S., Randall, V. G., Elsken, R. H. and Meneghelli, B. J. (1977). Mass spectral confirmation of aflatoxins, *J. Assoc. Off. Anal. Chem.*, **60**, 107–13.

Hald, B. and Krogh, P. (1975). Protection of ochratoxin A in barley, using silica gel minicolumns. *J. Assoc. Off. Anal. Chem.*, **58**, 156–8.

Hald, B., Christensen, D. H. and Krogh, P. (1983). Natural occurrence of the mycotoxin viomellein in barley and the associated quinone-producing *Penicillium*. *Appl. Environ. Microbiol.*, **46**, 1311–7.

Harris, C. C. and Sun, T. (1984). Multifactoral etiology of human liver cancer. *Carcinogenesis*, **5**, 697–701.

Hart, L. P. and Braselton, Jr., W. E. (1983). Distribution of vomitoxin in dry milled fractions of wheat infected with *Gibberella zeae*. *J. Agric. Food Chem.*, **31**, 657–9.

Hintikka, E.-L. (née Korpinen) (1977). The Genus *Stachybotrys*. In: *Mycotoxic Fungi, Mycotoxins, Mycotoxicoses*, Vol. I, *Mycotoxic Fungi and Chemistry of Mycotoxins*, T. D. Wyllie and L. G. Morehouse (Eds), Marcel Dekker, New York/Basel, pp. 91–8.

Howell, M. V. and Tayler, P. W. (1981). Determination of aflatoxins, ochratoxin A, and zearalenone in mixed feeds with detection by thin layer chromatography or high performance liquid chromatography. *J. Assoc. Off. Anal. Chem.*, **64**, 1356–63.

Hsieh, D. P. H. (1981). Mycotoxins: metabolism and transmission, *Proc. Int. Workshop and Symp. on Mycotoxins*, 6–16 September, Cairo.

Hsieh, D. P. H., and Ruebner, B. H. (1984). An assessment of cancer risk from aflatoxin B_1 and M_1. In: *Toxigenic Fungi: Their Toxins and Health Hazard*, H. Kurata and Y. Ueno (Eds), Elsevier, Amsterdam, pp. 332–8.

Hu, H. J., Hoychich, N. and Chu, F. S. (1983). Enzyme-linked immunosorbent assay of picogram quantities of aflatoxin M_1 in urine and milk. *J. Food Prot.*, **47**, 126–7.

Hult, K., Teiling, A. and Gatenbeck, S. (1976). Degradation of ochratoxin A by a ruminant. *Appl. Environ. Microbiol.*, **32**(3), 443–4.

Hult, K., Hokby, E., Gatenbeck, S. and Rutqvist, L. (1980). Ochratoxin A in blood from slaughter pigs in Sweden: use in evaluation of toxin content of consumed feed. *Appl. Environ. Microbiol.*, **39**(4), 828–30.

Hult, K., Plestina, R., Habazin-Novak, V., Radic, B. and Geovic, S. (1982). Ochratoxin A in human blood and Balkan endemic nephropathy. *Arch. Toxicol.*, **51**, 313–21.

Hutchison, R. D., Steyn, P. S. and Thompson, D. L. (1971). The isolation and structure of 4-hydroxyochratoxin A and 7-carboxy-3,4-dihydro-8-hydroxy-3-methylisocoumarin from *Penicillium viridicatum*. *Tetrahedron Lett.*, No. 43, 4033–6.

Ichinoe, M., Kurata, H., Sugiura, Y. and Ueno, Y. (1983). Chemotaxonomy of *Gibberella zeae* with special reference to production of trichothecenes and zearalenone. *Appl. Environ. Microbiol.*, **46**, 1364–9.

International Union against Cancer (1982). Hepatocellular carcinoma. In: *Workshops on the Biology of Human Cancer*, report No. 17, Geneva.

Itakura, H. (1982–3). Etiology of human primary hepatocellular carcinoma: is primary hepatocellular carcinoma caused by hepatitis viruses or mycotoxins? *J. Toxicol.: Toxin Rev.*, **1**, 309–16.

Jarvis, B. B. (1984). Trichothecene mycotoxins from the higher plant *Baccharis megapotamica*. In: *Toxigenic Fungi: Their Toxins and Health Hazard*, H. Kurata and Y. Ueno (Eds), Elsevier, Amsterdam, pp. 312–21.

Jones, B. D. (1957). *Proc. Conf. Animal Feeds of Tropical and Subtropical Origin*, Tropical Products Institute, London, pp. 273–90.

Jones, B. D. (1977*a*). Chemistry. In: *Mycotoxic Fungi, Mycotoxins, Mycotoxicoses* ed. by T. D. Wyllie and L. G. Morehouse, Marcell Dekker, New York, pp. 136–143.

Jones, B. D. (1977*b*). Occurrence in foods and feeds. In: *Mycotoxic Fungi, Mycotoxins, Mycotoxicoses*, Vol. I, Mycotoxic Fungi and Chemistry of Mycotoxins, T. D. Wyllie and L. G. Morehouse (Eds), Marcel Dekker, New York, pp. 190–237.

Jones, B. D. (1981). The occurrence of aflatoxins in edible nuts: sampling and analysis. 1st. Italian Meeting on Food Contaminations by Mycotoxins, Bologna, 3–4 September.

Kanisawa, M. and Suzuki, S. (1978). Induction of renal and hepatic carcinogenesis in mice by ochratoxin A, a mycotoxin. *Gann*, **69**, 599–600.

Karki, T. B., Bothast, R. J. and Stubblefield, L. (1979). Note on microbiological and aflatoxin analysis of cereal grains from the Tarai plain of southern Nepal. *Cereal Chem.*, **42**, 41–2.

Kawabata, Y., Tashiro, F. and Ueno, Y. (1982). Synthesis of a specific protein induced by zearalenone and its derivatives in rat uterus. *J. Biochem.* (Tokyo), **91**, 801–8.

Kensler, T. W., Egner, P. A., Trush, M. A., Bueding, E. and Groopman, J. D. (1985). Modification of aflatoxin B1 binding to DNA *in vivo* in rats fed phenolic antioxidants, ethoxyquin and dithiothione. *Carcinogenesis*, **6**(5), 759–63.

Kew, M. C. (1981). Clinical, pathological, and etiologic heterogeneity in hepatocellular carcinoma: evidence from South Africa. *Hepatology*, **1**(4), 366–9.

Kew, M. C., Rossouw, E., Hodgingson, J., Paterson, A., Dusheiko, G. M. and Whitcutt, J. M. (1983). Hepatitis B virus status of South African blacks with hepatocellular carcinoma: comparison between rural and urban patients. *Hepatology*, **3**, 65–8.

Kiermeier, F. (1985). Das Mykotoxin-Problem: Ergebnisse der Lebensmittel überwachung. *Z. Lebensm. Unters. Forsch.*, **180**, 389–93.

Kiermeier, F. and Mashalev, R. (1977). Einfluss der molkerei-technischen Behandlung der Rohmilk auf den Aflatoxin-M1-Gehalt der daraus hergestellten Produkte. *Z. Lebensm. Unters. Forsch.*, **164**, 183–7.

Kodama, M., Kamioka, Y., Nakayama, T., Nagata, C., Morooka, N. and Ueno, Y. (1987). Generation of free radicals and hydrogen peroxide from 2-hydroxyemodin, a direct-acting mutagen and DNA strand breaks by active oxygen. *Toxicol. Lett.*, in press.

Krishnamachari, K. A. V. R., Bhat, R. V., Nagarajan, V. and Tilak, T. B. (1975). Hepatitis due to aflatoxicosis: an outbreak in western India. *Lancet*, May 10, 1061–3.

Krogh, P. (1983). Diagnostic criteria for ochratoxin-induced nephropathy. In: *Current Research in Endemic (Balkan) Nephropathy*, S. Strahinjic and V. Stefanovic (Eds), Proc. 5th. Symp. on Endemic (Balkan) Nephropathy, NIS, pp. 11–4.

Krogh, P. (1977). Ochratoxins. In: *Mycotoxins in Human and Animal Health*, J. V. Rodricks, C. W. Hesseltine and M. A. Mehlman (Eds), Pathotox Publ., Park Forest South, Illinois, pp. 489–98.

Lafont, P. and Lafont, J. (1970). Contamination de produits cerealiers et d'aliments du betail par l'aflatoxine. *Food Cosmet. Toxicol.*, **8**, 403–8.

Lampiugh, S. M. and Hendrickse, T. (1983). Aflatoxins and Kwashiokor. *La Africa-Health*, **5**, 20–2.

Lee, U. S., Jang, H. S., Tanaka, T., Hasegawa, A., Oh, Y. J. and Ueno, Y. (1985). The coexistence of the *Fusarium* mycotoxins nivalenol, deoxynivalenol, and zearalenone in Korean cereals harvested in 1983. *Food Add. Contam.*, **2**, 185–92.

Lee, U.-S., Jang, H. S., Tanaka, T., Hasegawa, A., Oh, Y. J., Cho, C. M., Suguira, Y. and Ueno, Y. (1986). Further survey of the *Fusarium* mycotoxins in Korean cereals. *Food Add. Contam.*, **3**, 253–61.

Leistner, L. (1984). Toxigenic *Penicillia* occurring in feeds and foods. In: *Toxigenic Fungi: Their Toxins and Health Hazard*, H. Kurata and Y. Ueno (Eds), Elsevier, Amsterdam, pp. 162–71.

Levi, C. P., Trenk, H. L. and Mohr, H. K. (1974). Study of the occurrence of ochratoxin A in green coffee beans. *J. Assoc. Off. Anal. Chem.*, **57**, 866–70.

Linsell, A. (1984). Primary liver cancer: global epidemiology and main etiological factors. *Ann. Acad. Med.*, **13**(2), 185–9.

Liu, X. (1985). Studies on aflatoxin contamination in foods in China. *Proc. FAO/ UNEP/USSR Mycotoxin Workshop*, Elevan, June.

Macnab, G. M., Alexander, J. J., Lecatsas, G., Bey, E. M. and Urbanowicz, J. M. (1976). Hepatitis B surface antigen produced by a human cell line. *Brit. J. Cancer*, **34**, 509–15.

Manabe, M. and Tsuruta, O. (1975). Mycological damage of domestic brown rice during storage in warehouse under natural conditions. *Trans. Mycol. Soc. Japan*, **16**, 399 (in Japanese).

Marasas, W. F. O., Kriek, N. P. J., van Rosenburg, S. J., Steyn, M. and van Schalkwyk, G. C. (1977). Occurrence of zearalenone and deoxynivalenol, mycotoxins produced by *Fusarium graminearum* Schwabe in maize in southern Africa. *South Afr. Sci.*, **73**, 346–9.

Marasas, W. F. O., Nelson, P. E. and Toussoun, T. A. (Eds) (1984). *Toxigenic Fusarium Species*, Pennsylvania State University Press.

Martin, C. N., Gamer, R. C., Yursi, F., Gamer, J. V., Whittle, H. C., Ryder, R. W., Sizaret, P. and Montesano, R. (1985). An ELISA procedure for assaying aflatoxin B_1. In: *Monitoring Human Exposure to Carcinogenic and Mutagenic Agents*, A. Berlin, M. Draper, K. Hemmirki and H. Vauinio (Eds), IARC Scientific Publications, No. 59, International Agency for Research on Cancer, Lyon.

Masuda, T. and Ueno, Y. (1984). Microsomal transformation of emodin into a direct mutagen. *Mutat. Res.*, **125**, 135–44.

Masuda, T., Haraikawa, K., Morooka, N., Nakano, S. and Ueno, Y. (1985). 2-Hydroxyemodin, an active metabolite of emodin in the hepatic microsomes of rats. *Mutat. Res.*, **149**, 327–32.

Meisner, H. and Selenik, P. (1979). Inhibition of renal gluconeogenesis in rats by ochratoxin. *Biochem. J.*, **180**, 681–4.

Meisner, H., Cimbala, M. A. and Hanson, R. W. (1983). Decrease of renal phosphoenolpyruvate carboxykinase RNA and poly(A)$^+$ RNA level by ochratoxin A. *Arch. Biochem. Biophys.*, **223**, 264–70.

Miller, R. H. and Robinson, W. S. (1983). Integrated hepatitis B virus DNA sequences specifying the major viral core polypeptide are methylated in PLC/

PRF/5 cells. *Proc. Nat. Acad. Sci.*, **80**, 2534–6.

Moroi, K., Suzuki, S., Kuga, T., Yamazaki, M. and Kanisawa, M. (1985). Reduction of ochratoxin A toxicity in mice treated with phenylalanine and phenobarbital. *Toxicol. Lett.*, **25**, 1–5.

Munro, I. C. (1976). Naturally occurring toxicants in foods and their significance. *Clin. Toxicol.*, **9**, 647–63.

Nesheim, S., Hardin, N. F., Francis, O. J., Jr. and Langham, W. S. (1973). Analysis of ochratoxins A and B and their esters in barley, using partition and thin layer chromatography. I. Development of the method. *J. Assoc. Off. Anal. Chem.*, **56**, 819–21.

Newberne, P. M. (1984). Chemical carcinogenesis: mycotoxins and other chemicals to which humans are exposed. *Seminars Liver Dis.*, **4**(2), 122–35.

Ngindu, A., Johnson, B., Kenya, P. R., Ngira, J. A., Oscheng, D. M., Nandwa, H., Omondi, T. N., Jansen, A. J., Ngare, W., Kaviti, J. N., Gatei, D. and Sinogok, T. A. (1982). Outbreak of acute hepatitis caused by aflatoxin poisoning in Kenya. *Lancet*, June 12, 1346–84.

Nixon, J. E., Hendricks, J. D., Pawlowski, N. E., Pereira, V. B., Sinnhuber, R. O. and Bailey, G. S. (1984). Inhibition of aflatoxin B_1 carcinogenesis in rainbow trout by flavone and indole compounds. *Carcinogenesis*, **5**, 615–9.

Noda, K., Umeda, M. and Ueno, Y. (1981). Cytotoxic and mutagenic effects of sterigmatocystin in cultured Chinese hamster cells. *Carcinogenesis*, **2**, 945–9.

Novi, A. N. (1981). Regression of aflatoxin B_1-induced hepatocellular carcinomas by reduced glutathione. *Science*, **212**, 541–2.

Obara, T., Masuda, E., Takemodo, T. and Tatsuno, T. (1984). Immuno-suppressive effect of a trichothecene mycotoxin, fusarenon X. In: *Toxigenic Fungi: Their Toxins and Health Hazard*, H. Kurata and Y. Ueno (Eds), Elsevier, Amsterdam, pp. 301–11.

O'Brien, K., Moss, E., Judah, D. and Neal, G. (1983). Metabolic basis of the species difference to aflatoxin B_1 induced hepatotoxicity. *Biochem. Biophys. Res. Commun.*, **114**, 813–21.

Ohtani, K., Kawamura, O., Kajii, H., Chiba, J. and Ueno, Y. (1985). Development of enzyme-linked immunosorbent assay (ELISA) for T-2 toxin using monoclonal antibodies. *Proc. Jap. Assoc. Mycotoxicol.*, **22**, 31–2.

Omata, Y. and Ueno, Y. (1985). Fluorescence energy transfer measurements of the complexes of aflatoxin B_1 and cytochrome P-450. *Biochem. Biophys. Res. Commun.*, **129**, 493–8.

Oyeniran, J. O. (1973). *Rep. Nigerian Stored Product Res. Inst.*, p. 47.

Patterson, D. S. P. and Roberts, B. A. (1979). Mycotoxins in animal feedstuffs: sensitive thin layer chromatographic detection of aflatoxin, ochratoxin A, sterigmatocystin, zearalenone, and T-2 toxin. *J. Assoc. Off. Anal. Chem.*, **62**, 1265–7.

Pestka, J. J., Gaur, P. K. and Chu, F. S. (1980). Quantitation of aflatoxin B_1 and aflatoxin B_1 antibody by an enzyme-linked immunosorbent microassay. *Appl. Environ. Microbiol.*, **40**, 1027–31.

Pestka, J. J., Li, Y., Harder, W. O. and Chu, F. S. (1981*a*). Comparison of radioimmunoassay and enzyme-linked immunosorbent assay for determining aflatoxin M_1 in milk. *J. Assoc. Off. Anal. Chem.*, **64**, 294–301.

Pestka, J. J., Steinert, B. W. and Chu, F. S. (1981*b*). Enzyme-linked immunosorbent assay for detection of ochratoxin A. *Appl. Environ. Microbiol.*, **41**, 1472–4.

Peters, H., Dietrich, M. P. and Dose, L. (1982). Enzyme-linked immunosorbent assay for detection of T-2 toxin. *Hoppe-Seyler's Z. Physiol. Chem.*, **363**, 1437–41.

Petkova-Bocharova, T. and Castegnaro, M. (1985). Ochratoxin A contamination of cereals in an area of high incidence of Balkan endemic nephropathy in Bulgaria. *Food Add. Contam.*, **2**, 267–70.

Pettersson, H., Göransson, B., Kiessling, K. H., Tideman, K. and Johansson, T. (1978). Aflatoxin in a Swedish sample. *Nord. Vet. Med.*, **30**, 482–5.

Phillips, T. D., Stein, A. F., Ivie, G. W., Kubena, L. F., Hayes, A. W. and Heidelbaugh, N. D. (1983). High pressure liquid chromatographic determination of an O-methyl, methyl ester derivative of ochratoxin A. *J. Assoc. Off. Anal. Chem.*, **66**, 570–6.

Plattner, R. D., Bennett, G. A. and Stubblefield, R. D. (1984). Identification of aflatoxins by quadrupole mass spectrometry/mass spectrometry. *J. Assoc. Off. Anal. Chem.*, **67**, 734–8.

Pons, W. A. (1976). Resolution of aflatoxins B_1, B_2, G_1, and G_2 by high-pressure liquid chromatography. *J. Assoc. Off. Anal. Chem.*, **59**, 101–5.

Pons, W. A. and Franz, A. O. (1977). High performance liquid chromatography of aflatoxins in cottonseed products. *J. Assoc. Off. Anal. Chem.*, **60**, 89–96.

Prior, M. G. (1981). Ochratoxin A in animal feeds. *Can. J. Comp. Med.*, **45**, 116–9.

Rao, E. R., Basappa, S. C. and Murthy, V. S. (1979). Studies on the occurrence of ochratoxins in foodgrains. *J. Food Sci. Technol.*, **16**(3), 113–4.

Rascati, R. J. and McNeely, M. (1983). Induction of retrovirus gene expression by aflatoxin B_1 and 2-acetylaminofluorene. *Mutat. Res.*, **122**, 235–41.

Röschenthaler, R., Creppy, E. E., Dreismann, D. and Dirheimer, G. (1984). Ochratoxin A: on the mechanism of action. In: *Toxigenic Fungi: Their Toxins and Health Hazard*, H. Kurata and Y. Ueno (Eds), Elsevier, Amsterdam, pp. 255–64.

Rosen, R. T. and Rosen, J. D. (1984). Quantification and confirmation of four *Fusarium* mycotoxins in corn by gas chromatography/mass spectrometry/selected ion monitoring. *J. Chromatog.*, **283**, 223–30.

Rousseau, D. M., Slegers, G. A. and van Peteghem, C. H. (1985). Radio-immunoassay of ochratoxin A in barley. *Appl. Environ. Microbiol.*, **50**, 529–31.

Ryu, J.-C., Shiraki, N. and Ueno, Y. (1987). Effects of drugs and metabolic inhibitors on the acute toxicity of T-2 toxin in mice. *Toxicon*, in press.

Saito, M., Enomoto, M., Tatsuno, T. and Uraguchi, K. (1971). Yellowed rice toxins: luteoskyrin and related compounds, chlorine-containing compounds, citrinin, and citreoviridin. In: *Microbial Toxins*, Vol. VI, *Fungal Toxins*, A. Ciegler, S. Kadis and S. J. Ajl (Eds), Academic Press, New York, pp. 299–380.

Saito, K., Nishijima, M., Yasuda, K., Kamimura, H., Ibe, A., Nagayama, T., Ushijima, H. and Naoi, Y. (1979). Investigation of the natural occurrence of aflatoxins in beans used as a raw material for bean-jam ('An') and the effect of processing on their contents in 'An'. *J. Food Hyg. Soc. Jap.*, **20**, 358–62 (in Japanese).

Saito, K., Nishijima, M., Yasuda, K., Kamimura, H., Ibe, A., Nagayama, T., Ushiyama, H. and Naoi, Y. (1984). Investigation of the natural occurrence of aflatoxins and aflatoxicols in commercial pistachio nuts, corns and corn flours. *J.*

Food Hyg. Soc. Jap., **25**, 241–5 (in Japanese).

Salocks, C. B., Hsieh, D. P. H. and Byard, J. L. (1981). Butylated hydroxytoluene pretreatment protects against cytotoxicity and reduces covalent binding of aflatoxin B_1 in primary hepatocyte cultures. *Toxicol. Appl. Pharmacol.*, **59**, 331–45.

Sargent, K., Sheridan, A., O'Kelly, J. and Carnaghan, R. B. A. (1961). Toxicity associated with certain samples of groundnuts. *Nature*, **192**, 1096.

Schroeder, T., Zweifel, U., Sagelsdorff, P., Friederich, U., Luthy, J. and Schalatter, C. (1985). Ammoniation of aflatoxin-containing corn: distribution, *in vivo* covalent deoxyribonucleic acid binding, and mutagenicity of reaction products. *J. Agric. Food Chem.*, **33**, 311–6.

Schuller, P. L., Verhulsdonk, C. A. H. and Paulsch, W. E. (1970). Bestimmung von Aflatoxin B_1 durch Zweidimentionale Dunnschicht-Chromatographie mit fluorodensitometrichsche Auswertung. *Arzneim. Forsch.*, **20**, 1517–20.

Schuller, P. L., Stoloff, L. and van Egmond, H. P. (1982). Limits and regulations. In: *Environmental Carcinogens: Selected Methods of Analysis*, Vol. 5, *Some Mycotoxins*, H. Egan, L. Stoloff, M. Castegnaro, P. Scott, I. K. O'Neill and H. Bartsch (Eds), International Agency for Research on Cancer, Lyon, pp. 107–16.

Schuller, P. L., van Egmond, H. P. and Stoloff, L. (1983). Limits and regulation on mycotoxins. In: *Proc. Int. Symp. Mycotoxins*, National Res. Centre, Cairo, Egypt, 6–8 Sept. 1981, pp. 111–29.

Scott, P. M. (1982). Assessment of quantitative methods for determination of trichothecenes in grains and grain products. *J. Assoc. Off. Anal. Chem.*, **65**, 876–83.

Scott, P. M. (1984*a*). The occurrence of vomitoxin (deoxynivalenol, DON) in Canadian grains. In: *Toxigenic Fungi: Their Toxins and Health Hazard*, H. Kurata and Y. Ueno (Eds), Elsevier, Amsterdam/Oxford/New York/Tokyo, pp. 182–9.

Scott, P. M. (1984*b*). Effects of food processing on mycotoxins. *J. Food Protect.*, **47**, 489–99.

Scott, P. M., van Walbeek, W., Harwig, J. and Fennell, D. I. (1970). Occurrence of a mycotoxin, ochratoxin A, in wheat and isolation of ochratoxin A and citrinin producing strains of *Penicillium viridicatum*. *Can. J. Plant Sci.*, **50**, 583–5.

Scott, P. M., van Walbeek, W., Kennedy, B. and Anyeti, D. (1972*a*). Mycotoxins (ochratoxin A, citrinin, and sterigmatocystin) and toxigenic fungi in grains and other agricultural products. *J. Agric. Food Chem.*, **20**, 80–8.

Scott, P. M., Miles, W. F., Toft, P. and Dube, J. G. (1972*b*). Occurrence of patulin in apple juice. *J. Agric. Food Chem.*, **20**, 450–1.

Scott, P. M., Kanhere, S. R., Dexter, J. E., Brennan, P. W. and Trenholm, H. L. (1984). Distribution of the trichothecene mycotoxin deoxynivalenol (vomitoxin) during the milling of naturally contaminated hard red spring wheat and its fate in baking products. *Food Add. Contam.*, **1**, 313–23.

Seto, B. and Gerety, R. (1985). A glycoprotein associated with the non-A, non-B hepatitis agent(s): isolation and immunoreactivity. *Proc. Nat. Acad. Sci.*, **82**, 4934–8.

Shank, R. C., Wogan, G. N., Gibson, J. B. and Nondasuta, A. (1972). Dietary aflatoxins and human liver cancer. II. Aflatoxin in marker foods and foodstuffs of Thailand and Hong Kong. *Food Cosmet. Toxicol.*, **10**, 61–9.

Shinohara, Y., Arai, M., Sugihara, S., Nakanishi, K., Tsunoda, H. and Ito, N. (1976). Combination effect of citrinin and other chemicals on rat kidney tumorigenesis. *Gann*, **67**, 147–55.

Shotwell, O. L., Hesseltine, C. W., Burmeister, H. R., Kwolek, W. F., Shannon, G. M. and Hall, H. H. (1969*a*). Survey of cereal grains and soybeans for presence of aflatoxin. I. Wheat, grain, sorghum, and oats. *Cereal Chem.*, **46**, 446–54.

Shotwell, O. L., Hesseltine, C. W., Burmeister, H. R., Kwolek, W. F., Shannon, G. M. and Hall, H. H. (1969*b*). Survey of cereal grains and soybeans for presence of aflatoxin. II. Corn and soybeans. *Cereal Chem.*, **46**, 454–63.

Shotwell, O. L., Hesseltine, C. W. and Goulden, M. L. (1969*c*). Ochratoxin A: occurrence as natural contaminant of a corn sample. *Appl. Microbiol.*, **17**, 765–6.

Shotwell, O. L., Hesseltine, C. W. and Goulden, M. L. (1973). Incidence of aflatoxin in southern corn 1969–1970. *Cereal Sci. Today*, **18**, 192–5.

Shotwell, O. L., Goulden, M. L. and Hesseltine, C. W. (1976). Survey of U.S. wheat for ochratoxin and aflatoxin. *J. Assoc. Off. Anal. Chem.*, **59**, 122–4.

Shouval, D., Reid, L. M., Chakraborty, P. R., Ruiz-Opazo, N., Morecki, R., Gerber, M. A., Thung, S. N. and Shafritz, D. A. (1981). Tumorigenicity in nude mice of a human hepatoma cell line containing hepatitis B virus DNA. *Cancer Res.*, **41**, 1342–7.

Siraj, M. Y., Hayes, A. W., Unger, P. D., Hogen, G. R., Ryan, N. J. and Wray, B. B. (1981). Analysis of aflatoxin B_1 in human tissues with high pressure liquid chromatography. *Toxicol. Appl. Pharmacol.*, **58**, 422–30.

Smith, J. W. and Hamilton, P. B. (1970). Aflatoxicosis in the broiler chicken. *Poult. Sci.*, **49**, 207–15.

Snyder, R. L., Tyler, G. and Summers, J. (1982). Chronic hepatitis and hepatocellular carcinoma associated with woodchuck hepatitis virus. *Am. J. Pathol.*, **107**, 422–5.

Sphon, J. A., Dreifuss, P. A. and Schulten, H. (1977). Mycotoxins: field desorption mass spectrometry of mycotoxins and mycotoxin mixtures, and its application as a screening technique for foodstuffs. *J. Assoc. Off. Anal. Chem.*, **60**, 73–82.

Steyn, P. S. (1984). Ochratoxins and related dihydroisocoumarins. In: *Mycotoxins: Production, Isolation, Separation and Purification*, V. Betina (Ed.), Elsevier, Amsterdam, pp. 183–216.

Still, P. E., Macklin, A. W., Rebelin, W. E. and Smalley, E. B. (1971). Relation of ochratoxin A to fatal death in laboratory and domestic animals. *Nature*, **234**, 563–4.

Stoloff, L. (1976). Report on mycotoxins. *J. Assoc. Off. Anal. Chem.*, **59**, 317–23.

Stoloff, L. (1977). Aflatoxins: an overview. In: *Mycotoxins in Human and Animal Health*, J. V. Rodricks, C. W. Hesseltine and M. A. Mehlman (Eds), Pathotox Publ., Park Forest South, Illinois, pp. 7–28.

Stoloff, L. (1982). Analytical methods for aflatoxins: an overview. In: *Environmental Carcinogens: Selected Methods of Analysis*, Vol. 5, *Some Mycotoxins*, H. Egan, L. Stoloff, H. Castegnaro, P. Scott, I. K. O'Neill and H. Bartsch (Eds), IARC, Lyon, pp. 33–64.

Stoloff, L. (1983). Aflatoxin as a cause of primary liver-cell cancer in the United States: a probability study. *Nutrition and Cancer*, **5**, 165–86.

Storen, O., Holm, H. and Størmer, F. C. (1982). Metabolism of ochratoxin A by rats. *Appl. Environ. Microbiol.*, **44**, 785–9.

Størmer, F. C. and Pedersen, J. I. (1980). Formation of 4-hydroxyochratoxin A from ochratoxin A by rat liver microsomes. *Appl. Environ. Microbiol.*, **39**(5), 971–5.

Størmer, F. C., Hansen, C. E., Pedersen, J. I., Hvistendahl, G. and Aasen, A. J. (1981). Formation of (4R)- and (4S)-4-hydroxyochratoxin A from ochratoxin A by liver microsomes from various species. *Appl. Environ. Microbiol.*, **42**, 1051–6.

Sun, T. T. and Chu, Y. Y. (1984). Carcinogenesis and prevention strategy of liver cancer in areas of prevalence. *J. Cell Physiol. Suppl.*, **3**, 39–44.

Sun, T. and Wang, N. (1983). Studies on human carcinogenesis. In: *Human Carcinogenesis*, C. C. Harris and H. Autrup (Eds), Academic Press, New York, pp. 757–80.

Sun, T., Wu, Y. and Wu, S. (1983). Monoclonal antibody against aflatoxin B_1 and its potential applications. *Clin. J. Oncol.*, **5**, 401–5.

Takahashi, T., Onoue, Y. and Mori, M. (1982). Contamination of commercial corn flour with aflatoxin and citrinin. *J. Food Hyg. Soc. Jap.*, **23**, 73–80 (in Japanese).

Tanaka, T., Hasegawa, A., Matsuki, Y. and Ueno, Y. (1985*a*). A survey of the occurrence of nivalenol, deoxynivalenol and zearalenone in foodstuffs and health foods in Japan. *Food Add. Contam.*, **2**, 259–65.

Tanaka, T., Hasegawa, A., Matsuki, Y., Ishii, K. and Ueno, Y. (1985*b*). Improved methodology for the simultaneous detection of the trichothecene mycotoxins deoxynivalenol and nivalenol in cereals. *Food Add. Contam.*, **2**, 125–37.

Tanaka, T., Hasegawa, A., Matsuki, Y., Lee, U.-S. and Ueno, Y. (1985*c*). Co-contamination of the *Fusarium* mycotoxins, nivalenol, deoxynivalenol and zearalenone, in scabby wheat harvested in Hokkaido, Japan. *J. Food Hyg. Soc. Jap.*, **26**, 519–22.

Tanaka, T., Hasegawa, A., Matsuki, Y., Lee, U.-S. and Ueno, Y. (1985*d*). Rapid and sensitive determination of zearalenone in cereals by high-performance liquid chromatography with fluorescence detection. *J. Chromatog.*, **328**, 271–8.

Tanaka, T., Hasegawa, A., Matsuki, Y., Lee, U.-S. and Ueno, Y. (1986). A limited survey of *Fusarium* mycotoxins nivalenol, deoxynivalenol and zearalenone, in 1984 UK harvested wheat and barley. *Food Add. Contam.*, **3**, 247–52.

Tanaka, H., Morooka, N., Haraikawa, K. and Ueno, Y. (1987). Metabolic activation of emodin in the reconstituted cytochrome P-450 system of the hepatic microsomes of rats. *Mutation Res.*, **176**, 165–70.

Tashiro, F., Morimura, S., Hayashi, K., Makino, R., Kawamura, H., Horikoshi, N., Memoto, K., Ohtsubo, K., Sugimura, T. and Ueno, Y. (1986*a*). Expression of the c-*Ha-ras* and c-*myc* genes in aflatoxin B_1-induced hepatocellular carcinoma. *Biochem. Biophys. Res. Commum.*, **138**, 858–64.

Tashiro, F., Morimura, S., Hayashi, K., Makino, R., Kawamura, H., Horikoshi, N., Nemoto, K., Ohtsubo, K. and Ueno, Y. (1986*b*). Expression of proto-oncogenes in aflatoxin B_1-induced rat hepatocellular carcinomas and cultured cell line, Kagura-1. *Proc. Jpn. Assoc. Mycotoxicol.*, **23**, 29–33.

Tashiro, F., Horikoshi, N., Tanaka, N. and Ueno, Y. (1986*c*). Effects of aflatoxin B_1 and sterigmatocystin on the hormonal induction of liver-specific enzymes and glucocorticoid receptor. *Proc. Jpn. Assoc. Mycotoxicol.*, **23**, 35–40.

Tatsuno, Y., Saito, M., Enomoto, M. and Tsunoda, H. (1968). Nivalenol, a toxic principle of *Fusarium nivale*. *Chem. Pharm. Bull.*, **16**, 2519–20.

Terao, K. (1983). Sterigmatocystin: a masked potent carcinogenic mycotoxin. *J. Toxicol., Toxin Rev.*, **2**, 77–110.

Tiollais, P., Pourcel, C. and Dejean, A. (1985). The hepatitis B virus. *Nature*, **317**, 489–95.

Trucksess, M. W. and Stoloff, L. (1979). Extraction, cleanup, and quantitative determination of aflatoxin B_1 and M_1 in beef liver. *J. Assoc. Off. Anal. Chem.*, **62**, 1080–2.

Trucksess, M. W., Nesheim, S. and Eppley, R. (1984). Thin-layer chromatographic determination of deoxynivalenol in wheat and corn. *J. Assoc. Off. Anal. Chem.*, **67**(1), 40–3.

Tsuboi, S., Nakagawa, T., Tomita, M., Seo, T., Ono, H., Kawamura, K. and Iwamura, N. (1984). Detection of aflatoxin B_1 in serum samples of male Japanese subjects by radioimmunoassay and high performance liquid chromatography. *Cancer Res.*, **44**, 1231–4.

Ueno, Y. (1974). Citreoviridin from *Penicillium citreoviride* Biourge. In: *Mycotoxins*, I. F. H. Purchase (Ed.), Elsevier, Amsterdam, pp. 283–302.

Ueno, Y. (1977). Trichothecene overview. In: *Mycotoxins in Human and Animal Health*, J. V. Rodricks, C. W. Hesseltine and M. A. Mehlman (Eds), Pathotox Publ., Illinois, pp. 189–228.

Ueno, Y. (1980). Trichothecene mycotoxins: mycology, chemistry and toxicology. *Adv. Nutr. Res.*, **3**, 301–52.

Ueno, Y. (1982). Luteoskyrin and other *Penicillium islandicum* toxins. In: *Environmental Carcinogens: Selected Methods of Analysis*, Vol. 5, *Some Mycotoxins*, H. Egan, P. Scott, L. Stoloff, I. K. O'Neill, M. Castegnaro and H. Bartsch, IARC, Lyon, pp. 399–417.

Ueno, Y. (1983a). Citreoviridin. In: *CRC Handbook of Foodborne Diseases of Biological Origin*, M. Rechcigl, Jr. (Ed.), CRC Press, Boca Raton, Florida, pp. 181–92.

Ueno, Y. (1983b) (Ed.). *Trichothecenes: Chemical, Biological and Toxicological Aspects*, Developments in Food Science, No. 4, Elsevier, Amsterdam.

Ueno, Y. (1984a). Toxicological features of T-2 toxin and related trichothecenes. *Fund. Appl. Toxicol.*, **4**, S124–32.

Ueno, Y. (1984b). Hydroxyanthraquinones (skyrines). In: *Mycotoxins: Production, Separation and Purification*, V. Betina (Ed.), Elsevier, Amsterdam, pp. 329–50.

Ueno, Y. (1985a). Metabolism of mycotoxins in reconstituted cytochrome P-450 system. *Proc. Jap. Assoc. Mycotoxicol.*, **22**, 28–30.

Ueno, Y. (1985b). The toxicology of mycotoxins. *CRC Crit. Rev. Toxicol.*, **14**(2), 99–132.

Ueno, Y. (1986). Toxicology of microbial toxins. *Pure & Appl. Chem.*, **58**, 339–50.

Ueno, Y. and Ishii, K. (1985). Chemical and biological properties of trichothecenes from *Fusarium sporotrichioides*. In: *Trichothecenes and Other Mycotoxins*, J. Lacey (Ed.), John Wiley and Sons, Chichester, pp. 307–16.

Ueno, Y. and Kubota, K. (1976). DNA-attacking ability of carcinogenic mycotoxins in recombination-deficient mutant cells of *Bacillus subtilis*. *Cancer Res.*, **36**, 445–51.

Ueno, Y. and Tashiro, F. (1981). α-Zearalenol, a major hepatic metabolite in rats of zearalenone, an estrogenic mycotoxin of *Fusarium* species. *J. Biochem.*, **89**, 563–71.

Ueno, U., Ueno, I., Tatsuno, T., Ohkubo, K. and Tsunoda, H. (1969). Fusarenon X, a toxic principle of *Fusarium nivale* culture filtrate. *Experientia*, 25, 1062.

Ueno, Y., Ishii, K., Sakai, K., Kanaeda, S., Tsunoda, H., Tanaka, T. and Enomoto, M. (1972). Toxicological approaches to the metabolites of *Fusaria*. IV. Microbial survey on bean hulls poisoning of horses with the isolation of toxic trichothecenes, neosolaniol and T-2 toxin of *Fusarium solani* M-1-1. *Jap. J. Exp. Med.*, 42, 187–203.

Ueno, Y., Sato, N., Ishii, K., Sakai, K., Tsunoda, H. and Enomoto, M. (1973). Biological and chemical detection of trichothecene mycotoxins of *Fusarium* species. *Appl. Microbiol.*, 25(4), 699–704.

Ueno, Y., Kubota, K., Ito, T. and Nakamura, Y. (1978). Mutagenicity of carcinogenic mycotoxins in *Salmonella typhimurium*. *Cancer Res.*, 38, 536–42.

Ueno, Y., Ishii, K., Omata, Y., Kamataki, T. and Kato, R. (1983). Specificity of hepatic cytochrome P-450 isoenzymes from PCB-treated rats and participation of cytochrome b_5 in the activation of aflatoxin B_1. *Carcinogenesis*, 4, 1071–83.

Ueno, Y., Tashiro, F. and Nakaki, H. (1985). Mechanism of metabolic activation of aflatoxin B_1. *Gann Monograph Cancer Res.*, 30, 111–24.

Ueno, Y., Tanaka, T., Hasegawa, A., Hu, Z.-H. and Xu, D.-D. (1986a). Deoxynivalenol, nivalenol and zearalenone in scabby wheat from Shanghai, China. *J. Food Hyg. Soc. Jap.*, 27, 180–2.

Ueno, Y., Lee, U.-S., Tanaka, T., Hasegawa, A. and Matsuki, Y. (1986b). Examination of Chinese and USSR cereals for *Fusarium* mycotoxins, nivalenol, deoxynivalenol and zearalenone. *Toxicon*, 24, 618–21.

Ueno, Y., Lee, U.-S., Tanaka, T., Hasegawa, A. and Strzelecki, E. (1986c). Natural co-occurrence of nivalenol and deoxynivalenol in Polish cereals. *Microbiol.-Alim.-Nutr.*, 3, 321–6.

Uraguchi, K. (1969). Mycotoxic origin of cardiac beriberi. *J. Stored Prod. Res.*, 5, 227–36.

Uraguchi, K. (1971). Pharmacology of mycotoxins. In: *International Encyclopedia of Pharmacology and Therapeutics*, Section 71, H. Raskova (Ed.), Pergamon Press, Oxford, pp. 143–298.

van der Merwe, K. J., Steyn, P. S., Fourie, L., Scott, D. B. and Theron, J. J. (1965). Ochratoxin A, a toxic metabolite produced by *Aspergillus ochraceus* Wilhelm. *Nature*, 205, 1112–3.

van Rensburg, S. J., van der Watt, J. J., Purchase, I. F. H., Coutinho, L. P. and Markham, R. (1974). Primary liver cancer rate and aflatoxin intake in a high cancer area. *South Afr. Med. J.*, 48, 2508a–2058d.

van Rensburg, S. J., Kirshpuu, A., Coutinho, L. P. and van der Watt, J. J. (1975). Circumstances associated with the contamination of food by aflatoxin in a high primary liver cancer area. *South Afr. Med. J.*, 49, 877–83.

van Walbeek, W., Scott, P. M. and Thatcher, F. S. (1968). Mycotoxins from food-borne fungi. *Can. J. Microbiol.*, 14, 131–7.

van Walbeek, W., Scott, P. M., Harvig, J. and Lawrence, J. W. (1969). *Penicillium viridicatum* Westling: a new source of ochratoxin A. *Can. J. Microbiol.*, 15, 1281–5.

Vesonder, R. F. and Horn, B. W. (1985). Sterigmatocystin in dairy cattle feed contaminated with *Aspergillus versicolor*. *Appl. Environ. Microbiol.*, 49, 234–5.

Vesonder, R. F., Ciegler, A. and Jensen, A. H. (1973). Isolation of the emetic principle from *Fusarium*-infected corn. *Appl. Microbiol.*, 26, 1008–10.

Vesonder, R. F., Ciegler, A., Rogers, R. F., Burmeister, K. A., Bothast, R. J. and Jensen, A. H. (1978). Survey of 1977 crop year preharvest corn for vomitoxin. *Appl. Environ. Microbiol.*, **36**, 885–8.

Visconti, A. and Bottalico, A. (1983). High levels of ochratoxin A and B in moldy bread responsible for mycotoxicosis in farm animals. *J. Agric. Food Chem.*, **31**, 1122–3.

Wattenberg, L. W. (1985). Chemoprevention of cancer. *Cancer Res.*, **45**, 1–8.

Wattenberg, L. W. and Lam, L. T. (1981). Inhibition of chemical carcinogenesis by phenols, coumarines, aromatic isothiocyanates, flavones, and indoles. In: *Inhibition of Tumor Induction and Development.* M. S. Zedeck, and M. Lipkin (Eds), Plenum Press, New York, pp. 1–22.

Wei, C. I., Marshall, M. R. and Hsieh, D. P. H. (1985). Characterization of water-soluble glucuronide and sulfate conjugates of aflatoxin B_1. 1. Urinary excretion in monkey, rat and mouse. *Food Chem. Toxicol.*, **23**(9), 809–19.

Witham, M., Nixon, J. E. and Sinnhuber, R. O. (1982). Liver DNA bound *in vivo* with aflatoxin B_1 as a measure of hepatocarcinoma initiation in rainbow trout. *J. Nat. Cancer Inst.*, **68**, 623–8.

Wogan, G. N. (1977). Mycotoxins and other naturally occurring carcinogens. In: *Environmental Cancer*, Vol. 3, *Advances in Modern Toxicology*, H. F. Krybill and M. A. Mehlman (Eds), John Wiley and Sons, New York, pp. 263–90.

World Health Organization (1978). International histological classification of tumours. No. 20. *Histological Typing of Tumours of the Liver, Biliary Tract and Pancreas*, J. J. B. Gibson (Ed.), Geneva.

World Health Organization (1985). *Prevention of Liver Cancer*, WHO Technical Report Ser., 691, Geneva.

Wray, B. B. and Hayes, A. W. (1980). Aflatoxin B_1 in the serum of patient with primary hepatic carcinoma. *Environ. Res.*, **22**, 400–3.

Wyllie, T. S. and Morehouse, L. G. (1977). *Mycotoxic Fungi, Mycotoxins, Mycotoxicoses*, Vol. 1, *Mycotoxic Fungi and Chemistry of Mycotoxins*, Marcel Dekker, New York.

Yang, G., Nesheim, S., Benavides, J., Ueno, I., Campbell, A. D. and Pohland, A. (1980). Radioimmunoassay detection of aflatoxin B_1 in monkey and human urine. In: *Medical Mycology*, H. J. Preusser (Ed.), *Zentralblatt Bukt Suppl. 8*, 136–8.

Yang, S. S., Tuab, J. V., Modali, R., Vieira, W., Yasei, P. and Yang, G. C. (1985). Dose-dependency of aflatoxin B_1 binding on human high molecular weight DNA in the activation of a proto-oncogene. *Env. Health Perspect.*, **62**, 231–8.

Yoshizawa, T. (1983). Red-mold diseases and natural occurrence in Japan. In: *Trichothecenes: Chemical, Biological and Toxicological Aspects*, Y. Ueno (Ed.), Elsevier, Amsterdam, pp. 195–209.

Yoshizawa, T. and Morooka, N. (1973). Deoxynivalenol and its monoacetate, new mycotoxins from *Fusarium roseum* and moldy barley. *Agric. Biol. Chem.*, **37**, 2933–4.

Young, J. C., Fulcher, R. C., Hayhoe, J. H., Scott, P. M. and Dexter, J. E. (1984). Effect of milling and baking on deoxynivalenol (vomitoxin) content of eastern Canadian wheats. *J. Agric. Food Chem.*, **32**, 659–64.

Chapter 7

MUTAGENS AND CARCINOGENS IN HEAT-PROCESSED FOOD

JOHN CHR. LARSEN and E. POULSEN

Institute of Toxicology, National Food Agency, Søborg, Denmark

INTRODUCTION

During the last decade there has been a growing recognition that a causal relationship may exist between dietary components and several chronic diseases, especially cancer and cardiovascular disease. For cancer, concurrent estimates made by several expert groups have ascribed more than 30% of total cancers to dietary factors. Based on a large number of epidemiological studies, the best validated risk factor is high intake of fat, especially saturated fat, which correlates with an increased risk for colorectal cancer and breast cancer, and appears to increase the risk for

205

prostate cancer and possibly ovarian, renal and pancreatic cancer (Doll and Peto, 1981; Committee on Diet, Nutrition and Cancer, 1982; Willett and MacMahan, 1984). High consumption of meat has also been implicated as a risk factor in cancer by many investigators, although other studies have not been able to confirm this (Vuolo and Schuessler, 1985).

Tumour induction can be divided into at least two distinct stages, initiation and promotion. In animal experiments the initiation stage requires a single treatment with a carcinogen and is regarded as essentially irreversible. The initiation step involves a heritable modification in the genetic material of the cell. This can be brought about by compounds that bind covalently to DNA and other macromolecules. Such compounds are often detectable as mutagens in short-term *in vitro* assays. The promotional stage requires repeated treatments after initiation and probably can be divided into several phases, initially being reversible, later becoming irreversible. Many promoters are not detected as mutagens and do not bind to DNA. Many promoters are membrane-active agents, and this effect is therefore thought to be of importance. Recent observations that well-known promoters can cause DNA damage indirectly, observable as a clastogenic effect in *in vitro* systems, by generating active oxygen species within the cell, have led to speculations whether one or more steps in the promotional stage also require some kind of genetic alterations (Cerutti, 1985).

Much support is currently given to the theory that DNA damage, by covalent binding and/or by indirect active oxygen attack, activates oncogenes, which promote neoplastic transformation. The gene products of the oncogenes are thought to be related to growth factors, normally repressed in differentiated cells. Uncontrolled activation from a mutational event may result in synthesis of growth factors, leading to uncontrolled cellular growth and transformation (Marx, 1984). This hypothesis might explain why most initiating, mutagenic compounds are also normally able to promote cancer.

The dietary components so far recognized as risk factors in cancer, such as high fat intake, are thought mainly to act during tumour promotion. As regards initiators, great efforts have also been directed toward identifying such compounds in the diet. Until 1975 this search was essentially restricted to analytical chemical attempts to identify known carcinogens in the diet. Examples are the detection of polycyclic aromatic hydrocarbons (PAH) in charcoal-broiled and grilled meat (Lijinsky and Shubik, 1964) and nitrosamines in heated meat products containing nitrite and secondary amines (Pensabene *et al.*, 1974). After the introduction of short-term mutagenicity tests, especially the Ames test using *Salmonella typhimurium*, and the recognition that most genotoxic compounds could be detected as mutagens in these tests (McCann and Ames, 1976; Purchase *et al.*, 1976; Sugimura *et al.*, 1976), the task was greatly facilitated, as potentially initiating compounds could be easily detected in food. A better strategy could now be applied for their isolation, characterization, determination and subsequent toxicological testing in animal experiments.

Using this strategy a number of mutagenic and carcinogenic compounds have been identified in heat-processed food. The nearly exponential increase in scientific reports on processing-induced mutagens in food indicates that this will be an important challenge for safety evaluation in the future.

In the following sections we shall discuss the toxicological properties of different types of potentially harmful compounds that can be formed during heat processing of food. An initial brief consideration of the well-known formation of polycyclic aromatic hydrocarbons (PAH) is followed by a more thorough review of the recently discovered mutagenic compounds that are formed during heat processing of foods. Attention will be drawn to the conditions that favour their formation and the means by which they can be avoided or kept at a minimum. Such information must also be regarded as essential in the evaluation of future epidemiological studies.

POLYCYCLIC AROMATIC HYDROCARBONS IN GRILLED AND SMOKED FOODS

The polycyclic aromatic hydrocarbons (PAH) are ubiquitous in the environment as products of pyrolysis of organic matter. Benzo(a)pyrene and other PAH were recognized as potent carcinogens in mouse skin-painting experiments in the early 1930s (Phillips, 1983), and the carcinogenic properties of PAH have been intensively studied since. Numerous compounds belonging to this class have been identified in ambient air, environmental samples such as soil and water, and in foods. The major sources of PAH in the environment are heat and power generation (especially coal), refuse burning, coke production and motor vehicles (Lo and Sandi, 1978). In food more than 20 PAH have been identified, and more than 10 of these have been shown to be carcinogenic in experimental

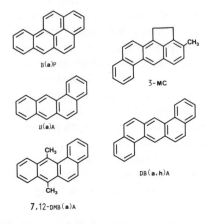

FIG. 1.**BaP** (benzo(*a*)pyrene), **BaA** (benzo(*a*)anthracene), **3-MC** (methylchol-anthrene), **DBahA** (dibenzo(*a,h*)anthracene), and **DMBaA** (dimethylbenzo(*a*)-anthracene).

animals using skin application and/or various forms of injection into the body of the animals. Studies using oral administration to rats and mice have so far identified benzo(*a*)pyrene (BaP), benzo(*a*)anthracene (BaA), 3-methylcholanthrene (3-MC), dibenzo(*a,h*)anthracene (DBahA) and dimethylbenzo(*a*)anthracene (DMBaA) as carcinogens by the oral route (Lo and Sandi, 1978) (Fig. 1). 3-MC and DMBaA are not normally found in food.

Analytical findings of PAH in food are in general expressed as BaP and ΣPAH. ΣPAH covers a variety of PAH many of which are not carcino-genic. The BaP content is considered a valuable expression of the carcinogenic potential of the mixture, although it may only account for up to 10% of the toxicity of the sample (Adrian *et al.*, 1984).

Two major sources exist for the occurrence of PAH in foods. The most important is the deposition and uptake of PAH from polluted air on food crops. This make cereals, vegetables, fruits and vegetable oils important contributors to man's intake of PAH. In particular, drying of cereals using direct application of combustion gases can result in 10 times higher PAH concentrations in the products than before treatment.

The other significant source is the formation and deposition of PAH on foods during heat processing using methods such as roasting, smoking and grilling. It is important to note that the formation of PAH is only significant at high temperatures. At temperatures below 400°C only small amounts of PAH are formed, while the amounts increase linearly in the range 400–1000°C (Tóth and Potthast, 1984).

PAH Formation during Grilling of Foods
Intensive heat treatment leads to the production of PAH. Grilling or broiling of meat and fish on an open fire leads to PAH contamination in several different ways. Firstly, the high temperatures lead to 'endogenous' formation of PAH on the surface of the food. Secondly, PAH can be formed during the combustion of the fuel used in the grilling. Thirdly, and perhaps most significantly, PAH is formed when melted fat drips down on the heat source. The PAH so formed during pyrolysis of the fat are spread to the atmosphere and partially deposited on the surface of the meat. PAH can be found both in the vapour phase and particle bound.

Lijinsky and Shubik (1964) identified BaP and other PAH in charcoal-broiled meat at an average level of 8 μg BaP per kg steak. Larsson *et al.* (1983) investigated several factors of importance for PAH contamination of frankfurters during grilling. As heating methods such as conduction in frying and radiation in electrical broiling only lead to minute amounts of PAH in food, the 'endogenous' formation of PAH in the meat seems to be of minor importance, under normal conditions. Only when the meat is placed directly in contact with the flames of a log fire are significant amounts of PAH (6–212 μg BaP/kg) formed, in spite of the fact that the embers of the log fire emit only moderate amounts of PAH (1–25 μg BaP/kg). Among the fuels normally used in grilling, charcoal yields only small amounts of PAH (0–1·0 μg BaP/kg). When smouldering spruce or pine cones are used as fuel, relatively high levels of PAH are found (2–31 μg BaP/kg).

The fat content of the meat seems to be very important. This is probably most evident when a 'clean' fuel is used, such as charcoal. The more fat drips on the fuel the more PAH may be formed and deposited on the meat (Lijinsky and Ross, 1967; Fritz, 1973; Tóth and Blaas, 1973; Doremire *et al.*, 1979). Increasing the fat content of charcoal-grilled ground beef patties from 15% to 40% led to an increase in BaP content from 16 to 121 μg/kg (Fretheim, 1983). Thus the contamination of grilled food with PAH can be avoided or minimized by using charcoal as fuel, by avoiding open flames, and by special grill constructions that prevent the fat from dripping onto the heat source.

PAH Formation during Smoking of Foods
Smoking, along with salting and drying, is one of the oldest procedures for preserving foods such as meat and fish. Today, where more effective preservation methods such as cooking, freezing and heat preservation are available, the main purpose of smoking is to give products a special desirable taste and palatability.

Curing smoke is normally produced from wood (sawdust) by the initial pyrolytic changes of lignin, hemicellulose and cellulose, followed by secondary reactions leading to the formation of a variety of different chemical compounds. The most important compounds formed are phenols, carbonyls, acids, furans, alcohols, esters, lactones and PAH. More than 300 compounds have been identified. The smoke is a complicated mixture of vapours (10%), and a dispersed phase of solid and liquid particles which contains the majority of the compounds generated (90%). In the smoke an equilibrium exists between the compounds in the gas phase and the particulate phase. The gas phase is thought to be of most importance in obtaining the characteristic taste of smoked products. The technological aspect of smoking has been reviewed by Tóth and Potthast (1984).

In traditional smoking methods the smoke is generated at the bottom of the oven and the products are placed directly over the smoking wood. In modern industrial ovens the smoke is normally generated in a separate chamber and led into the smoking chamber where the products are placed. This gives the possibility of better control of the smoke content by using various 'cleaning' methods such as washing the smoke which diminishes the PAH content, or using electrostatic filters which remove the particulates thus leading to less PAH in the smoke. Modern ovens also permit the regulation of such important parameters as smoke generation speed, circulation, temperature, humidity and smoke concentration in the chamber.

Phenols, carbonyls and acids are the important compounds for the desirable effect of the smoking process. Nitrogen oxides in the smoke can form nitrites/nitrates which are able to react with amines and amides in the products, yielding N-nitroso compounds. N-Nitrosodimethylamine is frequently detected in smoked products. In smoked fish levels up to $10 \mu g/kg$ can be found. In smoked meat the levels are more variable and normally lower than or about $1 \mu g/kg$. Only in very few cases are higher levels seen.

Low molecular weight PAH such as phenanthrene, anthracene and pyrene are frequently found in smoked food at levels of $10 \mu g/kg$. The higher molecular weight PAH such as BaP, BaA, benzo(b)fluoranthene, dibenzo(a,c)anthracene and DBahA are found in much lower concentrations. Smoked fish and meat normally contain less than $1 \mu g/kg$ and BaP is most often found at levels of $0 \cdot 1$–$0 \cdot 5 \mu g/kg$. Again, under special conditions higher levels can be found, especially on the outside of heavily smoked products (Adrian et al., 1984).

Metabolism of Polycyclic Aromatic Hydrocarbons

The PAH are oxidized by the cytochrome P-450 system to a complex mixture of phenols, dihydro-diols and quinones. Arene oxides are formed as intermediate metabolites, spontaneously being converted into phenols or further metabolized by epoxide hydrolase to dihydro-diols. These primary metabolites undergo further oxidative metabolism and conjugation reactions (Levin *et al.*, 1982).

The various arene oxides and other metabolites are mutagenic *in vitro*, but the majority do not display carcinogenicity, or are weaker than the parent compound, when tested *in vivo*. For BaP the 7,8-diol-9,10-epoxide has been shown to be highly mutagenic *in vitro* and to bind with much higher efficiency to DNA than BaP. It was also shown that *in vivo* (mouse skin) the 7,8-diol-9,10-epoxide gave rise to the same DNA adduct as did the parent compound BaP. Covalent binding to DNA was established between the C-10 position of BaP and the 2-amino group of guanine.

These findings with BaP, demonstrating that the ultimate carcinogen seems to be an epoxide situated in the 'bay region' (the angle between benzene rings in a non-linear arrangement), led to the development of the 'bay region' theory which predicted greater reactivity for 'bay region' diol-epoxides than for non-'bay region' diol-epoxides. This has actually been shown to be the case for many PAH. However, this characteristic alone does not predict the carcinogenicity of a hydrocarbon, as many other factors such as metabolic, sterochemical and conformational factors, as well as the biological reactivity of the metabolites, contribute to the marked differences in tumorigenicity of various PAH (Levin *et al.*, 1982; Pelkonen and Nebert, 1982; Phillips, 1983).

Carcinogenicity

The ability to produce skin tumours in the two-stage mouse skin carcinogenesis system and to produce local sarcomas at the injection site has been shown for a variety of PAH (IARC, 1983). Similarly, the ability to produce lung tumours after either intravenous injection or intratracheal instillation or inhalation has been shown for various PAH, in particular BaP. Mammary tumours induced by intragastric dosed DMBA have become an important model in the study of breast cancer.

Oral administration of PAH frequently results in papillomas and carcinomas in the forestomach of rodents. BaP, DBahA and DBcgC have been tested in mice, rats or hamsters. DMBaA and 3-MC also induce tumours of the stomach, and in addition ovarian, lymphoid, mammary and hepatic tumours. Gastric tumours, pulmonary adenomas and leukemia were induced in mice fed BaP at various levels. The effective daily doses seemed to be in the order of some mg/kg body weight (Lo and Sandi, 1978; IARC, 1983).

NEW MUTAGENS AND CARCINOGENS IN HEAT-PROCESSED FOOD

Since Nagao *et al.* (1977*a*) reported that substantial mutagenic activity was present in smoke condensates and extracts of the charred surface of broiled fish and meat, numerous reports have been published on the formation of mutagenic activity in a variety of food after heat treatment. The majority of investigations have used the Salmonella/mammalian microsome test of Ames *et al.* (1975). The *Salmonella typhimurium* tester strains normally used are the strains TA 98 and TA 1538 which detect frame-shift mutations, and to a lesser extent the strains TA 100 and TA 1535 detecting base-pair substitution mutations. Nagao *et al.* (1977*a*) noted that the activity from broiled fish and meat was especially pronounced in TA 98 with metabolic activation in the presence of a liver homogenate from Aroclor 1254 (PCB) treated rats (S9 Mix), and moreover they were able to show that the activity was not caused by benz(*a*)pyrene and other polycyclic aromatic hydrocarbons.

Amino Acid Pyrolysis Products

Occurrence
Following these initial observations it was shown that when pyrolysates (>300°C) from various proteins, carbohydrates, nucleic acids and fats were tested in Salmonella, significant mutagenic activity towards TA 98 with S9 was only detected in pyrolysates of protein, whereas pyrolysates from starch were directly mutagenic towards TA 100 without metabolic activation. A similar but rather weak effect in TA 100 was seen with pyrolysates of vegetable oil (Nagao *et al.*, 1977*b*). Subsequently it was shown that pyrolysates from various amino acids after heating at 300–600°C were mutagenic in TA 98 with S9. The highest specific activity was obtained after pyrolysis of tryptophan, and glutamic acid pyrolysate also showed high activity. Pyrolysates from most of the other amino acids were also active, but to a lesser extent (Matsumoto *et al.*, 1977; Kosuge *et al.*, 1978; Matsumoto *et al.*, 1978).

The principal mutagens, all heterocyclic amines (Fig. 2), were isolated

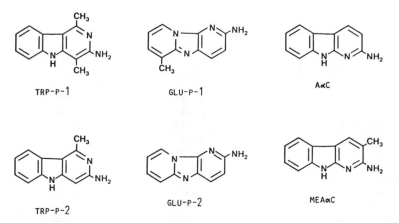

TRP-P-1   GLU-P-1   AαC

TRP-P-2   GLU-P-2   MEAαC

FIG. 2. Mutagens isolated from amino acid pyrolysates: **Trp-P-1** (3-amino-1,4-dimethyl-5*H*-pyrido[4,3-*b*]indole), **Trp-P-2** (3-amino-1-methyl-5*H*-pyrido[4,3-*b*]indole, **Glu-P-1** (2-amino-6-methyldipyrido[1,2-*a*:3',2'-*d*]imidazole), **Glu-P-2** (2-aminodipyrido[1,2-*a*:3',2'-*d*]imidazole), AαC (2-amino-9*H*-pyrido[2,3-*b*]indole), and **MeAαC** (2-amino-3-methyl-9*H*-pyrido[2,3-*b*]indole).

from pyrolysates of various amino acids. Trp-P-1 and Trp-P-2 were isolated from D,L-tryptophan pyrolysate (Sugimura *et al.*, 1977; Kosuge *et al.*, 1978), Glu-P-1 and Glu-P-2 were isolated from a pyrolysate of L-glutamic acid (Yamamoto *et al.*, 1978), and AαC and MeAαC were isolated from soy bean globulin pyrolysate (Yoshida *et al.*, 1978). The structures of these compounds are shown in Fig. 2, and the specific mutagenic activities in Ames tester strains TA 98 and TA 100 with the addition of S9 are shown in Table 1. Mutagenic substances were also isolated from L-phenylalanine (Tsuji *et al.*, 1978) and from L-lysine (Wakabayashi *et al.*, 1978). As can be seen, these pyrolysis products are potent inducers of frame-shift mutations.

Pyrolytic products of amino acids have been identified and quantified in various cooked foods. Trp-P-1 (13·3 ng/g) and Trp-P-2 (13·1 ng/g) have been found in sun-dried broiled sardine by Yamaizumi *et al.* (1980) and Trp-P-1 (53 ng/g) was isolated from broiled beef by Yamaguchi *et al.* (1980*a*). Glu-P-1 and Glu-P-2 as well as AαC and MeAαC were not detected. Glu-P-2 (280 ng/g) was, however, detected in broiled sun-dried cuttlefish by Yamaguchi *et al.* (1980*b*), but here Trp-P-1, Trp-P-2 and Glu-P-1 were not detected. AαC and MeAαC were found in various grilled foods by Matsumoto *et al.* (1981). In grilled chicken, grilled beef and

TABLE 1
Specific Mutagenic Activities of Amino Acid Pyrolysis Products and Muscle Food
Mutagens (after Sugimura, 1985)

Compound	TA 98	TA 100
MeIQ	661 000	30 000
IQ	433 000	7 000
4,8-DiMeIQ$_X$	183 000	9 000
7,8-DiMeIQ$_X$	163 000	8 000
MeIQ$_X$	145 000	14 000
Trp-P-2	104 000	1 800
Glu-P-1	49 000	3 200
Trp-P-1	39 000	1 700
Glu-P-2	1 900	1 200
AαC	300	20
MeAαC	200	120

grilled Chinese mushroom, 180, 650 and 47 ng/g of AαC and 15, 63 and 5·4 ng/g of MeAαC were found, respectively.

Metabolism
Covalent binding of Trp-P-2 to DNA *in vitro* in the presence of rat liver mircosomes from PCB-induced animals was first demonstrated by Hashimoto *et al.* (1978). A series of subsequent studies showed that the activation of these compounds to mutagenic and DNA-binding species was preferably performed by cytochrome P$_1$-450 (P-448). The highest degree of Trp-P-2 binding to calf thymus DNA *in vitro* was found when microsomes from 3-methylcholanthrene pretreated rat liver were used. PCB pretreatment was half as effective, whereas phenobarbital induction did not differ from the control situation (Nemoto *et al.*, 1979). Nebert *et al.* (1979) used benz(a)pyrene pretreated microsomes from 'responsive' and 'non-responsive' mice and showed that activation of Trp-P-1, Trp-P-2, Glu-P-1, Glu-P-2, AαC and MeAαC to TA 98 mutagens was most effective after cytochrome P-448 induction. Similar results were obtained by Yamazoe *et al.* (1980a). The efficiency of cytochrome P-448 in activating Trp-P-1 and Trp-P-2, Glu-P-1 and Glu-P-2 was convincingly demonstrated by Ishii *et al.* (1980, 1981) by comparing cytochromes P-450 and P-448 isolated from livers of PCB, 3-MC or PB pretreated animals. This was further confirmed in studies using antibodies against cytochromes P-450 (Watanabe *et al.*, 1982a).

The 3-hydroxylamine of Trp-P-2 and the 2-hydroxylamine of Glu-P-1 were shown as the active metabolites formed by rat liver microsomes, and when reacted with DNA *in vitro* the corresponding adducts to C-8 in guanine were identified (Hashimoto *et al.*, 1979*a,b*, 1980*a,b*). The reaction with DNA was limited in neutral media, whereas the *N–O*-acetylated hydroxylamines reacted readily. The significance of the *in vitro* findings was demonstrated when the same adducts with guanine were isolated from liver DNA of rats dosed intraperitoneally with Trp-P-1 or Glu-P-1 (Hashimoto *et al.*, 1982). Yamazoe *et al.* (1980*b*, 1981*a*) obtained similar results with Trp-P-2. Niwa *et al.* (1982) also suggested *N*-hydroxylation as the activation step for AαC. The cytosolic fraction of liver cells has been shown to enhance binding of Trp-P-2 to DNA (Nemoto *et al.*, 1979) and the involvement of seryl and prolyl tRNA synthetases was suggested in a further activation step for Trp-P-2 (Yamazoe *et al.*, 1981*b*, 1982, 1985). For Glu-P-1 and Glu-P-2, however, the sulphate ester of the *N*-hydroxy derivatives seemed to be more important (Nagao *et al.*, 1983*a*).

Glucuronide conjugation is known to play an important role in the detoxification of Trp-P-1 and Trp-P-2 whilst reduced glutathione (GSH) causes a decrease in mutagenic activity when intestinal S9 is used, but an increase when liver S9 is used (De Waziers and Decloître, 1984). Saito *et al.* (1983) found that the conjugation of *N*-OH-Trp-P-2 with GSH was catalysed by rat liver GSH transferase and a rat liver cytosolic fraction to yield three conjugates, one of which was even more mutagenic than *N*-OH-Trp-P-2.

After intravenous injection of ^{14}C-labelled Trp-P-1 in mice, uptake of radioactivity was seen in the lymphatic system, in the endocrine system, and in the liver, kidney medulla and brain. High radioactivity was present in the excretory pathways, especially bile and intestinal content. After 1–6 days most of the radioactivity had disappeared from the organism, except from the liver which still retained a high level. When animals were pretreated with the cytochrome P-448 inducer β-naphthoflavone a selective accumulation of radioactivity was seen in the lung parenchyma along with an increased uptake of radioactivity in the kidney cortex and small intestinal mucosa. This possibly reflects that induction of cytochrome P-448 in these organs leads to a higher persistent binding to macromolecules (Brandt *et al.*, 1983).

Mutagenesis

The pyrolysis products of amino acids, together with the muscle food mutagens to be mentioned later, have been tested in a variety of mutagenicity assays besides the Ames tests already mentioned in Table 1, and have nearly always been proven positive. Trp-P-2 and IQ were positive in a forward mutation assay for 8-azaguanine resistance in Salmonella and in a forward mutation assay for arabinose resistance in an ara D mutant of Salmonella (Felton *et al.*, 1983). Forward mutations in Chinese hamster lung (CHL) cells using diphtheria toxin resistance (DT^r) as a selective marker were induced with Trp-P-1, Trp-P-2, Glu-P-1, Glu-P-2, AαC, IQ, MeIQ and MeIQ$_X$ (Nakayasu *et al.*, 1983).

Trp-P-2 and IQ were tested in assays for cell killing, mutation of the hypoxanthine phosphoribosyltransferase (hprl) and adenine phosphoribosyltransferase (aprt) loci, sister chromatid exchanges, chromosomal aberrations, and micronuclei in Chinese hamster ovary (CHO) cells, UV-5 (hypersensitive to UV radiation because of a defect in excision repair). Trp-P-2 was found to be much more potent than IQ (Thompson *et al.*, 1983). Chromosomal aberrations and morphological transformation in hamster embryo cells were seen with Trp-P-1, Trp-P-2, Glu-P-1 and Glu-P-2 (Takayama *et al.*, 1978, 1979; Tsuda *et al.*, 1978). Trp-P-1, Trp-P-2, Glu-P-1 and AαC induced sister chromatid exchanges in a human lymphoblastoid cell line (Tohda *et al.*, 1980). Similarly, Trp-P-1, Trp-P-2, Glu-P-1, Glu-P-2, AαC and MeAαC induced structural chromosomal aberrations in a Chinese hamster lung fibroblast cell line (Ishidate *et al.*, 1981), and induction of 8-azoguanine and oubain resistance in CHL cells after treatment *in vivo* with the basic fraction of a tryptophan pyrolysate (Inui *et al.*, 1980). Finally, Trp-P-1, Trp-P-2, Glu-P-1 and Glu-P-2 induced DNA repair (UDS) in primary hepatocyte cultures (Loury and Byard, 1985), and Trp-P-2 and Glu-P-1 were positive in the mammalian spot test in mice (Jensen, 1983).

Inhibition of Mutagenicity

Yoshida and Matsumoto (1978) reported that treatment with nitrite in acidic solution to a large extent destroyed the mutagenic activity of various protein pyrolysates and of Trp-P-2. Tsuda *et al.* (1980) showed that the effect of nitrite on Trp-P-1, Trp-P-2 and Glu-P-1 was due to deamination to the corresponding hydroxy compounds. Tsuda *et al.* (1981) also noted that AαC was deaminated to the corresponding non-mutagenic hydroxy compound by nitrite, but on prolonged incubation a new mutagen not requiring S9 activation was formed. This compound was identified as 2-hydroxy-3-nitroso-α-carboline.

Other factors shown to inhibit the *in vitro* mutagenicity of pyrolysis products in the Ames test are haemin, biliverdin and chlorophyllin (Arimoto *et al.*, 1980), vitamin A (Busk *et al.*, 1982), cobaltous chloride

(Mochizuki and Kada, 1982), and extracts from a variety of vegetables such as cabbage, broccoli, green pepper, apple, pineapple and many others (Kada *et al.*, 1978; Morita *et al.*, 1978, 1982; Inoue *et al.*, 1981). It was suggested that the desmutagenic factor in cabbage is a peroxidase possessing NADPH-oxidase activity (Inoue *et al.*, 1981). The presence of a variety of polyphenols also inhibits the formation of mutagenic compounds during pyrolysis of albumin (Fukuhara *et al.*, 1981).

Carcinogenicity of Amino Acid Pyrolysis Products

Trp-P-1 and Trp-P-2. A basic fraction from a tryptophan pyrolysate was fed to groups of 5 Wistar rats for 20 months at levels of 0·2, 0·4, 0·6 and 0·8% in the diet. In the latter two groups the animals died due to toxicity. Among the rats fed 0·4%, one hepatocellular carcinoma and numerous hyperplastic nodules were found (Ishikawa *et al.*, 1979).

CDF$_1$ mice fed 0·02% Trp-P-1 or Trp-P-2 in the diet for 621 days developed hepatocellular carcinomas and adenomas. Female mice were more sensitive than male mice (Matsukura *et al.*, 1981) (Table 2). In F 344 rats fed 0·015% (male) or 0·02% (female) Trp-P-1 and 0·02% Trp-P-2, respectively, the most prominent tumours were hepatocellular carcinomas (Table 3) (Sugimura, 1985). Previously, Hosaka *et al.* (1981), feeding 0·01% of Trp-P-2 in the diet to 10 male and 10 female rats for up to 870 days, found 1 hemangioendothelial sarcoma of the liver and hyperplastic liver nodules in 6 female rats. No tumours were seen in male rats.

Glu-P-1 and Glu-P-2. CDF$_1$ mice fed 0·05% Glu-P-1 or Glu-P-2 developed hepatocellular adenomas and carcinomas (Table 2). The effect was much more prominent in females than in males. A high incidence of hemangioendothelial sarcoma, situated between the scapulae, was seen in either sex with both compounds (Ohgaki *et al.*, 1984a). In F 344 rats fed 0·05% Glu-P-1 or Glu-P-2 a high incidence of tumours was seen in several organs, notably the liver (hepatocellular adenomas and carcinomas), small and large intestine (adenomas and adenocarcinomas), zymbal gland (squamous cell carcinomas), and the clitoral gland (Table 3) (Sugimura, 1985).

AαC and MeAαC. In CDF$_1$ mice fed 0·08% of these compounds the pattern of tumour production was similar to that of the glutamic acid pyrolysis products, with tumours in the liver and blood vessels (Table 2). Half of the hemangioendothelial sarcomas induced by AαC were found in the abdominal cavity while those produced by MeAαC were situated between the scapulae (Ohgaki *et al.*, 1984a).

In F 344 rats fed 0·08% AαC for 2 years only a low incidence of cancer

TABLE 2

Carcinogenicity in CDF_1 Mice of Amino Acid Pyrolysis Products (after Sugimura, 1985)

Compound	Sex	Number of mice	Number of mice with tumours			
			Liver		Blood vessels	
			Hepatocellular adenoma	Hepatocellular carcinoma	Hemangioendo- thelioma	Hemangioendothelial sarcoma
Trp-P-1 (0·02%)	M	25	1	4	0	0
	F	24	2	14	0	0
Trp-P-2 (0·02%)	M	24	1	3	0	0
	F	26	0	22	0	0
Glu-P-1 (0·05%)	M	34	4	0	4	27
	F	38	13	24	3	28
Glu-P-2 (0·05%)	M	37	5	4	3	25
	F	36	6	30	3	19
AαC (0·08%)	M	38	6	9	2	17
	F	34	3	30	0	6
MeAαC (0·08%)	M	37	12	9	0	35
	F	33	13	15	0	28
Control	M	39 + 50 + 39	0	0	0	0
	F	40 + 50 + 40	0	0	0	0

TABLE 3
Carcinogenicity in F 344 Rats of Amino Acid Pyrolysis Products (after Sugimura, 1985)

Compound	Sex	Number of rats	Number of rats with tumours				
			Liver	Small intestine	Large intestine	Zymbal gland	Clitoral gland
Trp-P-1 (0·015%)	M	40	30	1	2	0	—
(0·02%)	F	40	37	1	0	0	0
Trp-P-2 (0·02%)	M	40	3	0	1	0	—
(0·02%)	F	40	5	2	2	2	5
Control	M	50	1	0	0	0	—
	F	50	0	0	0	0	0
Glu-P-1	M	42	35	26	19	18	—
(0·05%)	F	42	24	10	7	18	5
Glu-P-2	M	42	11	14	6	1	—
(0·05%)	F	42	2	8	8	7	11
Control	M	50	2	0	0	0	—
	F	50	0	0	0	0	0

was noted. Only 3 of 17 female rats had hepatic tumours. MeAαC at the same level showed high toxicity and the experiment was interrupted after 3 months. Severe atrophy of the salivary glands and of acinor cells of the pancreas was observed (Table 3). The experiments are being repeated using different dosage schedules (Sugimura, 1985).

It may thus be concluded that the pyrolysis products of amino acids are potent liver carcinogens in rats and mice, especially females, and that glutamic acid and soybean pyrolysates also produce tumours in various other organs.

MUTAGENS IN FOODS PROCESSED UNDER NORMAL HOUSEHOLD CONDITIONS

The Maillard Reaction

The Maillard reaction based on the non-enzymic browning reactions is essential for the development of flavours, texture and the brown pigments during heat processing of food. This is in contrast to the quality-detrimental enzymic browning reactions in fruits and vegetables where polymerization of phenols is catalysed by phenol oxidases. The palatability of cooked food is closely related to the Maillard reaction. This takes place in foods through the reaction of carbonylic compounds (e.g. aldehydes and ketones) such as reducing sugars (e.g. glucose and fructose) with compounds having free amino groups, such as amino acids, peptides and proteins. The reactions, which also take place during storage, are greatly facilitated by heat treatment of food. The chemistry is very complex and not fully understood in detail. A general scheme is shown in Figs 3–7.

The reactions can be divided into several main steps. An initial condensation of a reducing sugar with a compound having a free amino group (Fig. 3) is followed by the so-called Amadori rearrangement (Fig. 4), resulting in the formation of an Amadori compound, which readily reacts further in a series of decomposition reactions (Figs. 5, 6a, 6b). During these reactions the amine component is liberated again and can participate in new Maillard reactions. A variety of carbonylic compounds, cyclic structures and brown pigments are formed. When ammonia or hydrogen sulphide is present a variety of heterocyclic compounds are also formed. Heterocyclic structures are also formed during the so-called Strecker degradation as shown in Fig. 7.

The low molecular weight compounds formed are important for the

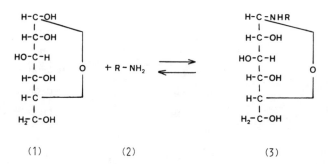

FIG. 3. Formation of aldosylamine (3) from glucose (1) and amino acid (2).

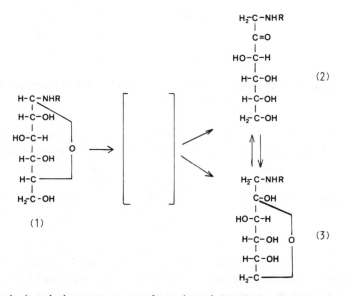

FIG. 4. Amadori rearrangement: formation of Amadori compound (2, 3) from aldosylamine (1).

flavour of cooked, baked and roasted foods. Furans, pyrones, cyclopentenes, carbonyl compounds and acids are derived from the degradation of sugar in the Maillard reaction. Simple amino acid degradation products are aldehydes and sulphur compounds. Volatile compounds formed during the subsequent reactions are pyrroles, pyridines, imidazoles, oxazoles, thiazoles and many others. A significant feature of these reactions is the

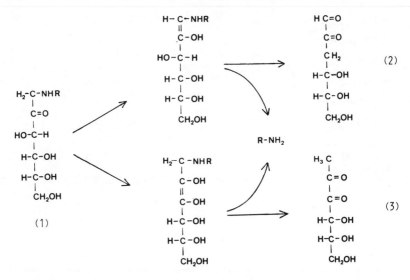

FIG. 5. Formation of enediols, 3-deoxyhexosone (2) and 1-deoxyhexosone (3), from Amadori compound (1).

ultimate formation of red/brown insoluble polymers called melanoidines. These pigments give baked, roasted and fried foods their characteristic colours. The structures of the polymers are not fully understood. The Maillard reaction has been reviewed by Baltes (1982).

The nutritive aspects of the non-enzymic browning reactions have been the object of many investigations (Björk, 1982), because amino acids are lost from the food during the reactions. The content of free amino acids in food is normally low, and does not play any significant role in nutrition. However, the nutritive value of proteins can be decreased partly due to destruction of amino acids and partly due to cross-linking which reduces the rate of protein digestion. The most vulnerable essential amino acid is lysine. Only at extreme processing conditions, leading to non-edible foods, do the losses approach 50%. During drying of milk, losses of 10–30% have been seen, but modern technology has substantially minimized the problem (Mauron, 1985).

The toxicological implication of the browning reaction recently attracted attention when Kimiagar (1979) reported changes in blood biochemistry, increased relative organ weights, and brown-black pigmentation in liver cells after feeding rats on 10% browned egg albumin for 12 months. Pintauro et al. (1983), however, did not find any toxicological effects in an

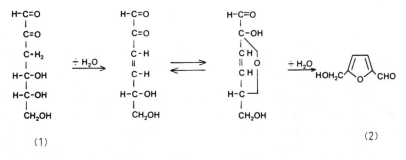

FIG. 6a. Formation of 5-hydroxymethylfurfural (2) from 3-deoxyhexosone (1).

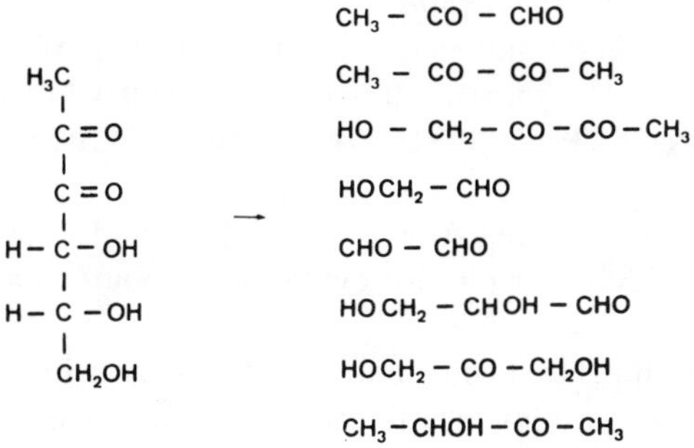

CH$_3$ – CO – CHO

CH$_3$ – CO – CO – CH$_3$

HO – CH$_2$ – CO – CO – CH$_3$

HOCH$_2$ – CHO

CHO – CHO

HOCH$_2$ – CHOH – CHO

HOCH$_2$ – CO – CH$_2$OH

CH$_3$ – CHOH – CO – CH$_3$

(1)   (2)

FIG. 6b. Formation of carbonyl compounds (2) from 1-deoxyhexosone (1).

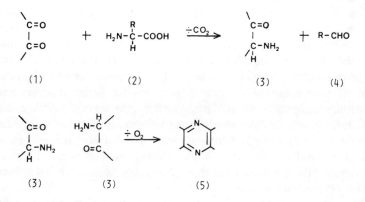

FIG. 7. Strecker degradation: formation of α-aminocarbonyl compound (3) and Strecker aldehyde (4) from dicarbonyl (1) and α-amino acid (2). Formation of pyrazine (5) from α-aminocarbonyl compound (3).

18 months rat feeding study using 3% browned egg albumin, and moreover explained the earlier observed changes as a result of nutritive or dietary imbalance. Furthermore, extracts of the browned egg albumin used by Pintauro *et al.* (1983) did not show any mutagenic activity in the Ames test (Pintauro *et al.*, 1980).

A commercial thermally processed flavour product prepared by heating wheat gluten hydrolysate, glucose or xylose and L-cysteine was claimed to be non-carcinogenic when fed to rats and mice (Wilson, 1982). A flavour product based on protein, amino acids, carbohydrates and fats was also shown to lack carcinogenicity in rats (Wilson, 1982).

Mutagenicity of Maillard Reaction Products
A number of short-term mutagenicity tests has been performed on model browning systems. The short-term toxicity of Maillard reaction products has been reviewed by Elias (1982), Powrie *et al.* (1982), Shibamoto (1982) and Barnes *et al.* (1983).

Results obtained in the Ames test with model browning systems incubated at 90–120°C for one to several hours point to a very complex situation.

When the testing has been done directly on the incubated mixture without extractions, a tendency towards activity in tester strain TA 100 without addition of S9 has been observed. This was demonstrated by Omura *et al.* (1983) using model browning systems with glucose and a variety of different amino acids (Table 4). Direct activity towards TA 100 was also seen by Powrie *et al.* (1981) who treated fructose with various amino acids (arginine, lysine, serine, glutamine, glutamic acid) at 121°C for 1 h. Bjeldanes and Chew (1979) found that 1,2-dicarbonyl compounds such as glyoxal and diacetyl, known to be formed during the Maillard reaction, were mutagenic in TA 100 without S9. Powrie *et al.* (1981) suggested that reductones, such as enediol, enaminol, enediamine, thiol-enol and enamine-thiol, intermediates in the Strecker degradation reaction, may have contributed to the activity. Omura *et al.* (1983) isolated 3 mutagenic substances: 5-hydroxymethylfurfural (glucose and phenyl-alanine), α-(2-formyl-5-hydroxymethylpyrrol-7-yl)norleucine (glucose and lysine) and 2-methylthiazolidine (glucose and cysteine). Mihara and Shibamoto (1980) also isolated mutagenic thiazolidine derivatives from a glucose–cysteamine system.

When the model browning systems have been subjected to extraction with dichloromethane in order to obtain volatile fractions, the impression is that the major mutagenic compounds present in these fractions were the

TABLE 4
Mutagenicity of Glucose (1M) and Amino Acid (1M) Model Browning Systems[a]
(after Omura et al., 1983)

Amino acid	TA 100		TA 98	
	−S9	+S9	−S9	+S9
Glutamic acid	103	153	37	25
Glutamine	309	138	60	49
Lysine	739	297	16	32
Arginine	754	235	34	97
Phenylalanine	253	365	21	36
Tryptophan	139	153	16	9
Tyrosine	178	142	19	19
Cysteine	213	1 669	76	159
Cystine	198	131	24	82
Methionine	262	179	20	26
Proline	183	153	30	37
Glycine	451	130	47	240
Alanine	566	133	23	36
Valine	277	138	0	87
Leucine	269	167	29	52
Isoleucine	319	224	30	36
Serine	257	161	14	37
Threonine	315	103	15	0
Aspartic acid	173	86	41	56
Asparagine	146	164	27	39
Control	129	136	28	33

[a] 10 h reflux at 100°C; 0·2 ml/plate.

frame-shift type, active in Ames tester strain TA 98, and often requiring activation with S9 mix. Spingarn and Garvie (1979) found mutagenic activity in TA 98 with S9 in the dichloromethane extracts of model systems each containing one of various sugars (arabinose, 2-deoxyglucose, galactose, glucose, rhamnose, xylose) and ammonia. The systems had been refluxed for 2 h or 6 h. The development of mutagenic activity followed the formation of pyrazines, but the simple alkylpyrazines were not mutagenic in the assay. Stich et al. (1980) also found no mutagenic activity in the Ames test with pyrazine and four of its alkyl derivatives (2-methyl-2-ethyl-, 2,5-dimethyl-, 2,6-dimethyl-pyrazine), but the compounds were highly active in inducing chromosomal aberrations in Chinese hamster ovary (CHO) cells.

Shibamoto et al. (1981) obtained mutagenic activity towards TA 98 with S9 activation in dichloromethane extracts of a maltol–ammonia browning model system at 100°C for 5 h. Toda et al. (1981) similarly found TA 98 + S9 positive activity in an L-rhamnose–ammonia–hydrogen sulphide system kept at 90°C for 5 h. Approximately 300 different compounds were detected using GLC. The fraction containing alkylimidazoles was the most active, but authentic reference compounds did not show mutagenic activity.

1,5(or 7)-Dimethyl-2,3,6,7-tetrahydro-1H,5H-biscyclopentapyrazine, mutagenic towards TA 98 without S9 mix, was isolated by Shibamoto (1980) from a dichloromethane extract of a cyclotene–ammonia system kept at 90°C for 2 h.

Powrie et al. (1981), in their investigation of glucose and fructose model systems with arginine, lysine, histidine, serine, glutamic acid and glutamine at 121°C for 1 h, besides the mutagenic activity in TA 100 without S9, also found mutagenic and recombinogenic activity in Saccharomyces cerevisiae D5 and potent clastogenic activity in CHO cells. Again the addition of S9 was not required. As mentioned earlier, a series of alkylpyrazines were clastogenic in CHO cells without being active in the Ames test (Stich et al., 1980), and furthermore it was shown that a series of furan derivatives also present in browning mixtures was clastogenic in CHO cells without showing activity in the Ames test (Stich et al., 1981a).

Clastogenic activity was found in caramelized sugars (sucrose, glucose, mannose, arabinose, maltose, fructose) as well as in a commercial ammonia caramel powder (Stich et al., 1981b). Mutagenic activity toward TA 100 without S9 addition was also found in a commercial ammonia caramel sample. The activity was strongly enhanced when preincubation was introduced into the Ames assay, and moreover the activity only showed up very late in the manufacturing process at the same time as the brown colour developed (Jensen et al., 1983).

All these results indicate that a diversity of compounds with differing genotoxic activities in various short-term test systems can be formed during the non-enzymic browning of food, and that their detection should not rely on one single test only.

The genotoxic effects in S. cerevisiae of a glucose–lysine system and of a commercial ammonia caramel powder were depressed by trace metals (Cu II and Fe III) in concentrations normally present in body fluids. Several cellular enzymic systems (horse-radish peroxidase, beef liver catalase and rat liver S9) also inhibited the activity (Rosin et al., 1982). Furthermore, Chan et al. (1982) were able to show significant suppression by a lysine–fructose mixture (121°C for 2 h) and caramelized sucrose (180°C for 1·5 h) of the mutagenic activity of N-methyl-N^1-nitro-N-nitrosoguanidine in TA 1535 and aflatoxin B_1 in TA 98+ S9.

Although the N-nitroso compounds are not included in this review, it should be mentioned that it has been shown that some members of this important class of carcinogens can be formed during the nitrosation of certain Maillard reaction products, the Amadori compounds. The Amadori compounds contain secondary amino groups easily nitrosated by the reaction with nitrite. The N-nitroso derivatives of several D-fructose-amino acids have been tested in Ames tests. Among the compounds tested, the alanine, phenylalanine and aspartic acid compounds were not mutagenic, the glycine and serine compounds showed low activity in TA 1535 without S9, while nitrosated D-fructose-L-tryptophan (NO-Trp-Fru) was mutagenic in all strains tested both with and without S9. Trp-Fru can be nitrosated at three different sites, so the exact composition of the mutagenic component is not known (Pool et al., 1984). Similar results were obtained with NO-Trp-Fru by Russel (1983). NO-Trp-Fru also caused a large increase in DNA repair in HeLa S3 cells even at concentrations below 1 μM (Lynch et al., 1983). Other products of the Maillard reaction, the thiazolidines, are known to be easily nitrosated to mutagenic compounds. Sekizawa and Shibamoto (1980) demonstrated mutagenic activity of N-nitrosothiazolidine and several 2-alkyl-N-nitrosothiazolidines in TA 98 and TA 100. A series of 2-hydroxyalkyl-N-nitrosothiazolidines was not mutagenic towards TA 98, while a few showed activity in TA 100 (Umano et al., 1984). N-Nitrosothiazolidine also showed positive responses in the rec assay in Bacillus subtilis, and induced DNA repair in primary rat hepatocyte cultures (Loury et al., 1984).

It seems that several N-nitroso compounds, not detectable with the analytical methods currently used in nitrosamine analysis of foods, can be easily formed during cooking and smoking of cured meat and fish by nitrosation of Maillard reaction products.

Mutagenic Activity in Heat-processed Food

When broiled cuttlefish was analysed for the amino acid pyrolysis products it was discovered that these compounds could account for only 5% of the total mutagenic activity (Yamaguchi *et al.*, 1980*b*). Similar results were obtained with broiled beef and sun-dried sardines (Yamaguchi *et al.*, 1980*a*; Kasai *et al.*, 1980*a*).

While the formation of the pyrolysis products seemed to depend on rather high temperatures (more than 300°C) not normally used in the cooking of foods, Commoner *et al.* (1978) found mutagenic activity towards TA 1538 when they tested dichloromethane extracts of the *basic fractions* from pan-fried ground beef (plate temperature 200°C) and from commercial beef extract. The activity required metabolic activation by S9 fraction from PCB treated rats. In a series of experiments using an aqueous beef stock solution, Dolara *et al.* (1979) predicted a sharp rise in the rate of mutagen formation in beef between 140°C and 180°C. This was confirmed by frying ground beef patties at different temperatures. Patties cooked at 100°C in a microwave oven for 5–10 min contained no frame-shift mutagens, whereas frying at 190–210°C for 3–6 min yielded significant mutagenic activity in the surface crust.

The influence of cooking times and temperatures on mutagen formation in ground beef has been studied in more detail by Spingarn and Weisburger (1979) and Pariza *et al.* (1979*a*). Using Ames tester strain TA 98, Spingarn and Weisburger (1979) showed that pan-frying of beef patties did not lead to mutagen formation until the surface temperature of the patties after a lag period of 5 min exceeded 100°C. Thereafter a sharp rise in temperature (up to 250°C) and mutagen formation occurred. Broiling over charcoal showed a lag period of 35 min before a sharp rise in the mutagenic activity occurred, and the surface temperature only reached 130°C. Pariza *et al.* (1979*a*) showed temperature to be the most important parameter for mutagen production in pan-fried hamburger. Frying at 143°C for 20 min only produced low activity, whereas 191°C and 210°C for up to 10 min gave high activities. Lag periods of 4–6 min were noted. The lag period occurs while water is evaporated from the surface of the meat.

A considerable amount of data now exists on the TA 98 or TA 1538 mutagenic activity in heat-processed foods (Pariza *et al.*, 1979*b*; Spingarn *et al.*, 1980*a*; Krone and Iwaoka, 1981; Bjeldanes *et al.*, 1982*a,b*;

Hargraves and Pariza, 1984). From these studies it appears that the formation of frame-shift mutagens in high activity occurs almost only in muscle foods, such as fried ground beef, broiled beef steak, fried ham, fried pork chops, fried sausages, broiled chicken and broiled lamb. Egg and egg products produce mutagens only after cooking at very high temperatures. Seafood samples show varying results; high temperatures are normally required for mutagen formation.

Many other heat-processed foods such as crackers, corn flakes, rice cereals, bread crust, biscuit, pancake and fried potato contain TA 98 mutagens in their basic fractions, but always in low activity, well below that in muscle foods. However, when it was investigated (Springarn et al., 1980a), notable activity towards TA 100 appeared in starchy foods.

Regarding cooking methods, it appears that only low levels of TA 98 mutagenic activity are produced when ground beef is microwaved, stewed, simmered, boiled or deep-fat fried. Baking, roasting and broiling produce moderate activity, while frying produces the highest activity.

Mutagens in Heat-processed Muscle Food

A new class of mutagenic heterocyclic amines, the amino-imidazo azarenes (Fig. 8), have been isolated from heat-processed muscle food. IQ and MeIQ were isolated from broiled sun-dried sardines and $MeIQ_x$ was together with IQ isolated from fried beef (Kasai et al., 1979, 1980a,b,c; 1981a,b,c; Springarn et al., 1980b; Sugimura and Iitaka, 1980).

Recently, Felton et al. (1985) isolated, as major mutagens in fried ground beef, $4,8\text{-DiMeIQ}_x$ (2-amino-3,4,8-trimethylimidazo[4, 5-f]quinoxaline), PIP (2-amino-6-phenyl-N-methylimidazo[4,5-b]pyridine), and an aminotrimethyl-imidazopyridine called TIP, where the exact positions of the methyl groups have not yet been fully clarified.

The isolation and quantification of the small amounts of these mutagens present in heat-processed food are an extremely difficult analytical chemical task. Consequently, there is as yet little quantitative data on their presence in cooked food.

In the studies performed in Japan, 158 ppb of IQ and 72 ppb of MeIQ were determined in sun-dried sardines cooked over an open flame, and 0·6 ppb of IQ and 2·4 ppb of $MeIQ_x$ were found in beef cooked on an electric hot plate (Nagao et al., 1983b). The most thorough studies on fried ground beef have been performed by Hargraves and Pariza (1983) and in particular by Felton et al. (1984a, 1985). From these studies it appears that $MeIQ_x$ $4,8\text{-DiMeIQ}_x$, TIP and PIP are the major mutagens, comprising approximately 75% of the total mutagenic activity and more than 90% of

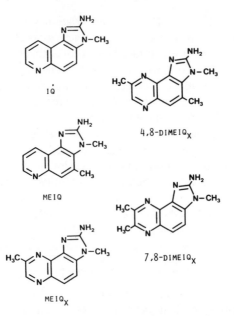

FIG. 8. Structures of **IQ** (2-amino-3-methylimidazo[4,5-*f*]quinoline), **MeIQ** (2-amino-3,4-dimethylimidazo[4,5-*f*]quinoline), **MeIQ**x (2-amino-3,8-dimethyl-imidazo[4,5-*f*]quinoxaline), **4,8-DiMeIQx** (2-amino-3,4,8-trimethyl-imidazo[4,5-*f*]quinoxaline), and **7,8-DiMeIQx** (2-amino-3,7,8-trimethyl-imidazo[4,5-*f*]quinoxaline).

the mass of mutagenic constituents in fried beef. Smaller amounts of IQ and MeIQ were isolated (<10% of the mutagenicity). The remaining mutagenicity was made up by a number of polar compounds (approx. 3%) and an oxygen-containing non-polar compound (approx. 12%). These compounds have not yet been identified. Felton *et al.* (1985) estimate that the total mutagenic activity in TA 1538 of approximately 300 000 revertants per kg in fried ground beef (fresh weight) is due to approximately 20 μg of mutagenic amino-imidazo azarenes. IQ and MeIQ$_x$ have so far been found in the highest amounts in certain types of commercial beef extracts, where IQ levels in the range 18–141 μg/kg and MeIQ$_x$ levels of 34–527 μg/kg have been reported (Hargraves and Pariza, 1984).

In many countries pork is a more important food than beef. Mutagenic activity has been detected in fried pork at a rate comparable to fried beef (Baker *et al.*, 1982; Bjeldanes *et al.*, 1982a; Gocke *et al.*, 1982, Övervik *et al.*, 1984). Fried bacon, both nitrite-free and nitrite-treated, also contained considerable mutagenic activity towards TA 98 + S9 when the alkaline dichloromethane extract was tested; volatile nitrosamines were not detected (Miller and Buchanan, 1983). In a series of experiments performed at our institute, Vahl *et al.* (1985) have shown, using extraction and isolation procedures similar to Felton *et al.* (1984*a*), that the mutagenic profile in fried ground pork is very similar to that found by Felton *et al.* (1985) in fried ground beef, both qualitatively and quantitatively.

Several factors are known to modify the mutagenic activity of the basic extract of fried ground beef.

Oleic acid is able to inhibit the mutagenic activity in fried beef. Hayatsu *et al.* (1981) ascribed the inhibitory action of the acidic fraction of cooked beef to its content of oleic acid.

Spingarn *et al.* (1981) showed that the fat content in ground beef was of importance for the formation of mutagenic activity after pan-frying at 180–185°C. 0–35% of surrounding fat was added to carefully trimmed lean meat. Mutagenicity reached a peak at 10% added fat and thereafter decreased, but at 15–35% added fat it was still an order of magnitude above samples with 0–5% fat. It should be noted that most other studies on mutagenicity formation in ground beef have been on meat containing between 15% and 25% of fat.

Decreased formation of mutagens during frying was seen by Wang *et al.* (1982) when soy protein concentrate was added, and the food additive BHA also suppressed the mutagen formation.

Model Studies on the Formation of the Amino-imidazo Azarenes
Spingarn and Weisburger (1979) suggested that the Maillard reaction (non-enzymic browning reactions) was important for the formation of mutagens in fried ground beef. Later, Jägerstad *et al.* (1982) suggested that creatinine and Maillard reaction products were important precursors for IQ, MeIQ and MeIQ$_x$. It was proposed that MeIQ$_x$ could be formed from creatinine, 2,5-dimethylpyrazine (formed in the Maillard reaction from reducing sugars such as glucose or fructose) and glycine. The active principle from glycine was thought to be formaldehyde or the corresponding Schiff base formed in the Strecker degradation of glycine (Fig. 9). By analogy, the formation of IQ would require creatinine, 2-methylpyridine and glycine, while the formation of MeIQ required creatinine, 2-methylpyridine and alanine. Thus the theory was that the quinoline structure (IQ, MeIQ) would arise from a condensation between pyridines and aldehydes, and the quinoxaline structure (MeIQ$_x$) as a result of condensation between pyrazines and aldehydes. Condensation with

creatinine would then account for the imidazo structure. Creatinine is readily formed in muscle food from creatine. Using a model system where creatinine, glucose and various free amino acids were refluxed for 2 h at 128°C in aqueous diethylene glycol, Jägerstad et al. (1983) could easily detect mutagenic activity towards TA 98 and S9. Threonine, glycine, lysine and alanine were the amino acids that produced the highest activities.

Jägerstad et al. (1984) isolated MeIQ$_x$ from such a model system after heating a mixture of creatinine, glucose and glycine, and MeIQ$_x$ accounted for 90% of the total mutagenic activity. Later, Negishi et al. (1984) showed

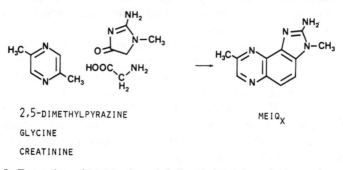

2,5-DIMETHYLPYRAZINE

GLYCINE

CREATININE

MEIQ$_x$

FIG. 9. Formation of **MeIQ$_x$** from 2,5-dimethylpyrazine, glycine and creatinine (after Jägerstad et al., 1983).

that the other mutagen present was 7,8-DiMeIQ$_x$. Substituting threonine for glycine in the model system yielded MeIQ$_x$ (25%) and 4,8-DiMeIQ$_x$ (75%), and the total mutagenic activity was 6 times higher than in the previous study (Jägerstad et al., 1985). 4,8-DiMeIQ$_x$ was also produced as the main mutagenic component with a mixture of creatinine, fructose and alanine (Grivas et al., 1986).

From these studies it appears that an important factor, besides the cooking temperature and time, is the content in the meat of possible precursors such as creatinine, reducing sugars and free amino acids. The naturally occurring concentrations of these compounds in fresh muscle amount to approximately 4200 ppm of glucose and glucose phosphates, 600 ppm of fructose-6-phosphate, 4000 ppm of creatine and 1000–3000 ppm of total free amino acids (Jägerstad et al., 1985). The low yield of mutagens in the model systems, and the fact that the reaction only takes place at the surface of the meat, favoured by the high temperatures and low water content, may explain why these compounds are only formed in ppb quantities in heat-processed foods.

Toxicological Studies with Basic Fractions from Cooked Muscle Foods
Dolara *et al.* (1980) did not find mutagenic activity in the intrasanguine host-mediated assay (TA 98) in mice dosed with the basic fraction of fried ground beef, nor was mutagenic activity detected in urine of mice following oral or intraperitoneal administration. Felton *et al.* (1980) have reported that the basic fraction from grilled hamburger, at a level which was highly mutagenic towards Salmonella, induced toxicity in various mouse hepatoma cell lines and in CHO cells. Sister chromatid exchanges, however, were not seen in the bone marrow of mice.

Basic fractions from ground pork sausages fried at temperatures up to 230°C for various periods (2–25 min) were found to be highly mutagenic in TA 1538 and TA 98 assays (Gocke *et al.*, 1982). In the intrasanguine host-mediated assay (TA 98) in PCB-pretreated NMRI mice, only low activity was observed, whereas borderline activity on SCE induction was seen in V 79 Chinese hamster cells. No activity was found in the assay for thioguanine resistance with V 79 cells, in Drosophila sex-linked recessive lethal test, in micronucleus test (single i.p. injection) in NMRI mice, and in the mouse spot test using female C57BL6 mice.

Mutagenic activity toward TA 98 and TA 1538 + S9 was detected by Baker *et al.* (1982) in human urine after ingestion of 150 g of either fried bacon or pork. The bacon and pork were fried at 150–190°C until well done, but not charred. Urine samples were concentrated using XAD-2. The majority of mutagenic activity was recovered within 2–4 h after eating the fried meat, but activity could be demonstrated for up to 24 h. Incubation of urine with β-glucuronidase did not enhance the activity. The activity in urine had chemical and biological characteristics similar to those found in the basic fractions of fried bacon or pork. The total mutagenic activity recovered in urine accounted for one-third of the total mutagenic activity ingested.

Toxicological Studies with Amino-imidazo Azarenes

Metabolism
Using liver microsomes from PCB-pretreated rats, Okamoto *et al.* (1981) identified a reactive metabolite of IQ as 2-hydroxyamino-3-methyl-imidazo[4,5-*f*]quinoline, the *N*-hydroxylated derivative of IQ. The compound was very unstable, and could only be detected after short incubation times, the half-life being about 1 min at room temperature. *N*-OH-IQ was synthesized, and was found readily to bind covalently to calf thymus DNA under neutral conditions. Watanabe *et al.* (1982*a*), by using

specific antibodies, showed that IQ is activated by cytochrome P-448. Watanabe et al. (1982b) also showed that IQ, MeIQ and MeIQ$_x$ without metabolic activation show strong non-covalent binding (intercalation) to DNA, and that the binding correlates well with the mutagenicity in TA 98 assays.

Yamazoe et al. (1983) further showed the mutagenic metabolite of IQ formed in rat liver microsomes to be 2-hydroxyamino-3-methylimidazo[4, 5-f]quinoline. The N-hydroxylation and mutagenicity were demonstrated to be catalysed by a high-spin form of cytochrome P-450, P-448 II-a, induced by 3-MC and PCB in the rat (Yamazoe et al., 1984).

There is evidence that in the Salmonella strain TA 98 the ultimate reactive species of IQ, MeIQ and MeIQ$_x$ are the sulphate esters of their N-hydroxy derivatives (Nagao et al., 1983a). In primary monolayer cultures of rat hepatocytes the involvement of sulphate conjugation in IQ activation seems to be much less than in Salmonella (Loretz and Pariza, 1984). In these cells glutathione provided a strong protective effect against the covalent binding of IQ to macromolecules, thus implicating gluta-thione conjugation as an important detoxification pathway.

An important study was conducted by Felton and Healy (1984) who used human liver microsomes in the Ames/Salmonella assay (TA 1538) to activate the basic fraction from fried ground beef, known to contain MeIQ$_x$ and 4,8-DiMeIQ$_x$ as the major mutagens. Microsomes from all six human livers were significantly more active than microsomes from uninduced rats or mice, with microsomes from one person being almost as active as PCB-induced rodent liver microsomes. The activation was inhibited by β-naphthoflavone, thus showing that the human liver microsomes con-tained the inducible form(s) of cytochrome P-448.

Sjödin and Jägerstad (1984), using 2-^{14}C-labelled IQ and MeIQ, have shown that after oral intubation in rats more than 90% of the radioactivity is excreted within 24 h. After 72 h the faecal excretion accounted for 50–60% of both compounds in males and 40–50% in female rats. The urinary excretion amounted to 37–48%. Only 1–2% was left in the carcass after 72 h. In a separate experiment in male rats where bile was collected, about 70% of IQ and 80% of MeIQ were found in the bile. Mutagenicity was found in the bile closely following the excretion of radioactivity while no mutagenicity was detected in the urine, but the presence of several metabolites was indicated. It thus appears that IQ and MeIQ are readily absorbed, undergo metabolism and enterohepatic circulation, and are rapidly excreted in urine and faeces. Essentially similar results have been obtained using 2-^{14}C-MeIQ$_x$ (Sjödin and Jägerstad, 1985; Sjödin et al., 1985).

When beef extract or the basic fraction of beef extract was dosed orally to rats, mutagenicity (TA 1538 + S9) could be easily detected in the stomach content, the bile and the urine. No mutagenicity was detected in blood samples (Münzner and Wever, 1984).

The distribution of intravenously injected ^{14}C-labelled IQ and MeIQ was investigated by whole-body autoradiography in mice (Bergman, 1984, personal communication). The compounds showed a similar distribution pattern. Shortly after administration, radioactivity began to accumulate in metabolic and excretory organs (liver, kidney, urine, gastric and intestinal contents), as well as in lymphomyeloid tissues (bone marrow, thymus, spleen, lymph nodes) and endocrine and reproductive tissues. After longer time periods non-extractable radioactivity was retained only in the liver and kidney. IQ and MeIQ passed the placenta, but were not retained in foetal tissues.

Mutagenicity

These compounds are potent frame-shift mutagens in Salmonella (TA 1538, TA 98, TA 97). IQ gives only weak response in TA 96, a frame-shift strain which is specific for changes in adenine or thymine, not guanine or cytosine. It thus appears that IQ is specific for G/C change (Felton *et al.*, 1984*b*). Comparing the activity in Salmonella strains TA 1538 (a uvr B repair deficient strain) and TA 1978 (a strain sufficient for uvr B repair), the TA 1538 strain was 30–50-fold more active (Thompson *et al.*, 1983). The result indicates that the excision repair operates on the type of damage produced by IQ.

When the effect of IQ and Trp-P-2 was compared in normal CHO cells it was shown that Trp-P-2 in concentrations below 1 μg/ml produced dose-dependent increases in cell killing, gene mutations, sister chromatid exchanges and chromosomal aberrations, whereas IQ in concentrations from 10 to more than 100 μg/ml produced some cell killing but no genotoxic effect. A clear-cut response on the genetic end-point was only seen when IQ in concentrations above 10 μg/ml was tested in an excision repair deficient mutant strain (UV-5) (Thompson *et al.*, 1983). It appears that CHO cells are much more resistant to the genetic effects of IQ than bacterial cells. Most probably the active metabolite of IQ is too reactive to reach the nuclear target in the CHO cells. This postulate is supported by DNA binding studies in CHO cells, which show that IQ and Trp-P-2 have roughly the same mutagenic efficiency (4 mutations per 1000 adducts bound), but that IQ binding is very low compared to Trp-P-2 binding (Brookman *et al.*, 1985).

In CHL cells, IQ, MeIQ and MeIQ$_x$ showed mutagenic activity when diphtheria toxin resistance was used as a marker. In the same system Trp-P-2 and Trp-P-1 showed higher activity, while Glu-P-1 and Glu-P-2 showed lower activity (Nakayasu *et al.*, 1983). Caderni *et al.* (1983) found a dose-related genotoxic effect of IQ in radiation-induced mouse leukaemia cells as judged by alkaline elution of DNA. Several studies have also demonstrated that IQ and MeIQ are potent inducers of unscheduled DNA synthesis (repair) in primary cultures of rat hepatocytes (Barnes *et al.*, 1985; Loury and Byard, 1985).

At rather high doses (200–800 mg/kg), single oral doses of IQ and MeIQ induced nuclear damage to colon epithelial cells. In this respect these compounds were more potent than the pyrolysates of amino acids (Bird and Bruce, 1984). The ability to induce this effect has been observed with various known colon carcinogens, whereas carcinogens with different organ specificities generally have not induced the lesion (Wargovich *et al.*, 1983).

In vivo cytogenetic effects (sister chromatid exchanges and chromosomal aberrations) of IQ and Trp-P-2 were investigated by Minkler and Carrano (1984) in mouse bone marrow. Trp-P-2 significantly induced both lesions, while IQ produced only a weak (but significant) increase in sister chromatid exchanges.

Inhibition of Mutagenicity

Chlorinated tap water inactivates the mutagenic activity of the amino-imidazo azarenes and the amino acid pyrolysis products (Tsuda *et al.*, 1983) but, in contrast to the pyrolysis products, the mutagenic activity of the former compounds is not inhibited by nitrous acid (Hatch *et al.*, 1982). Sjödin *et al.* (1985) have shown that IQ, MeIQ and $MeIQ_x$ are bound to various vegetable fibres *in vitro*.

Carcinogenicity of the Amino-imidazo Azarenes

The chemical synthesis of these mutagens, especially the quinoxaline type of compounds, is difficult and the yields are rather low. Therefore, amounts large enough to perform long-term animal experiments have been difficult to obtain, and furthermore are expensive. The only carcinogenicity studies to have been completed so far are studies with IQ in F 344 rats and CDF_1 mice. As seen from Tables 5 and 6, IQ was found to be a multipotent carcinogen in both mice and rats. In the rat in particular, tumours were seen at many sites after a daily dose corresponding to approximately 15 mg/kg body weight (Ohgaki *et al.*, 1984*b*; Sugimura, 1985).

TABLE 5
Carcinogenicity of IQ in Mice (after Ohgaki et al., 1984b)

Compound	Sex	Number of animals	Hepatocellular adenoma	Hepatocellular carcinoma	Forestomach papilloma	Forestomach squamous cell carcinoma	Lung adenoma	Lung carcinoma
						Number of mice with tumours		
IQ (0·03%)	M	39	8	8	11	5	13	14
	F	36	5	22	8	3	7	8
Control	M	33	2	0	1	0	4	3
	F	38	0	0	0	0	3	4

TABLE 6
Carcinogenicity of IQ in the Rat (after Sugimura, 1985)

Compound	Sex	Number of rats	Number of rats with tumours							
			Liver	Large intestine	Small intestine	Zymbal gland	Skin	Clitoral gland	Oral cavity
IQ	M	40	27	25	12	36	17	—	2
(0·03%)	F	40	18	9	1	27	3	20	1
Control	M	50	1	0	0	0	0	—	0
	F	50	0	0	0	0	0	0	0

IQ was given to female rats at a dose of approximately 80 mg/kg body weight 3 times a week for 4 weeks, then twice a week in weeks 5–8 followed by once a week for the next 23 weeks. The animals were killed 52 weeks after the first dose. The diet contained 15% added corn oil (total fat 20%). Out of 32 rats, 14 developed mammary carcinomas. Tumours were also seen in the liver and ear duct (Barnes *et al.*, 1984, personal communication).

Carcinogenicity studies on MeIQ and MeIQ$_x$ are in progress (Sugimura, 1985). In mice fed 0·04% MeIQ the development of forestomach tumours and hepatic tumours has so far been observed. With MeIQ$_x$ at a dose of 0·06% in the diet, intestinal tumours have already been noted.

DISCUSSION

It is now well established that heat-processing of a variety of foods leads to the formation of mutagenic compounds. In particular, frying, grilling and broiling of protein-rich foods, especially meat derived from animal muscle tissue, result in the formation of extremely potent Salmonella mutagens (amino acid pyrolysis products and amino-imidazo azarenes).

When tested in animal carcinogenesis assays the compounds so far investigated have proven carcinogenic in mice and rats. They therefore deserve serious attention as a potential hazard to human health.

The TA 1538 and TA 98 positive mutagens have as yet only been found in trace quantities (at the ppb level) in heat-processed food, while the carcinogenesis assays have been conducted with much higher amounts in single dose level experiments. This makes a quantitative risk evaluation extremely difficult. Another complicating factor is that the muscle food mutagens initially isolated and subsequently tested in mutagenesis and carcinogenesis assays (IQ and MeIQ) do not seem to be the major mutagens present in cooked meat. Recent analytical chemical progress has revealed the presence of other mutagens. Therefore the final evaluation must await developments in the difficult chemical synthesis of such compounds as MeIQ$_x$, DiMeIQ$_x$s, TIP and PIP, in order to provide enough material to perform further toxicological studies. These might be carcinogenic and toxico-kinetic studies using graduated dose schedules, and should hopefully also include realistic mixtures of the compounds in question.

In order to fulfil the latter requirement, more knowledge is also needed on the amounts and composition of mutagens present in several different heat-processed foods. This will require the development of simple but nevertheless reliable analytical procedures. The procedures currently used are highly time-consuming, require the use of sophisticated analytical equipment, and are not suitable for screening of heat-processed foods.

An important area of research will be the toxico-kinetic properties of the compounds in question, with special attention paid to the various factors in our daily diet that potentially could modify the action of the mutagens. Such factors of importance could be dietary fibres, fats, enzyme inducing agents, antioxidants, desmutagenic factors in vegetables, and many others.

Although the current interest in relation to heat-processed mutagens is concentrated on the amino-imidazo azarenes formed in muscle food, the possible presence of the N-nitroso compounds and the pyrolysis products including PAH should not be forgotten. All these compounds must ultimately be evaluated together. As judged from the mutagenicity data and animal carcinogenicity data, they all seem to be potent initiators of cancer, and they may well act together in this respect in the human situation.

The theory that initiation is followed by promotion in the carcinogenic process puts an important question on the predictive value of the results from long-term animal experiments with the cooked food mutagens. Is the potency recorded in such assays predictive for the situation in humans? Are, for instance, the amino-imidazo azarenes very potent initiators, but at the same time only weak promoters? If so, the outcome of the animal studies may lead to an underestimation of their significance in human diet through which man is also exposed to other promotional factors, such as high fat, not normally included in the animal studies.

When discussing mutagens in heat-processed foods there is a tendency to forget or exclude the TA 100 mutagenic compounds that are formed during the Maillard reactions. This is probably due to the fact that they do not possess extreme potency, and perhaps also that model systems such as the food additive ammonia caramel have not shown carcinogenicity in rodent studies. However, from a scientific point of view it seems important to take a closer look at these mutagens. It is noteworthy that several Maillard reaction model systems have been shown to possess potent clastogenic activity in mammalian *in vitro* systems. This poses the question whether this effect is mediated via active oxygen species. The generation of active oxygen within the cells is now thought to have an important role in tumour promotion. It would therefore be of great interest to investigate whether the Maillard reaction mutagens play any role *in vivo*. If this is the case, it should be clarified whether the natural defence systems against active oxygen species in the organism are sufficient to counteract any potential promotional effect from heat-processed foods.

Although a substantial part of the food we eat undergoes culinary, palatability increasing, heat-processing, such as boiling, baking, broiling, roasting, frying or smoking, this aspect has not been emphasized in the majority of the epidemiological studies carried out. Therefore no definitive conclusions are available regarding the health significance of heat-processing practices in human disease.

However, the presence of potent mutagens in heat-processed foods is a challenge to the risk evaluation of foods, but there is a long way to go, analytically, toxicologically and epidemiologically, before a final answer can be given.

REFERENCES

Adrian, J., Billaud, C. and Rabache, M. (1984). Part of technological processes in the occurrence of benzo(a)pyrene in foods. *World Rev. Nutr. Diet*, **44**, 155–84.

Ames, B. N., McCann, J. and Yamasaki, E. (1975). Methods for detecting carcinogens and mutagens with the Salmonella/mammalian microsome test. *Mutat. Res.*, **31**, 347–64.

Arimoto, S., Ohara, Y., Namba, T., Negishi, T. and Hayatsu, H. (1980). Inhibition of the mutagenicity of amino acid pyrolysis products by hemin and other biological pyrrole pigments. *Biochem. Biophys. Res. Commun.*, **92**(2), 662–8.

Baker, R., Arlauskas, A., Bonin, A. and Ancus, D. (1982). Detection of mutagenic activity in human urine following fried pork or bacon meals. *Cancer Lett.*, **16**, 81–9.

Baltes, W. (1982). Chemical changes in food by the Maillard reaction. *Food Chem.*, **9**, 59–73.

Barnes, W., Spingarn, N. E., Garvie-Gould, C., Vuolo, L. L., Wang, Y. Y. and Weisburger, J. H. (1983). Mutagens in cooked foods: possible consequences of the Maillard reaction. In: *The Maillard Reaction in Foods and Nutrition*, ACS Symposium Series 215, G. R. Waller and M. Feather (Eds), American Chemical Society, Washington, DC, pp. 485–506.

Barnes, W. S., Lovelette, C. A., Tong, C., Williams, G. M. and Weisburger, J. H. (1985). Genotoxicity of the food mutagen 2-amino-3-methylimidazo[4,5-f]quinoline (IQ) and analogs. *Carcinogenesis*, **6**(3), 441–4.

Bird, R. P. and Bruce, W. R. (1984). Damaging effect of dietary components to colon epithelial cells in vivo: effect of mutagenic heterocyclic amines. *J. Nat. Cancer Inst.*, **73**(1), 237–40.

Bjeldanes, L. F. and Chew, H. (1979). Mutagenicity of 1,2-dicarbonyl compounds: maltol, kojic acid, diacetyl and related substances. *Mutat. Res.*, **67**, 367–71.

Bjeldanes, L. F., Morris, M. M., Felton, J. S., Healy, S., Stuermer, D., Berry, P., Timourian, H. and Hatch, F. (1982a). Mutagens from the cooking of food. II.

Survey by Ames/Salmonella test of mutagen formation in the major protein-rich foods of the American diet. *Food Chem. Toxicol.*, **20**, 357–63.

Bjeldanes, L. F., Morris, M. M., Felton, J. S., Healy, S., Stuermer, D., Berry, P., Timourian, H. and Hatch, F. (1982*b*). Mutagens from the cooking of food. III. Survey by Ames/Salmonella test of mutagen formation in secondary sources of cooked dietary protein. *Food Chem. Toxicol.*, **20**, 365–9.

Björk, I. (1982). Inverkan på proteinnäringsvärdet. *Livsmedelteknik*, **4**, 166–7.

Brandt, I., Gustafsson, J.-Å. and Rafter, J. (1983). Distribution of the carcinogenic tryptophan pyrolysis product Trp-P-1 in control, 9-hydroxyellipticine and β-naphthoflavone pretreated mice. *Carcinogenesis*, **4**(10), 1291–6.

Brookman, K. W., Salazar, E. P. and Thompson, L. H. (1985). Comparative mutagenic efficiencies of the DNA adducts from the cooked-food-related mutagens Trp-P-2 and IQ in CHO cells. *Mutat. Res.*, **149**, 249–55.

Busk, L., Ahlborg, U. G. and Albanus L. (1982). Inhibition of protein pyrolysate mutagenicity by retinol (vitamin A). *Food Chem. Toxicol.*, **20**, 535–9.

Caderni, G., Kreamer, B. L. and Dolara, P. (1983). DNA damage of mammalian cells by the beef extract mutagen 2-amino-3-methylimidazo[4,5-f]quinoline. *Food Chem. Toxicol.*, **21**, 641–3.

Cerutti, P. A. (1985). Prooxidant states and tumor promotion. *Science*, **227**, 375–81.

Chan, R. I. M., Stich, H. F., Rosin, M. P. and Powrie, W. D. (1982). Antimutagenic activity of browning reaction products. *Cancer Lett.*, **15**, 27–33.

Committee on Diet, Nutrition and Cancer (1982). Assembly of Life Sciences, National Research Council. *Diet, Nutrition and Cancer*, National Academy Press, Washington, DC.

Commoner, B., Vithayathil, A. J., Dolara, P., Nair, S., Madyastha, P. and Cuca, G. C. (1978). Formation of mutagens in beef and beef extract during cooking. *Science*, **201**, 913–6.

De Waziers, I. and Decloître, F. (1984). Effect of glutathione and uridine-5′-diphosphoglucuronic acid on the mutagenicity of tryptophan pyrolysis products (Trp-P-1 and Trp-P-2) by rat-liver and -intestine S9 fraction. *Mutat. Res.*, **139**, 15–9.

Dolara, P., Commoner, B., Vithayathil, A., Cuca, G., Tuley, E., Madyastha, P., Nair, S. and Kriebel, D. (1979). The effect of temperature on the formation of mutagens in heated beef stock and cooked ground beef. *Mutat. Res.*, **60**, 231–7.

Dolara, P., Barale, R., Mazzoli, S. and Benetti, D. (1980). Activation of the mutagens of beef extract in vitro and in vivo. *Mutat. Res.*, **79**, 213–21.

Doll, R. and Peto, R. (1981). The causes of cancer: quantitative estimates of avoidable risks of cancer in the United States today. *J. Nat. Cancer Inst.*, **66**, 1191–1308.

Doremire, M. E., Harmon, G.E. and Pratt, D. E. (1979). 3,4-Benzopyrene in charcoal grilled meats. *J. Food Sci.*, **44**, 622–3.

Elias, P. (1982). Short-term toxicity of Maillard reaction products. Paper presented at the Interdisciplinary Conference on Food Toxicology, Zürich, 13–15 October.

Felton, J. S. and Healy, S. K. (1984). Activation of mutagens in cooked ground beef by human-liver microsomes. *Mutat. Res.*, **140**, 61–5.

Felton, J. S., Carrano, T., Carver, J., Thompson, L., Stuermer, D., Timourian, H., Hatch, F., Bjeldanes, L. and Morris, M. (1980). Evaluation of mutagens from cooked hamburger with several short-term mammalian bioassays. *Environ. Mutagen.*, **2**, 303–4.

Felton, J. S., Healey, S., Avalos, L. and Wuebbles, B. (1983). Comparison of mutagenicity of two cooking mutagens with three microbial bioassays. *Environ. Mutagen.*, **5**, 446.

Felton, J. S., Knize, M. G., Wood, C., Wuebbles, B. J., Healy, S. K., Stuermer, D. H., Bjeldanes, L. F., Kimble, B. J. and Hatch, F. T. (1984*a*). Isolation and characterization of new mutagens from fried ground beef. *Carcinogenesis*, **5**, 95–102.

Felton, J. S., Bjeldanes, L. F. and Hatch, F. T. (1984*b*). Mutagens in cooked foods: metabolism and genetic toxicity. In: *Nutritional and Toxicological Aspects of Food Safety*, M. Friedman (Ed.), Plenum Publishing Corporation, pp. 555–66.

Felton, J. S., Knize, M. G., Shen, N., Healy, S. K., Andersen, B. D., Bjeldanes, L. F. and Hatch, F. T. (1985). Cooked beef mutagens: isolation and identification of new mutagens from fried ground beef. Poster presented at the symposium on Genetic Toxicology of the Diet, Copenhagen, June 19–21.

Fretheim, K. (1983).Polycyclic aromatic hydrocarbons in grilled meat products: a review. *Food Chem.*, **10**, 129–39.

Fritz, W. (1973). Zur Bildung kanzerogener Kohlenwasserstoffe bei der thermischen Behandlung von Lebensmitteln. 5. Untersuchungen zur Kontamination beim Grillen über Holzkohle. *Deutsch. Lebensm. Rundsch.*, **69**, 119–22.

Fukuhara, Y., Yoshida, D. and Goto, F. (1981). Reduction of mutagenic products in the presence of polyphenols during pyrolysis of protein. *Agric. Biol. Chem.*, **45**, 1061–6.

Gocke, E., Eckhardt, K., King, M.-T. and Wild, D. (1982). Mutagenicity study of fried sausages in Salmonella, Drosophila and mammalian cells in vitro and in vivo. *Mutat. Res.*, **101**, 293–304.

Grivas, S., Nyhammer, T., Olsson, K. and Jägerstad, M. (1986). Formation of a new mutagenic DiMeIQ$_X$ compound in a model system by heating creatinine, alanine and fructose. *Mutat. Res.*, **151**, 171–83.

Hargraves, W. A. and Pariza, M. W. (1983). Purification and mass spectral characterization of bacterial mutagens from commercial beef extracts. *Cancer Res.*, **43**, 1467–72.

Hargraves, W. A. and Pariza, M. W. (1984). Mutagens in cooked foods. *J. Environ. Sci. Health*, **C2**(1), 1–49.

Hashimoto, Y., Takeda, K., Shudo, K., Okamoto, T., Sugimura, T. and Kosuge, T. (1978). Rat liver microsome mediated binding to DNA of 3-amino-1-methyl-5H-pyrido[4,3-b]indole, a potent mutagen isolated from tryptophan pyrolysate. *Chem. Biol. Interact.*, **23**, 137–40.

Hashimoto, Y., Shudo, K. and Okamoto, T. (1979*a*). Structural identification of a modified base in DNA covalently bound with mutagenic 3-amino-1-methyl-5H-pyrido[4,3-b]indole. *Chem. Pharm. Bull.*, **27**(4), 1058–60.

Hashimoto, Y., Shudo, K. and Okamoto, T. (1979*b*). Structure of a base in DNA modified by Glu-P-1. *Chem. Pharm. Bull.*, **27**(10), 2532–4.

Hashimoto, Y., Shudo, K. and Okamoto, T. (1980*a*). Metabolic activation of a mutagen, 2-amino-6-methyldipyrido[1,2-a:3′,2′-d]imidazole and its reaction with DNA. *Biochem.Biophys. Res. Commun.*, **92**, 971–6.

Hashimoto, Y., Shudo, K. and Okamoto, T. (1980b). Activation of a mutagen, 3-amino-1-methyl-5H-pyrido[4,3-b]indole; identification of 3-hydroxyamino-1-methyl-5H-pyrido[4,3-b]indole and its reaction with DNA. *Biochem. Biophys. Res. Commun.*, **96**(1), 355–62.

Hashimoto, Y., Shudo, K. and Okamoto, T. (1982). Modification of nucleic acids with muta-carcinogenic heteroaromatic amines in vivo; identification of modified bases in DNA extracted from rats injected with 3-amino-1-methyl-5H-pyrido[4,3-b]indole and 2-amino-6-methyldipyrido[1,2-a:3',2'-d]imidazole. *Mutat. Res.*, **105**, 9–13.

Hatch, F. T., Felton, J. S. and Bjeldanes, L. F. (1982). Mutagens from the cooking of food: thermic mutagens in beef. In: *Carcinogens and Mutagens in the Environment*, Vol. 1, *Food Products*, H. F. Stich (Ed.), CRC Press, Boca Raton, Florida, pp. 147–63.

Hayatsu, H., Inoue, K., Ohta, H., Namba, T., Togawa, K., Hayatsu, T., Makita, M. and Wataya, Y. (1981). Inhibition of the mutagenicity of cooked beef basic fraction by its acidic fraction. *Mutat. Res.*, **91**, 437–42.

Hosaka, S., Matsushima, T., Hirono, I. and Sugimura, T. (1981). Carcinogenic activity of 3-amino-1-methyl-5H-pyrido[4,3-b]indole (Trp-P-2), a pyrolysis product of tryptophan. *Cancer Lett.*, **13**, 23–8.

IARC (1983). *Polynuclear Aromatic Compounds*, Part 1, *Chemical, Environmental and Experimental Data*, Vol. 32. Monographs on the evaluation of the carcinogenic risk of chemicals to humans, International Agency for Research on Cancer, Lyon, France.

Inoue, T., Morita, K. and Kada, T. (1981). Purification and properties of a plant desmutagenic factor for the mutagenic principle of tryptophan pyrolysate. *Agric. Biol. Chem.*, **45**(2), 345–53.

Inui, N., Nishi, Y. and Hasegawa, M. (1980). Induction of 8-azaguanine or oubain resistant somatic mutation of Chinese hamster lung cells by treatment with tryptophan pyrolysis products. *Cancer Lett.*, **9**, 185–9.

Ishidate, M., Jr., Sofuni, T. and Yoshikawa, K. (1981). Chromosomal aberration tests in vitro as a primary screening tool for environmental mutagens and/or carcinogens. *Gann Monograph Cancer Res.*, **27**, 95–108.

Ishii, K., Ando, M., Kamataki, T., Kato, R. and Nagao, M. (1980). Metabolic activation of mutagenic tryptophan pyrolysis products (Trp-P-1 and Trp-P-2) by a purified cytochrome P-450 dependent monooxygenase system. *Cancer Lett.*, **9**, 271–6.

Ishii, K., Yamazoe, Y., Kamataki, T. and Kato, R. (1981). Metabolic activation of glutamic acid pyrolysis products, 2-amino-6-methyldipyrido[1,2-a:3',2'-d]imidazole and 2-aminodipyrido[1,2-a:3',2'-d]imidazole, by purified cytochrome P-450. *Chem. Biol. Interact.*, **38**, 1–13.

Ishikawa, T., Takayama, S., Kitagawa, T., Kawachi, T., Kinebuchi, M., Matsukura, N., Uchida, E. and Sugimura, T. (1979). In vivo experiments on tryptophan pyrolysis products. In: *Naturally Occurring Carcinogens: Mutagens and Modulators of Carcinogenesis*, E. G. Miller, J. A. Miller, I. Hirono, T. Sugimura and S. Takayama (Eds), Japan Sci. Soc. Press, Tokyo/Univ. Park Press, Baltimore, pp. 159–67.

Jägerstad, M., Laser Reuterswärd, A., Öste, R., Dahlqvist, A., Grivas, S., Olsson, K. and Nyhammer, T. (1982). Creatinine and Maillard reaction products as precursors of mutagenic compounds formed in fried beef. In: *The Maillard Reaction in Foods and Nutrition*, ACS Symposium Series 215, G. R. Waller and M. Feather (Ed.), American Chemical Society, Washington, DC, pp. 507–19.

Jägerstad, M., Laser Reuterswärd, A., Olsson, R., Grivas, S., Nyhammer, T., Olsson, K. and Dahlqvist, A. (1983). Creatin(in)e and Maillard reaction products as precursors of mutagenic compounds: effects of various amino acids. *Food Chem.*, **12**, 255–64.

Jägerstad, M., Olsson, K., Grivas, S., Negishi, C., Wakabayashi, K., Tsuda, M., Sato, S. and Sugimura, T. (1984). Formation of 2-amino-3,8-dimethylimidazo[4,5-f]quinoxaline in a model system by heating creatinine, glycine and glucose. *Mutat. Res.*, **126**, 239–44.

Jägerstad, M., Grivas, S., Olsson, K., Laser Reuterswärd, A., Negishi, C. and Sato, S. (1985). Formation of food mutagens via Maillard reactions. Paper presented at the symposium on Genetic Toxicology of the Diet, Copenhagen, June 19–22.

Jensen, N. J. (1983). Pyrolytic products from tryptophan and glutamic acid are positive in the mammalian spot test. *Cancer Lett.*, **20**, 241–4.

Jensen, N. J., Willumsen, D. and Knudsen, I. (1983). Mutagenic activity at different stages of an industrial ammonia caramel process detected in Salmonella typhimurium TA 100 following pre-incubation. *Food Chem. Toxicol.*, **21**(5), 527–30.

Kada, T., Morita, K. and Inoue, T. (1978). Antimutagenic action of vegetable factor(s) on the mutagenic principle of tryptophan pyrolysate. *Mutat. Res.*, **53**, 351–3.

Kasai, H., Nishimura, S., Nagao, M., Takahashi, Y. and Sugimura, T. (1979). Fractionation of a mutagenic principle from broiled fish by high-pressure liquid chromatography. *Cancer Lett.*, **7**, 343–8.

Kasai, H., Yamaizumi, Z., Wakabayashi, K., Nagao, M., Sugimura, T., Yokoyama, S., Miyazawa, T., Spingarn, N. E., Weisburger, J. H. and Nishimura, S. (1980a). Potent novel mutagens produced by broiling fish under normal conditions. *Proc. Japan Acad.*, **56**(B), 278–83.

Kasai, H., Yamaizumi, Z., Wakabayashi, K., Nagao, M., Sugimura, T., Yokoyama, S., Miyazawa, T. and Nishimura, S. (1980b). Structure and chemical synthesis of MeIQ, a potent mutagen isolated from broiled fish. *Chem. Lett.*, 1391–4.

Kasai, H., Nishimura, S., Wakabayashi, K., Nagao, M. and Sugimura, T. (1980c). Chemical synthesis of 2-amino-3-methylimidazo[4,5-f]quinoline (IQ), a potent mutagen isolated from broiled fish. *Proc. Japan Acad.*, **56**(B), 382–4.

Kasai, H., Yamaizumi, Z., Nishimura, S., Wakabayashi, K., Nagao, M., Sugimura, T., Spingarn, N. E., Weisburger, J. H., Yokoyama, S. and Miyazawa, T. (1981a). A potent mutagen in broiled fish. Part 1. 2-Amino-3-methyl-3H-imidazo[4,5-f]quinoline. *J. Chem. Soc. Perkin Trans. 1*, 2290–3.

Kasai, H., Yamaizumi, Z., Shiomi, T., Yokoyama, S., Miyazawa, T., Wakabayashi, K., Nagao, M., Sugimura, T. and Nishimura, S. (1981b). Structure of a potent mutagen isolated from fried beef. *Chem. Lett.*, 485–8.

Kasai, H., Shiomi, T., Sugimura, T. and Nishimura, S. (1981c). Synthesis of 2-amino-3,8-dimethylimidazo[4,5-f]quinoxaline (MeIQ$_x$), a potent mutagen isolated from fried beef. *Chem. Lett.*, 675–8.

Kimiagar, M. (1979). Long-term feeding effects of Maillard brown products to rats. *Diss. Abstr. Internat.*, **40**(6), 2612-B.

Kosuge, T., Tsuji, K., Wakabayashi, K., Okamoto, T., Shudo, K., Iitaka, Y., Itai, A., Sugimura, T., Kawashi, T., Nagao, M., Yahagi, T. and Seino, Y. (1978). Isolation and structure studies of mutagenic principles in amino acid pyrolysates. *Chem. Pharm. Bull.*, **26**(2), 611–9.

Krone, C. A. and Iwaoka, W.T. (1981). Mutagen formation during the cooking of fish. *Cancer Lett.*, **14**, 93–9.

Larsson, B. K., Sahlberg, G. P., Eriksson, A. T. and Busk, L. Å. (1983). Polycyclic aromatic hydrocarbons in grilled food. *J. Agric. Food Chem.*, **31**, 867–73.

Levin, W., Wood, A., Chang, R., Ryan, D., Thomas, P., Yagi, H., Thakker, D., Vyas, K., Boyd, C., Chu, S.-Y., Conney, A. and Jerina, D. (1982). Oxidative metabolism of polycyclic hydrocarbons to ultimate carcinogens. *Drug Metab. Rev.*, **13**(4), 555–80.

Lijinsky, W. and Ross, A. E. (1967). Production of carcinogenic polynuclear hydrocarbons in the cooking of food. *Food Cosmet. Toxicol.*, **5**, 343–7.

Lijinsky, W. and Shubik, P. (1964). Benzo(a)pyrene and other polynuclear hydrocarbons in charcoal-broiled meat. *Science*, **145**, 53–5.

Lo, M.-T. and Sandi, E. (1978). Polycyclic aromatic hydrocarbons in foods. *Residue Rev.*, **69**, 35–86.

Loretz, L. J. and Pariza, M. W. (1984). Effect of glutathione levels, sulfate levels, and metabolic inhibitors on covalent binding of 2-amino-3-methylimidazo[4,5-f]quinoline and 2-acetylaminofluorene to cell macromolecules in primary monolayer cultures of adult rat hepatocytes. *Carcinogenesis*, **5**, 895–9.

Loury, D. J. and Byard, J. L. (1985). Genotoxicity of the cooked-food mutagens IQ and MeIQ in primary cultures of rat, hamster, and guinea pig hepatocytes. *Environ. Mutagen.*, **7**, 245–54.

Loury, D. J., Byard, J. E. and Shibamoto, T. (1984). Genotoxicity of N-nitroso-thiazolidine in microbial and hepatocellular test systems. *Food Chem. Toxicol.*, **22**(12), 1013–4.

Lynch, S. C., Gruenwedel, D. W. and Russell, G. F. (1983). Mutagenic activity of a nitrosated early Maillard product: DNA synthesis (DNA repair) induced in HeLa S3 carcinoma cells by nitrosated 1-(*N*-L-tryptophan)-1-deoxy-D-fructose. *Food Chem. Toxicol.*, **21**(5), 551–6.

Marx, J. L. (1984). What do oncogenes do? *Science*, **223**, 673–6.

Matsukura, N., Kawachi, T., Morino, K., Ohgaki, H. and Sugimura, T. (1981). Carcinogenicity in mice of mutagenic compounds from a tryptophan pyrolysate. *Science*, **213**(17), 346–7.

Matsumoto, T., Yoshida, D., Mizusaki, S. and Okamoto, H. (1977). Mutagenic activity of amino acid pyrolysates in Salmonella typhimurium TA 98. *Mutat. Res.*, **48**, 279–86.

Matsumoto, T., Yoshida, D., Mizusaki, S. and Okamoto, H. (1978). Mutagenicities of the pyrolyzates of peptides and proteins. *Mutat. Res.*, **56**, 281–8.

Matsumoto, T., Yoshida, D. and Tomita, H. (1981). Determination of mutagens, amino-α-carbolines in grilled foods and cigarette smoke condensate. *Cancer Lett.*, **12**, 105–10.

Mauron, J. (1985). Influence of processing on protein quality. *Bibl. Nutr. Dieta*, **34**, 56–81.

McCann, J. and Ames, B. N. (1976). Detection of carcinogens as mutagens in the Salmonella/microsome test: assay of 300 chemicals; discussion. *Proc. Nat. Acad. Sci.*, **73**, 950–4.

Mihara, S. and Shibamoto, T. (1980). Mutagenicity of products obtained from cysteamine-glucose browning model systems. *J. Agric. Food. Chem.*, **28**, 62–6.

Miller, A. J. and Buchanan, R. L. (1983). Detection of genotoxicity in fried bacon by the Salmonella/mammalian microsome mutagenicity assay. *Food Chem. Toxicol.*, **21**, 319–23.

Minkler, J. L. and Carrano, A. V. (1984). In vivo cytogenetic effects of the cooked food related mutagens Trp-P-2 and IQ in mouse bone marrow. *Mutat. Res.*, **140**, 49–53.

Mochizuki, H. and Kada, T. (1982). Antimutagenic action of cobaltous chloride on Trp-P-1 induced mutations in Salmonella typhimurium TA 98 and TA 1538. *Mutat. Res.*, **95**, 145–57.

Morita, K., Hara, M. and Kada, T. (1978). Studies on natural desmutagen: screening for vegetable and fruit factors active in inactivation of mutagenic pyrolysis products from amino acids. *Agric. Biol. Chem.*, **42**(6), 1235–8.

Morita, K., Yamada, H., Iwamoto, S., Sotomura, M. and Suzuki, A. (1982). Purification and properties of desmutagenic factor from broccoli (Brassica Olerancea var. Italica Plenck) for mutagenic principle of tryptophan pyrolysate. *J. Food Safety*, **4**(3), 139–50.

Münzner, R. and Wever, J. (1984). Investigations on the detection of mutagenic activity of beef extract in rats after oral administration. *Cancer Lett.*, **23**, 109–14.

Nagao, M., Honda, M., Seino, Y., Yahagi, T. and Sugimura, T. (1977*a*). Mutagenicities of smoke condensates and the charred surface of fish and meat. *Cancer Lett.*, **2**, 221–6.

Nagao, M., Honda, M., Seino, Y., Yahagi, T., Kawachi, T. and Sugimura, T. (1977*b*). Mutagenicities of protein pyrolysates. *Cancer Lett.*, **2**, 335–40.

Nagao, M., Fujita, Y., Wakabayashi, K. and Sugimura, T. (1983*a*). Ultimate forms of mutagenic and carcinogenic heterocyclic amines produced by pyrolysis. *Biochem. Biophys. Res. Commun.*, **114**, 626–31.

Nagao, M., Sato, S. and Sugimura, T. (1983*b*). Mutagens produced by heating foods. In: *The Maillard Reaction in Foods and Nutrition*, ACS Symposium Series 215, G. R. Waller and M. Feather (Eds), American Chemical Society, Washington, DC, pp. 521–36.

Nakayasu, M., Nakasato, F., Sakamoto, H., Terada, M. and Sugimura, T. (1983). Mutagenic activity of heterocyclic amines in Chinese hamster lung cells with diphtheria toxin resistance as a marker. *Mutat. Res.*, **118**, 91–102.

Nebert, D. W., Bigelow, S., Okey, A. B., Yahagi, T., Mori, Y., Nagao, M. and Sugimura, T. (1979). Pyrolysis products from amino acids and proteins: highest mutagenicity requires cytochrome P_1-450. *Proc. Nat. Acad. Sci.*, **76**(11), 5929–33.

Negishi, C., Wakabayashi, K., Tsuda, M., Sato, S., Sugimura, T., Saitô, H., Maeda, M. and Jägerstad, M. (1984). Formation of 2-amino-3,7,8-trimethyl-imidazo[4,5-f]quinoxaline, a new mutagen, by heating a mixture of creatinine, glucose and glycine. *Mutat. Res.*, **140**, 55–9.

Nemoto, N., Kusumi, S., Takayama, T., Nagao, M. and Sugimura, T. (1979). Metabolic activation of 3-amino-5H-pyrido[4,3-b]indole, a highly mutagenic principle in tryptophan pyrolysate, by rat liver enzymes. *Chem. Biol. Interact.*, **27**, 191–8.

Niwa, T., Yamazoe, Y. and Kato, R. (1982). Metabolic activation of 2-amino-9H-pyrido[2,3-b]indole by rat liver microsomes. *Mutat. Res.*, **95**, 159–70.

Ohgaki, H., Matsukura, N., Morino, K., Kawachi, T., Sugimura, T. and Takayama, S. (1984a). Carcinogenicity in mice of mutagenic compounds from glutamic acid and soy bean globulin pyrolysates. *Carcinogenesis*, **5**, 815–9.

Ohgaki, H., Kusama, K., Matsukura, N., Morino, K., Hasegawa, H., Sato, S., Takayama, S. and Sugimura, T. (1984b). Carcinogenicity in mice of a mutagenic compound, 2-amino-3-methylimidazo[4,5-f]quinoline, from broiled sardine, cooked beef and beef extract. *Carcinogenesis*, **5**, 921–4.

Okamoto, T., Shudo, K., Hashimoto, Y., Kosuge, T., Sugimura, T. and Nishimura, S. (1981). Identification of a reactive metabolite of the mutagen 2-amino-3-methylimidazo[4,5-f]quinoline. *Chem. Pharm. Bull.*, **29**(2), 590–3.

Omura, H., Jahan, N., Shinohara, K. and Murakami, H. (1983). Formation of mutagens by the Maillard reaction. In: *The Maillard Reaction in Foods and Nutrition*, ACS Symposium Series 215, G. R. Waller and M. Feather (Eds), American Chemical Society, Washington, DC, pp. 537–63.

Övervik, E., Nilsson, L., Fredholm, L., Levin, Ö., Nord, C.-E. and Gustafsson, J.-Å. (1984). High mutagenic activity formed in pan-broiled pork. *Mutat. Res.*, **135**, 149–57.

Pariza, M. W., Ashoor, S. H., Chu, F. S. and Lund, D. B. (1979a). Effect of temperature and time on mutagen formation in pan-fried hamburgers. *Cancer Lett.*, **7**, 63–9.

Pariza, M. W., Ashoor, S. H. and Chu, F. S. (1979b). Mutagens in heat-processed meat, bakery and cereal products. *Food Cosmet. Toxicol.*, **17**, 429–30.

Pelkonen, O. and Nebert, D. W. (1982). Metabolism of polycyclic aromatic hydrocarbons: etiologic role in carcinogenesis. *Pharmacol. Rev.*, **34**(2), 189–222.

Pensabene, J. W., Fiddler, W., Gates, R. A., Fagan, J. C. and Wasserman, A. E. (1974). Effect of frying and other cooking conditions on nitrosopyrrolidine formation in bacon. *J. Food Sci.*, **39**, 314–6.

Phillips, D. H. (1983). Fifty years of benzo(a)pyrene. *Nature*, **303**, 468–72.

Pintauro, S. J., Page, G. V., Solberg, M., Lee, T.-C. and Chichester, C. O. (1980). Absence of mutagenic response from extracts of Maillard browned egg albumin. *J. Food Sci.*, **45**, 1442–3.

Pintauro, S. J., Lee, T.-C. and Chichester, C. O. (1983). Nutritional and toxicological effects of Maillard browned protein ingestion in the rat. In: *The Maillard Reaction in Foods and Nutrition*, ACS Symposium Series 215, G. R. Waller and M. Feather (Eds), American Chemical Society, Washington, DC, pp. 467–83.

Pool, B. L., Röper, H., Röper, S. and Romruen, K. (1984). Mutagenicity studies on N-nitrosated products of the Maillard browning reaction: N-nitroso-fructose-amino acids. *Food Chem. Toxicol.*, **22**(10), 797–801.

Powrie, W. D., Wu, C. H., Rosin, M. P. and Stich, H. F. (1981). Clastogenic and mutagenic activities of Maillard reaction model systems. *J. Food Sci.*, **46**, 1433–45.

Powrie, W. D., Wu, C. H. and Stich, H. F. (1982). Browning reaction systems as sources of mutagens and modulators. In: *Carcinogens and Mutagens in the Environment*, Vol. 1, *Food Products*, H. F. Stich (Ed.), CRC Press, Boca Raton, Florida, pp. 121–33.

Purchase, I. F. H., Longstaff, E., Ashby, J., Styles, J. A., Anderson, D., Lefevre, P. A. and Westwood, F. R. (1976). Evaluation of six short-term tests for detecting organic chemical carcinogens and recommendations for their use. *Nature*, **264**, 624–7.

Rosin, M. P., Stich, H. F., Powrie, W. D. and Wu, C. H. (1982). Induction of mitotic gene conversion by browning reaction products and its modulating by naturally occurring agents. *Mutat. Res.*, **101**, 189–97.

Russel, G. F. (1983). Nitrite interactions in model Maillard browning systems. In: *The Maillard Reaction in Foods and Nutrition*, ACS Symposium Series 215, G. R. Waller and M. Feather (Eds), American Chemical Society, Washington, DC, pp. 84–90.

Saito, K., Yamazoe, Y., Kamataki, T. and Kato, R. (1983). Activation and detoxification of N-hydroxy-Trp-P-2 by glutathione and glutathione transferases. *Carcinogenesis*, **4**, 1551–7.

Sekizawa, J. and Shibamoto, T. (1980). Mutagenicity of 2-alkyl-N-nitrosothiazolidines. *J. Agric. Food Chem.*, **28**, 781–3.

Shibamoto, T. (1980). Mutagenicity of 1,5(or 7)-dimethyl-2,3,6,7-tetrahydro-1H,5H-biscyclopentapyrazine obtained from a cyclotene/NH$_3$ browning model system. *J. Agric. Food Chem.*, **28**, 883–4.

Shibamoto, T. (1982). Occurrence of mutagenic products in browning model systems. *Food Technol.*, March, 59–62.

Shibamoto, T., Nishimura, O. and Mihara, S. (1981). Mutagenicity of products obtained from a maltol-ammonia model system. *J. Agric. Food Chem.*, **29**, 643–6.

Sjödin, P. and Jägerstad, M. (1984). A balance study of ^{14}C-labelled 3H-imidazo[4,5-f]quinoline-2-amines (IQ and MeIQ) in rats. *Food Chem. Toxicol.*, **22**, 207–10.

Sjödin, P. and Jägerstad, M. (1985). A balance study of labelled food mutagens (IQ, MeIQ, MeIQ$_X$) in rats. Poster presented at the symposium on Genetic Toxicology of the Diet, Copenhagen, June 19–22.

Sjödin, P., Nyman, M., Nielsson, L., Asp, N.-G. and Jägerstad, M. (1985). Binding of ^{14}C-labelled food mutagens (IQ, MeIQ, MeIQ$_X$) by dietary fiber *in vitro*. Poster presented at the symposium on Genetic Toxicology of the Diet, Copenhagen, June 19–22.

Spingarn, N. E. and Garvie, C. T. (1979). Formation of mutagens in sugar-ammonia model systems. *J. Agric. Food Chem.*, **27**, 1319–21.

Spingarn, N. E. and Weisburger, J. H. (1979). Formation of mutagens in cooked foods. I. Beef. *Cancer Lett.*, **7**, 259–64.

Spingarn, N. E., Slocum, L. A. and Weisburger, J. H. (1980a). Formation of mutagens in cooked foods. II. Foods with high starch content. *Cancer Lett.*, **9**, 7–12.

Spingarn, N. E., Kasai, H., Vuolo, L., Nishimura, S., Yamaizumi, Z., Sugimura, T., Matsushima, T. and Weisburger, J. H. (1980b). Formation of mutagens in cooked foods. III. Isolation of a potent mutagen from beef. *Cancer Lett.*, **9**, 177–83.

Spingarn, N. E., Garvie-Gould, C., Vuolo, L. L. and Weisburger, J. H. (1981). Formation of mutagens in cooked foods. IV. Effect of fat content in fried beef patties. *Cancer Lett.*, **12**, 93–7.

Stich, H. F., Stich, W., Rosin, M. P. and Powrie, W. D. (1980). Mutagenic activity of pyrazine derivatives: a comparative study with Salmonella typhimurium, Saccharomyces cerevisiae and Chinese hamster ovary cells. *Food Cosmet. Toxicol.*, **18**, 581–4.

Stich, H. F., Rosin, M. P., Wu, C. H. and Powrie, W. D. (1981a). Clastogenicity of furans found in food. *Cancer Lett.*, **13**, 89–95.

Stich, H. F., Stich, W., Rosin, M. P. and Powrie, W. D. (1981b). Clastogenic activity of caramel and caramelized sugars. *Mutat. Res.*, **91**, 129–36.

Sugimura, T. (1985). Carcinogenicity of mutagenic heterocyclic amines formed during the cooking process. *Mutat. Res.*, **150**, 33–41.

Sugimura, T. and Iitaka, Y. (1980). Crystal and molecular structures of 2-amino-3-methylimidazo[4,5-f]quinoline, a novel potent mutagen found in broiled food. *FEBS Lett.*, **122**, 261–3.

Sugimura, T., Sato, S., Nagao, M., Yahagi, T., Matsushima, T., Seino, Y., Takeuchi, M. and Kawachi, T. (1976). Overlapping of carcinogens and mutagens. In: *Fundamentals of Cancer Prevention*, P. N. Magee, S. Takayama, T. Sugimura and T. Matsushima (Eds), Japan Scientific Societies Press, Tokyo, pp. 191–215.

Sugimura, T., Kawachi, T, Nagao, M., Yahagi, T., Seino, Y., Okamoto, T., Shudo, K., Kosuge, T., Tsuji, K., Wakabayashi, K., Iitaka, Y. and Itai, A. (1977). Mutagenic principle(s) in tryptophan and phenylalanine pyrolysis products. *Proc. Japan Acad.*, **53**(1), 58–61.

Takayama, S., Katoh, Y., Tanaka, M., Nagao, M., Wakabayashi, K. and Sugimura, T. (1977). In vitro transformation of hamster embryo cells with tryptophan pyrolysis products. *Proc. Japan Acad.*, **53B**, 126–9.

Takayama, S., Hirakawa, T. and Sugimura, T. (1978). Malignant transformation in vitro by tryptophan pyrolysis products. *Proc. Japan Acad.*, **54B**, 418–22.

Takayama, S., Hirakawa, T., Tanaka, M., Kawachi, T. and Sugimura, T. (1979). In vitro transformation of hamster embryo cells with a glutamic acid pyrolysis product. *Toxicol. Lett.*, **4**, 281–4.

Takayama, S., Nakatsura, Y., Masuda, M., Ohgaki, H., Sato, S. and Sugimura, T. (1984). Demonstration of carcinogenicity in F344 rats of 2-amino-3-methyl-imidazo[4,5-f]quinoline from broiled sardine, fried beef and beef extract. *Gann*, **75**, 467–70.

Thompson, L. H., Carrano, A. V., Salazar, E., Felton, J. S. and Hatch, F. T. (1983). Comparative genotoxic effects of the cooked food-related mutagens Trp-P-2 and IQ in bacteria and cultured mammalian cells. *Mutat. Res.*, **117**, 243–57.

Toda, H., Sekizawa, J. and Shibamoto, T. (1981). Mutagenicity of the L-rhamnose-ammonia-hydrogen sulfide browning reaction mixture. *J. Agric. Food Chem.*, **29**, 381–4.

Tohda, H., Oikawa, A., Kawachi, T. and Sugimura, T. (1980). Induction of sister-chromatid exchanges by mutagens from amino acid and protein pyrolysates. *Mutat. Res.*, **77**, 65–9.

Tóth, L. and Blaas, W. (1973). Der Gehalt gegrillter Fleischerzeugnisse an cancerogenen Kohlenwasserstoffen. *Fleischwirtschaft*, **53**, 1456–9.

Tóth, L. and Potthast, K. (1984). Chemical aspects of the smoking of meat and meat products. *Adv. Food Res.*, **29**, 87–158.

Tsuda, H., Kato, K., Matsumoto, T., Yoshida, D. and Mizusaki, S. (1978). Chromosomal aberrations and morphological transformation of hamster embryonic cells induced by L-tryptophan pyrolysate in vitro. *Mutat. Res.*, **49**, 145–8.

Tsuda, M., Takahashi, Y., Nagao, M., Hirayama, T. and Sugimura, T. (1980). Inactivation of mutagens from pyrolysates of tryptophan and glutamic acid by nitrite in acidic solution. *Mutat. Res.*, **78**, 331–9.

Tsuda, M., Nagao, M., Hirayama, T. and Sugimura, T. (1981). Nitrite converts 2-amino-α-carboline, an indirect mutagen, into 2-hydroxy-α-carboline, a non-mutagen, and 2-hydroxy-3-nitroso-α-carboline, a direct mutagen. *Mutat. Res.*, **83**, 61–8.

Tsuda, M., Wakabayashi, K., Hirayama, T., Kawachi, T. and Sugimura, T. (1983). Inactivation of potent pyrolysate mutagens by chlorinated tap water. *Mutat. Res.*, **119**, 27–34.

Tsuji, K., Yamamoto, T., Zenda, H. and Kosuge, T. (1978). Studies on active principles of tar. VII. Production of biologically active substances in pyrolysis of amino acids. (2) Antifungal constituents in pyrolysis products of phenylalanine. *Yakugaku Zasshi*, **98**, 910–3.

Umano, K., Shibamoto, T., Fernando, S. Y. and Wei, C.-I. (1984). Mutagenicity of 2-hydroxyalkyl-N-nitrosothiazolidines. *Food Chem. Toxicol.*, **22**(4), 253–9.

Vahl, M., Andersen, P. H. and Gry, J. (1985). Comparison of HPLC profiles of mutagens in pork and beef fried under household conditions. Poster presented at the symposium on Genetic Toxicology of the Diet, Copenhagen, June 19–22.

Vuolo, L. L. and Schuessler, G. J. (1985). Review: Putative mutagens and carcinogens in foods. VI. Protein pyrolysate products. *Environ. Mutagen.*, **7**, 577–98.

Wakabayashi, K., Tsuji, K., Kosuge, T., Takeda, K., Yamaguchi, K., Shuda, K., Iiaka, T., Okamoto, T., Yahagi, T., Nagao, M. and Sugimura, T. (1978). Isolation and structure determination of a mutagenic substance in L-lysine pyrolysate. *Proc. Japan Acad.*, **54**(B), 569–71.

Wang, Y. I. Y., Vuolo, L. L., Spingarn, N. E. and Weisburger, J. H. (1982). Formation of mutagens in cooked foods. V. The mutagen reducing effect of soy protein concentrates and antioxidants during frying of beef. *Cancer Lett.*, **16**, 179–89.

Wargovich, M. J., Goldberg, M. T., Newmark, H. L. and Bruce, W. R. (1983). Nuclear aberrations as short-term test for genotoxicity to the colon: evaluation of nineteen agents. *J. Nat. Cancer Inst.*, **71**, 133–7.

Watanabe, J., Kawajiri, K., Yonekawa, H., Nagao, M. and Tagashira, Y. (1982*a*). Immunological analysis of the roles of two major types of cytochrome P-450 in mutagenesis of compounds isolated from pyrolysates. *Biochem. Biophys. Res. Commun.*, **10**(1), 4193–9.

Watanabe, T., Yokoyama, S., Hayashi, K., Kasai, H., Nishimura, S. and Miyazawa, T. (1982*b*). DNA-binding of IQ, MeIQ and MeIQ$_X$, strong mutagens found in broiled foods. *FEBS Lett.*, **150**(2), 434–8.

Willett, W. C. and MacMahan, B. (1984). Diet and cancer: an overview. *New Engl. J. Med.*, **310**, 633–8, 697–703.

Wilson, R. (1982). Rodent studies on thermal processed (Maillard reaction) flavours. Paper presented at the Interdisciplinary Conference on Food

Toxicology, Zürich, October 13–15.
Yamaguchi, K., Shudo, K., Okamoto, T., Sugimura, T. and Kosuge, T. (1980a).
Presence of 3-amino-1,4-dimethyl-5H-pyrido[4,3-b]indole in broiled beef.
Gann, 71, 745–6.
Yamaguchi, K., Shudo, K., Okamoto, T., Sugimura, T. and Kosuge, T. (1980b).
Presence of 2-aminodipyrido[1,2-a:3′,2′-d]imidazole in broiled cuttlefish. *Gann*,
71, 743–4.
Yamaizumi, Z., Shiomi, T., Kasai, H., Nishimura, S., Takahashi, Y., Nagao, M.
and Sugimura, T. (1980). Detection of potent mutagens, Trp-P-1 and Trp-P-2, in
broiled fish. *Cancer Lett.*, 9, 75–83.
Yamamoto, T., Tsuji, K., Kosuge, T., Okamoto, T., Shudo, K., Takeda, K.,
Iitaka, Y., Yamaguchi, K., Seino, Y., Yahagi, T., Nagao, M. and Sugimura, T.
(1978). Isolation and structure determination of mutagenic substances in L-
glutamic acid pyrolysate. *Proc. Japan Acad.*, 54(B), 248–50.
Yamazoe, Y., Yamaguchi, N., Kamataki, T. and Kato, R. (1980a). Metabolic
activation of Trp-P-2, a mutagenic amine from tryptophan-pyrolysate, by liver
microsomes from 3-methylcholanthrene-responsive and non-responsive mice.
Xenobiotica, 10(7,8), 483–94.
Yamazoe, Y., Ishii, K., Kamataki, T., Kato, R. and Sugimura, T. (1980b).
Isolation and characterization of active metabolites of tryptophan-pyrolysate
mutagen Trp-P-2, formed by rat liver microsomes. *Chem. Biol. Interact.*, 30,
125–38.
Yamazoe, Y., Ishii, K., Kamataki, T. and Kato, R. (1981a). Structural elucidation
of a mutagenic metabolite of 3-amino-1-methyl-5H-pyrido[4,3-b]indole. *Drug
Metab. Dispos.*, 9(3), 292–6.
Yamazoe, Y., Tada, M., Kamataki, T. and Kato, R. (1981b). Enhancement of
binding of N-hydroxy-Trp-P-2 to DNA by seryl tRHA synthetase. *Biochem.
Biophys. Res. Commun.*, 102, 432–9.
Yamazoe, Y., Shimada, M., Kamataki, T. and Kato, R. (1982). Covalent binding
of N-hydroxy-Trp-P-2 to DNA by cytosolic proline dependent system. *Biochem.
Biophys. Res. Commun.*, 107, 165–72.
Yamazoe, Y., Shimada, M., Kamataki, T. and Kato, R. (1983). Microsomal
activation of 2-amino-3-methylimidazo[4,5-f]quinoline, a pyrolysate of sardine
and beef extracts, to a mutagenic intermediate. *Cancer Res.*, 43, 5768–74.
Yamazoe, Y., Shimada, M., Maeda, K., Kamataki, T. and Kato, R. (1984).
Specificity of four forms of cytochrome P-450 in the metabolic activation of
several aromatic amines and benzo(a)pyrene. *Xenobiotica*, 14(7), 549–52.
Yamazoe, Y., Shimada, M., Shinohara, A., Saito, K., Kamataki, T. and Kato, R.
(1985). Catalysis of the covalent binding of 3-hydroxyamino-1-methyl-5H-
pyrido[4,3-b]indole to DNA by an L-proline and adenosine triphosphate-
dependent enzyme in rat hepatic cytosol. *Cancer Res.*, 45, 2495–500.
Yoshida, D. and Matsumoto, T. (1978). Changes in mutagenicity of protein
pyrolyzates by reaction with nitrite. *Mutat. Res.*, 58, 35–40.
Yoshida, D., Matsumoto, T., Yoshimura, R. and Matsuzaki, T. (1978).
Mutagenicity of amino-α-carbolines in pyrolysis products of soybean globulin.
Biochem. Biophys. Res. Commun., 83(3), 915–20.

Chapter 8

MODIFICATION OF THE CARCINOGENIC RESPONSE BY ANTIOXIDANTS

Nobuyuki Ito, Shoji Fukushima and Masao Hirose

First Department of Pathology, Nagoya City University Medical School, Nagoya, Japan

INTRODUCTION

Antioxidants have been widely used as food additives in various processed foods, and many investigators have examined the toxicology of antioxidants. In particular, previous studies on the subchronic or chronic toxicity and carcinogenicity of butylated hydroxyanisole (BHA) (Allen, 1976; Branen, 1975; Brown *et al.*, 1959; Hodge *et al.*, 1964, 1966; Kohn, 1971) and butylated hydroxytoluene (BHT) (Deichmann *et al.*, 1955; DHEW publication, 1979; Hirose *et al.*, 1981; Shirai *et al.*, 1982) did not show any evidence of chronic toxic or carcinogenic effects. Mutagenic activities of BHA and BHT were not demonstrated in short-term tests including bacterial and mammalian cell mutagenesis and chromosome aberration tests (Epstein and Shafner, 1968; Joner, 1977; Kawachi, 1979).

Additionally, two studies found that BHA had antimutagenic activity (Batzinger et al., 1978; Cumming and Walton, 1973). Furthermore, several investigators reported that BHA (Clegg, 1965; Hansen and Meyer, 1978; Telford et al., 1962; Vorhees et al., 1981) and BHT (Ames et al., 1956; Clegg, 1965; Johnson, 1965; Telford et al., 1962) had no teratogenic activity in rodents. Studies on absorption and metabolism demonstrated that the antioxidants are rapidly metabolized, excreted in the urine and moreover excreted in faeces because of entry into the enterohepatic circulation (Astill et al., 1962; Dacre and Denz, 1956; Daniel and Gage, 1965; Daniel et al., 1973a,b,c; Hathway, 1966; Holder et al., 1970; Ladomery et al., 1967; Matsuo et al., 1984; Minegishi et al., 1981). According to their results, the use of these compounds has generally been thought to be without hazard.

In addition, some antioxidants have been demonstrated to have anti-carcinogenic activities when given before and/or concurrently with carcinogens (Wattenberg, 1976, 1978, 1980). For instance, BHA and BHT inhibited the induction of tumors in the intestine of mice and also the intestine, liver and mammary glands of rats, when given before or concomitantly with carcinogen (Clapp et al., 1979; King et al., 1979, 1981; Reddy et al., 1983; Ulland et al., 1973; Weisburger et al., 1977). Earlier studies on the mechanism of carcinogenesis have shown that various carcinogens, such as polycyclic aromatic hydrocarbons, and poly-chlorinated biphenyls, inhibited induction of liver tumors by hepato-carcinogens when these compounds were administered simultaneously with the carcinogen (Miller et al., 1958; Richardson et al., 1952). In these studies, the inhibitory action depends on the fact that polycyclic aromatic hydrocarbons or polychlorinated biphenyls increase drug-metabolizing enzymes in rat liver. The inhibitory effects of these compounds on carcino-genesis may be related to their ability to prevent the in vivo activation of carcinogens to proximate or ultimate forms, or to increased detoxification of the reactive intermediate by inducing relevant enzymes such as epoxide hydrase and glutathione S-transferase or decreasing the amount of aryl hydrocarbon hydroxylase activity (Benson et al., 1978, 1979; Cha et al., 1978; Kahe and Wulff, 1979; Lam and Wattenberg, 1979; Sparnins et al., 1982; Speier and Wattenberg, 1975). Therefore, antioxidants including BHA and BHT have been generally considered to inhibit chemical carcinogenesis.

BHA (Creaven et al., 1966; Cumming and Walton, 1973; Martin and Gilbert, 1968) and BHT (Crampton et al., 1977), however, have also been shown to induce liver enlargement and mixed-function oxidase activities. One study reported that BHT caused hemorrhagic death in rats

(Takahashi and Hiraga, 1978). Recently, induction of squamous cell carcinomas of the forestomach in rats and hamsters given BHA was detected in our laboratory (Ito *et al.*, 1983*a,b*). We further demonstrated that the induction of proliferative and neoplastic lesions of the forestomach in male rats treated with BHA is dose-dependent (Ito *et al.*, 1986). It has also been reported that BHT induced hepatocellular carcinoma in rats exposed to the compound *in utero* (Olsen *et al.*, 1983), and there are several recent publications on the enhancement of tumor formation in animals by antioxidants, when given concomitantly with carcinogens (Cook and McNamara, 1980; Maeura *et al.*, 1984; Toth and Patil, 1983; Williams *et al.*, 1983; Witschi, 1981). Therefore, antioxidants may have a wide variety of hazardous and non-hazardous effects in rodents, and possibly also in humans.

The two-stage process of chemical carcinogenesis, with qualitatively different 'initiation' and 'promotion' steps, is now thought to be applicable to many different organs (Berenblum and Shubik, 1947; Peraino *et al.*, 1971). For example, sodium saccharin has been found to have promoting effects on urinary bladder carcinogenesis (Cohen *et al.*, 1979; Hicks *et al.*, 1975; Ito *et al.*, 1983*c*), while phenobarbital (Ito *et al.*, 1983*d*; Peraino *et al.*, 1971; Tsuda *et al.*, 1983) or nephrotoxic agents (Hiasa *et al.*, 1983) are thought to promote liver or kidney carcinogenesis. The characteristic nature of promoting agents has also been investigated in many systems *in vivo* and *in vitro* (Weinstein and Troll, 1977). Since various agents and chemical contaminants in food may be important in tumorigenesis in man, special consideration should be paid to evaluation of the activities of food additives, including antioxidants, in chemical carcinogenesis.

This chapter focuses on recent studies in our laboratory on the ability of several antioxidants to modify the tumor promotion stage of chemical carcinogenesis in various organs of rats, and discusses the outcome of these investigations.

MODIFICATION OF STOMACH CARCINOGENESIS

Since there is a possible relation between salty food and stomach cancer, several experimental approaches have been used to examine the role of NaCl in gastric carcinogenesis. Although no clear promoting action of NaCl in the stomach has been demonstrated, NaCl acts as a cocarcinogen when administered together with a carcinogen (Takahashi *et al.*, 1983, 1984; Tatematsu *et al.*, 1975).

An investigation was undertaken to clarify the promoting effects of

BHA, BHT and NaCl on gastric carcinogenesis in F344 rats (Shirai *et al.*, 1984). The synergistic effects of BHA and NaCl, and BHT and NaCl, were also investigated. BHA, BHT and NaCl were added to the basal diet at concentrations of 0·5, 1·0 and 5·0%, respectively, and these diets were formed into pellets. The rats were divided into 11 groups as shown in Table 1. Rats in groups 1 to 6 (20 animals per group) were given N-methyl-N'-nitro-N-nitrosoguanidine at a dose of 150 mg/kg body weight dissolved in DMSO at a concentration of 3·75% (150 mg MNNG/4 mg DMSO) by gastric intubation on day 1 of the experiment. One week after MNNG administration, the animals were placed on basal diet for 51 weeks with the following additions: group 1, 0·5% BHA; group 2, 1·0% BHT; group 3, 5·0% NaCl; group 4, 0·5% BHA plus 5·0% NaCl; group 5, 1·0% BHT plus 5·0% NaCl; group 6, no addition. Groups 7 to 11 (15 rats each) were the respective controls for groups 1 to 5 and were given the vehicle (DMSO) instead of MNNG followed by BHA, BHT and/or NaCl. All animals were sacrificed at week 52 of the experiment.

Although no significant differences in food intakes of groups were noted, body weight gain was less in groups given BHT and/or NaCl throughout the experiments. The average water consumption was about 40 ml/rat/day in groups on diet containing NaCl. This volume is about 2·5 times the control value.

A single dose of MNNG by intragastric instillation resulted in development of tumors in the forestomach and glandular stomach after 52 weeks. The incidences of tumors and epithelial hyperplasias in the forestomach are summarized in Table 1. After initiation with MNNG, administration of BHA significantly increased the incidences of both papillomas and squamous cell carcinomas in the forestomach (Figs 1 and 2), while NaCl increased only that of papillomas relative to the incidences in controls. BHT did not increase the incidence of either papillomas or carcinomas. Interestingly, when BHA or BHT were given together with NaCl after MNNG treatment, the incidences of papillomas and carcinomas were higher than in the groups given BHA or BHT alone. The combination of BHA and NaCl was especially effective, raising the incidence of papilloma and carcinoma to 100% and 70%, respectively. In groups 7 to 11 which were not given MNNG, no tumors were observed, and the incidence of hyperplasia was highest in the groups treated with BHA plus NaCl. Some squamous cell carcinomas in groups 3 to 5 given NaCl were located in the limiting ridge and had the characteristic of a semi-circular crater in the fundic region.

Various lesions, including tumors of the glandular stomach, were

TABLE 1

Proliferative and Neoplastic Lesions of the Forestomach of Rats Treated with N-Methyl-N'-nitro-N-nitrosoguanidine (MNNG) Followed by Test Chemical

Group	Treatment[a]	Effective no. of rats	Number of rats with:[b] Hyperplasia	Papilloma	Squamous cell carcinoma	Sarcoma[c]
1	MNNG→BHA	20	20 (100)	18 (90)[d]	9 (45)[e]	0
2	MNNG→BHT	19	19 (100)	13 (68·4)	3 (15·8)	0
3	MNNG→NaCl	20	20 (100)	17 (85)[e]	6 (30)	1
4	MNNG→BHA + NaCl	17	20 (100)	20 (100)[f]	14 (70)[f]	1
5	MNNG→BHT + NaCl	17	17 (100)	16 (94·1)[g]	9 (52·9)[g]	1
6	MNNG	18	18 (100)	10 (55·6)	2 (11·1)	0
7	BHA	14	5 (35·7)	0	0	0
8	BHT	14	3 (21·4)	0	0	0
9	NaCl	15	4 (26·7)	0	0	0
10	BHA + NaCl	15	14 (93·3)	0	0	0
11	BHT + NaCl	12	11 (91·7)	0	0	0

[a] Groups 7–11 received initial treatment with DMSO.
[b] Numbers in parentheses represent percentages.
[c] Leiomyosarcoma.
[d] Significantly different from control (group 6) at $p < 0.02$.
[e] Significantly different from control (group 6) at $p < 0.05$.
[f] Significantly different from control (group 6) at $p < 0.001$.
[g] Significantly different from control (group 6) at $p < 0.01$.

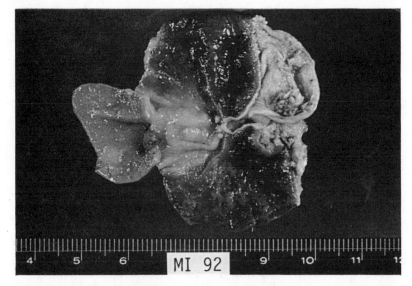

FIG. 1. Macroscopic appearance of tumors in the forestomach of a rat given MNNG followed by BHT plus NaCl.

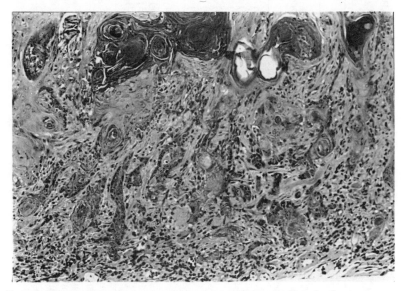

FIG. 2. Histologic appearance of the tumor shown in Fig. 1; the tumor was squamous cell carcinoma characterized by cornification; H&E; ×100.

TABLE 2
Incidences of Non-neoplastic and Neoplastic Lesions of the Glandular Stomach in Rats Treated with MNNG Followed by Test Chemical

Group	Treatment[a]	Effective no. of rats	Fundus Pyloric metaplasia	Fundus Dys-plasia	Fundus Ade-noma	Fundus Carci-noma	Fundus Sar-coma	Pylorus Hyper-plasia	Pylorus Dys-plasia	Pylorus Ade-noma	Pylorus Carci-noma	Pylorus Sar-coma
1	MNNG→BHA	20	16[b]	8	0	0	0	11	2	2	3	0
2	MNNG→BHT	19	10	4	1	1	0	12	2	0	0	0
3	MNNG→NaCl	20	19[c]	9	2	0	1	19	8[d]	1	1[e]	0
4	MNNG→BHA + NaCl	20	18[c]	9	1	0	0	17	9[d]	2	1	1
5	MNNG→BHT + NaCl	17	16[c]	4	0	1	0	12	8[f]	0	0	0
6	MNNG	18	7	3	0	0	0	14	2	0	3[g]	0

[a] Data on groups 7–11 were not included.
[b] Significantly different from the control value (group 6) at $p < 0.01$.
[c] Significantly different from the control value (group 6) at $p < 0.001$.
[d] Significantly different from the control value (group 6) at $p < 0.05$.
[e] Undifferentiated carcinoma.
[f] Significantly different from the control value (group 6) at $p < 0.02$.
[g] One well-differentiated adenocarcinoma, one mucinous adenocarcinoma and one signet ring cell carcinoma.

located in the pylorus as well as in the fundus. The incidences of neoplastic lesions and non-neoplastic lesions in the glandular stomach are shown in Table 2. The numbers and types of carcinoma were not affected by any subsequent treatment. No tumors of the stomach developed in groups given BHA, BHT or NaCl without MNNG pretreatment. Clear increases in the appearance of pyloric metaplasia after subsequent treatment with BHA, NaCl, BHA plus NaCl or BHT plus NaCl were apparent. Dysplasia in the pylorus was also increased by NaCl administration, but the incidence of hyperplasia was not affected by subsequent treatment. Intestinal metaplasia was also observed sporadically in the pylorus, but its incidence was not influenced by any of the treatments tested.

Thus, the present study revealed that NaCl, BHA but not BHT exerted a promoting activity on MNNG-induced forestomach carcinogenesis in rats and that, when BHA or BHT are given together with NaCl, additive effects of these compounds on tumor promotion occur.

EFFECTS ON COLON CARCINOGENESIS

To our knowledge, there has been only a single report about the effects of antioxidants on colon carcinogenesis under two-stage experimental conditions (Weisburger et al., 1977). In the study we now describe, the influence of five antioxidants, BHA, BHT, sodium L-ascorbate (SA), ethoxyquin (EQ) and propyl gallate (PG), given after initiation with 1,2-dimethylhydrazine (DMH), on colon tumorigenesis was investigated in rats (Shirai et al., 1985).

Male F344 rats were 6 weeks old at the beginning of the experiments and all the antioxidants were mixed into their basal diet. In one experiment, rats were divided into 10 groups. Rats in groups 1–5 (20 animals per group) were injected subcutaneously with DMH at a dose of 20 mg/kg body weight in physiological saline once a week for 4 weeks. One week after the last injection of DMH, these animals were placed on the following diets for 36 weeks: group 1, 5·0% SA; group 2, 0·5% BHA; group 3, 0·8% EQ; group 4, 1·0% PG; group 5, the basal diet alone. Groups 6–10 (15 rats each) were the corresponding controls to groups 1–5 and were given the vehicle (0·9% NaCl) instead of DMH followed by SA, BHA, EQ and PG. The effect of 0·5% BHT was investigated separately under the same conditions. All animals were killed and autopsied 40 weeks after the beginning of the experiment.

DMH administration did not affect body weight gain. Animals fed antioxidants grew less than control animals, an approximate 14–20% body weight suppression being evident with EQ throughout the experiment.

Table 3 summarizes the incidence of colon tumors in rats treated with DMH and antioxidants (data on non-initiated groups are not shown). Rats given only antioxidant had no intestinal tumors. All colon tumors were histologically of the epithelial type, i.e. adenomas and carcinomas.

The incidence of adenoma in animals given DMH followed by SA was significantly higher than that in animals given DMH alone. However, there were no significant differences in the incidences of carcinoma and in overall incidences of colon tumors among groups. Colon carcinomas were histologically divided into three types: tubular adenocarcinoma, signet ring cell carcinoma and mucinous adenocarcinoma. There was a tendency for signet ring cell carcinoma to arise in the proximal colon and well differentiated adenocarcinoma in the distal colon. The total number of carcinomas was similar in the groups, and no shifts to any specific type of carcinoma due to subsequent treatment with antioxidant were found.

The numbers of colon tumors and their locations are summarized in Table 4. Compared with the group given DMH alone, the number of colon tumors per rat was significantly increased in the groups given DMH followed by SA. This increase was due to heightened development of tumors in the transverse and descending colon. Subsequent treatment with EQ after DMH induced significantly more tumors in the descending colon than did DMH alone, while the DMH-BHT group had fewer tumors in the descending colon than the control.

Five tumors of the small intestine were present: three signet ring cell carcinomas and two tubular adenocarcinomas, all of which were located in the ileum. No statistical differences in the incidence of these tumors were detected among the groups.

Thus, modification of tumor development by SA, EQ and BHT was apparent, mainly in the distal colon. No modification of tumor development was observed with BHA or PG.

DOSE-DEPENDENT EFFECTS ON DEVELOPMENT OF ENZYME ALTERED FOCI IN THE LIVER

The effects of BHA, BHT and EQ on induction of glutathione S-transferase P (GST-P) (Kitahara *et al.*, 1984) and γ-glutamyl-transpeptidase (γ-GT) positive foci in the liver were assayed in an *in vivo* assay for the detection of promoting activity for liver carcinogenesis

TABLE 3
Mean Final Body Weight and Incidences of Colon Tumors

Group	Treatment	Effective no. of rats	Final body weight	Number of rats with (%): Adenoma	Carcinoma	Tumor[a]
Experiment I						
1	DMH → SA	20	390·3	6 (30)[b]	7 (35)	10 (50)
2	DMH → BHA	20	392·3	2 (10)	8 (40)	8 (40)
3	DMH → EQ	18	324·3	4 (22)	7 (39)	8 (44)
4	DMH → PG	20	364·0	5 (25)	6 (30)	10 (50)
5	DMH	20	430·7	1 (5)	6 (30)	7 (35)
Experiment II						
1	DMH → BHT	19	341·9	4 (21)	9 (48)	9 (47)
2	DMH	18	405·3	5 (28)	7 (39)	10 (56)

[a] Adenoma or carcinoma.
[b] Significantly different from DMH alone at $p < 0.05$.

TABLE 4
Numbers of Colon Tumors and Their Locations

Treatment	Number of colon tumors					
	Total	Per rat	Cecum	Ascending colon	Transverse colon	Descending colon
Experiment I						
DMH → SA	16	0·80 ± 1·00[b] (20)[a]	1	3	3	9
DMH → BHA	11	0·55 ± 0·76 (20)	0	6	0	5
DMH → EQ	12	0·67 ± 0·91 (18)	0	1	0	11[b]
DMH → PG	11	0·55 ± 0·60 (20)	0	2	2	7
DMH	7	0·35 ± 0·49 (20)	1	3	0	3
Experiment II						
DMH → BHT	12	0·56 ± 0·62 (19)	0	8	0	3[b]
DMH	16	0·94 ± 0·87 (18)	0	7	0	9

[a]Numbers in parentheses indicate the effective number of rats.
[b]Significantly different from DMH alone at $p < 0.05$.

developed in this laboratory (Ito *et al.*, 1982; Thamavit *et al.*, 1985).

Four hundred and seventy five 6-week-old rats were divided into 19 groups. Nine groups were treated with combinations of diethylnitrosamine (DEN) and 2, 1 and 0·5% BHA, 1, 0·5 and 0·25% BHT, or 0·5, 0·25 and 0·125% EQ, respectively (Table 5). Nine groups were treated with the same doses of the test chemicals without DEN, and one group received DEN alone. DEN was given as a single intraperitoneal injection of 200 mg of DEN per kg body weight on 0·9% NaCl solution, and control animals were given only 0·9% NaCl solution. After 2 weeks on basal diet, all groups of animals received their respective diets for 6 weeks. All animals were subjected to partial hepatectomy 3 weeks after DEN administration.

At the time of sacrifice, the livers were fixed in acetone or formalin and processed for histochemical examination of γ-GT, for immunohisto-chemical examination of GST-P by the unlabeled antibody peroxidase-antiperoxidase staining technique and for staining with hematoxylin and eosin as described previously (Imaida *et al.*, 1983; Ito *et al.*, 1982). A color image processor (VIP-21C) was used for quantitative analysis of GST-P- and γ-GT-positive foci. Foci less than 0·2 mm in diameter were not included in the analysis.

BHA, BHT and EQ, with or without DEN initiation, dose-dependently induced intense staining for γ-GT in hepatocytes of zone I (periportal area). Extension of staining from hepatic triads to central veins was seen in about one-half of the lobules with 2% BHA, about one-third with 1 and 0·5% BHA, two-thirds with 1% BHT, one-third to one-half with 0·5% BHT, less than one-third with 0·25% BHT, one-third to one-half with 0·5% EQ, one-third with 0·25% EQ and less than one-third with 0·125% EQ. In both nodular hyperplastic and non-nodular periportal cells, γ-GT staining was positive only at the membrane of the hepatocytes.

The three doses of BHA with or without DEN initiation also caused dose-dependent non-nodular scattered staining for GST-P in periportal and subcapsular cells. The higher the dose of BHA, the greater the extent of background staining, with GST-P staining induced by 1% BHT alone being similar in location and intensity to that of 1% BHA. Induction of heterogeneous periportal GST-P staining was not seen with 0·5 or 0·25% BHT, or any of the EQ doses tested. Staining of both nodular and non-nodular hepatocytes was evident in the cytoplasm and in most nuclei, the strongest staining being seen in preneoplastic foci.

With regard to γ-GT- and GST-P-positive foci in DEN-treated animals, BHA showed a clear dose-dependent inhibition of the number and the total area of foci positive for the two markers, although the degrees of

TABLE 5

Average Liver Weight and Quantitative Values for γ-GT- and GST-P-positive Foci in the Liver of F344 Rats Initiated with DEN and Subsequently Treated with Various Doses of BHA, BHT or EQ and Partial Hepatectomy

Treatment[a]	No. of animals	Liver weight[b]		γ-GT-positive foci[b]		GST-P-positive foci[b]	
		g	% body weight	No./cm²	Area (mm²)/cm²	No./cm²	Area (mm²)/cm²
DEN→BHA 2·0%	21	9·1 ± 1·2[c]	3·7 ± 0·4[c]	0·56 ± 0·50[c]	0·03 ± 0·03[c]	0·75 ± 0·61[c]	0·06 ± 0·06[c]
DEN→BHA 1·0%	25	9·0 ± 1·5[c]	3·3 ± 0·6[c]	0·67 ± 0·61[c]	0·07 ± 0·08[c]	1·52 ± 1·45[c]	0·11 ± 0·12[c]
DEN→BHA 0·5%	23	8·5 ± 1·1[c]	3·0 ± 0·3[c]	1·65 ± 1·09[c]	0·14 ± 0·12[c]	3·08 ± 1·41[d]	0·26 ± 0·14[d]
DEN→BHT 1·0%	24	13·3 ± 1·5[c]	5·5 ± 0·5[c]	3·00 ± 1·62[d]	0·25 ± 0·16[d]	4·28 ± 1·96	0·41 ± 0·23
DEN→BHT 0·5%	23	11·5 ± 1·5[c]	4·2 ± 0·5[c]	3·18 ± 1·15[d]	0·32 ± 0·12[e]	4·77 ± 2·15	0·51 ± 0·26
DEN→BHT 0·25%	21	9·8 ± 1·2[c]	3·5 ± 0·3[c]	3·81 ± 1·78[e]	0·38 ± 0·20	6·18 ± 3·21	0·64 ± 0·36
DEN→EQ 0·5%	22	12·1 ± 1·8[c]	4·5 ± 0·5[c]	1·82 ± 0·73[c]	0·16 ± 0·07[c]	4·69 ± 1·85	0·43 ± 0·15
DEN→EQ 0·25%	20	10·0 ± 1·3[c]	3·5 ± 0·4[c]	3·17 ± 1·25[d]	0·27 ± 0·14[d]	3·50 ± 1·64[e]	0·39 ± 0·21
DEN→EQ 0·125%	19	8·9 ± 1·5[c]	3·1 ± 0·4[c]	3·25 ± 1·23[d]	0·31 ± 0·13[e]	3·92 ± 1·67	0·41 ± 0·22
BHA 2·0%	25	9·0 ± 1·0[c]	3·5 ± 0·4[c]	—	—	—	—
BHA 1·0%	24	9·1 ± 0·5[c]	3·2 ± 0·1[c]	—	—	—	—
BHA 0·5%	21	8·9 ± 0·9[c]	3·1 ± 0·4[c]	—	—	—	—
BHT 1·0%	21	13·9 ± 1·0[c]	5·4 ± 0·3[c]	—	—	—	—
BHT 0·5%	20	11·3 ± 0·7[c]	4·1 ± 0·2[c]	—	—	—	—
BHT 0·25%	22	10·0 ± 0·8[c]	3·5 ± 0·2[c]	—	—	—	—
EQ 0·5%	23	12·4 ± 1·1[c]	4·4 ± 0·3[c]	—	—	—	—
EQ 0·25%	22	10·0 ± 1·0[c]	3·5 ± 0·4[c]	—	—	—	—
EQ 0·125%	22	8·7 ± 0·7[c]	3·0 ± 0·2[c]	—	—	—	—
DEN	22	7·0 ± 0·9	2·4 ± 0·3	4·98 ± 2·06	0·41 ± 0·20	4·75 ± 2·12	0·54 ± 0·34

[a] DEN = diethylnitrosamine; BHA = butylated hydroxyanisole; BHT = butylated hydroxytoluene; EQ = ethoxyquin.
[b] Values are means ± SD.
[c,d,e] Significantly different from the DEN-treated group at $P<0·001$, $P<0·01$ and $P<0·05$, respectively.

inhibition of the numbers of γ-GT foci with 2% and the 1% BHA were not significantly different (Table 5). All doses of BHT significantly decreased the number of γ-GT foci, but only 1% and 0·5% BHT decreased the area of the foci assayed using this marker (Fig. 3). There was no significant difference in either the number or the area of GST-P foci in any BHT group relative to those in controls treated with DEN (Fig. 4). The three EQ-treated groups also showed decreased numbers and areas of γ-GT positive foci. A dose-dependent effect of 0·5% EQ over those of 0·25% and 0·125% EQ was also seen. EQ at 0·25% slightly decreased the number, but not the area, of GST-P-positive foci. In zone I in each group, γ-GT-positive foci were difficult to distinguish from γ-GT-positive, otherwise normal looking hepatocytes. The GST-P values were higher than the corresponding γ-GT ones. No γ-GT- or GST-P-positive foci were detected in the control groups treated with antioxidants but not DEN.

Results with both markers demonstrated a dose-dependent decrease of foci in BHA-treated rats relative to those in carcinogen only control rats. Morphometric analysis of γ-GT-positive lesions also revealed decrease in both the number and area of foci in BHT- and EQ-treated groups. The discrepancy between results of quantitation of γ-GT- and GST-P-positive foci was attributable to the induction of a background, periportal zone staining for γ-GT, which made differentiation of smaller foci difficult (Figs 3 and 4). Comparison of results with the two markers from 13 quantitative studies on enzyme altered foci in rat liver suggested that GST-P is the more accurate marker. Thus, the activities of various doses of BHA, BHT and EQ to modify DEN-initiated hepatocarcinogenesis in rats have been investigated in our *in vivo* system.

MODIFICATION OF LIVER AND KIDNEY CARCINOGENESIS

The effects of BHA and EQ on the development of preneoplastic and neoplastic lesions in the liver and kidney of rats pretreated with N-ethyl-N-hydroxyethylnitrosamine (EHEN) have been investigated in our laboratory. (Tsuda *et al.*, 1984.)

In these investigations, 60 rats (group 1) were given 0·1% EHEN in their drinking water for 2 weeks and then 1 week later they were divided into subgroups and were given powdered basal diet containing 2·0% BHA or 0·8% EQ. Twenty-five rats (group 2) were treated with EHEN as in group 1 and then given tap water. They were given basal diet throughout the experiment. Groups of 25 rats were given BHA and EQ, respectively,

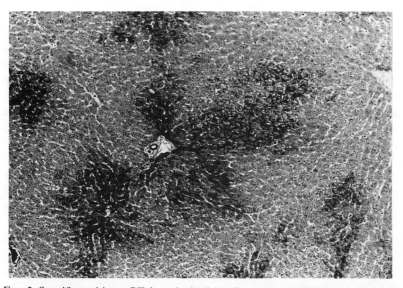

FIG. 3. Specific positive γ-GT-focus in the liver of a rat given DEN followed by BHT that was difficult to differentiate from the surrounding non-specific positive foci; γ-GT staining; ×100.

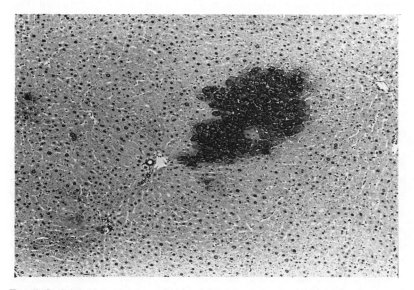

FIG. 4. Serial section of the preparation for Fig. 3; a specific positive GST-P-focus is seen; GST-P staining; ×100.

from week 3 to the end of the experiment. All animals were killed for examination at the end of week 32. Sections of liver were processed for demonstration and quantitative analysis of γ-GT positive foci. The numbers and areas of hyperplastic nodules were measured in sections stained with hematoxylin and eosin. All types of hyperplastic nodules were included in quantitative analyses in this study. The kidneys were cut sagittally with a razor blade into 2 or 3 sections and embedded, and sections were routinely stained with hematoxylin and eosin. Atypical cell foci and adenomas were measured in the same manner as lesions in the liver.

The liver weight was significantly less in groups given BHA or EQ than in controls, except the subgroup given BHA after EHEN. The greater weight in the group given EHEN alone was caused by development of hyperplastic nodules and hepatocellular carcinoma. The kidney weight was significantly increased in rats given EQ with or without EHEN.

Table 6 summarizes the incidences, numbers and areas of γ-GT positive foci, hyperplastic nodules and hepatocellular carcinomas in the liver. All rats treated with EHEN had γ-GT positive foci. In animals given BHA or EQ with or without EHEN, hepatocytes in periportal areas throughout the liver stained positively for γ-GT. The numbers and areas of γ-GT positive foci were significantly less in groups given BHA or EQ after EHEN than in rats given EHEN alone.

The number of hyperplastic nodules in the group given BHA after EHEN and the area of hyperplastic nodules in groups given either of these chemicals were significantly less than those in animals given EHEN alone (Fig. 5). Similarly, the incidences of hepatocellular carcinomas were significantly lower in all groups given these chemicals than in the control group (Fig. 6). No animals given BHA or EQ without prior treatment with EHEN had γ-GT positive foci, hyperplastic nodules or hepatocellular carcinomas.

Foci of tubular proliferation in the kidney composed of cells with clear or mostly basophilic cytoplasm and a round, slightly enlarged nucleus with prominent nucleoli were tentatively named atypical cell foci in this study (Fig. 7). The cells of atypical cell foci were usually tall and columnar and arranged linearly on dilated tubules. In some atypical cell foci, the cells showed proliferation into the lumen and were packed in papillary structures or cords of two or more cells thickness. The foci showed slight compression of surrounding tubules. For quantitative analysis, atypical cell foci of more than 0·15 mm mean diameter, which is approximately the diameter of a glomerulus, were included. The incidences of atypical cell foci in the groups given EHEN and EQ were significantly higher than those

TABLE 6

Incidences and Quantitative Values of Preneoplastic and Neoplastic Lesions in the Liver

Group	Treatment	No. of rats	γ-GT$^+$ foci			Hyperplastic nodules			Hepatocellular carcinoma incidence (%)
			No. of rats (%)	No./cm²^a	Area^a (mm²/cm²)	No. of rats (%)	No./cm²^a	Area^a (mm²/cm²)	
1	EHEN→BHA	24	24 (100)	1·7 ± 1·2^d	8·63 ± 14·24^c	22 (91·7)	0·6 ± 0·5^d	3·02 ± 4·54^b	2 (8·3)^c
	EHEN→EQ	27	27 (100)	1·0 ± 3·6^d	9·94 ± 11·29^c	27 (100)	1·5 ± 0·9	2·25 ± 3·71^c	3 (11·1)^b
2	EHEN	23	23 (100)	20·8 ± 8·3	21·98 ± 13·15	22 (95·8)	1·9 ± 1·0	6·98 ± 7·06	11 (47·8)
3	BHA	25	0	—	—	0	—	—	0
	EQ	25	0	—	—	0	—	—	0

^{a}Values are mean ± SD.
^{b}Significantly different from group 2 at $p < 0.05$.
^{c}Significantly different from group 2 at $p < 0.01$.
^{d}Significantly different from group 2 at $p < 0.001$.

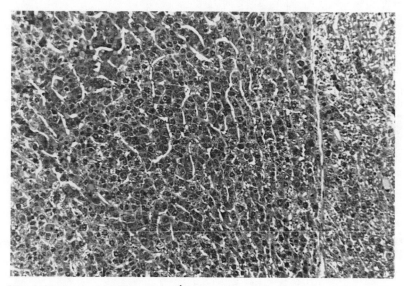

FIG. 5. Hyperplastic nodule in the liver of a rat given EHEN alone; H&E; ×100.

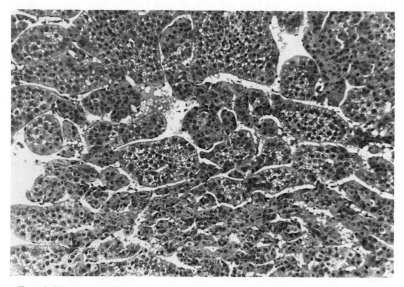

FIG. 6. Hepatocellular carcinoma in a rat given EHEN alone; H&E; ×100.

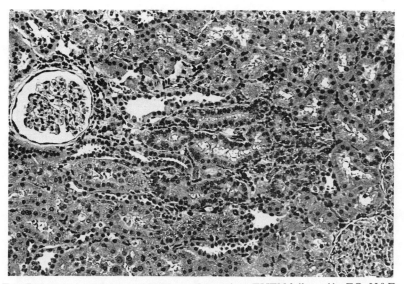

FIG. 7. Atypical cell focus in the kidney of a rat given EHEN followed by EQ; H&E; ×100.

in the group given EHEN alone (Table 7). The number and area of atypical cell foci were also significantly higher in this group. Renal cell adenomas composed of sheets of epithelial cells, mostly with slightly basophilic or clear cytoplasm and round nuclei, were observed in the groups given EHEN (groups 1 and 2) (Fig. 8). The incidences and numbers of renal cell adenomas were significantly higher in rats given EHEN followed by EQ than in those given EHEN alone. Three rats in the group given EQ after EHEN had renal cell carcinomas, whereas rats given EHEN alone had none. This difference, however, was not significant.

Thus, BHA and EQ inhibited the induction of preneoplastic and neoplastic lesions in the liver when given during the second stage of carcinogenesis. In contrast, EQ enhanced the induction of preneoplastic and neoplastic lesions in the kidney.

EFFECT ON URINARY BLADDER CARCINOGENESIS

Modification by Sodium L-Ascorbate, L-Ascorbic Acid, Sodium Erythorbate and EQ

The promoting effect of four antioxidants, sodium L-ascorbate (SA), L-ascorbic acid (AA), sodium erythorbate (SE) and EQ, on the develop-

TABLE 7
Incidences and Quantitative Values of Neoplastic Lesions in the Kidney

Group	Treatment	No. of rats	Atypical cell foci			Adenoma			Adeno-carcinoma (%)	Nephro-blastoma (%)
			No. of rats (%)	No./cm²	Area (×10⁻² mm²/cm²)	No. of rats (%)	No./cm²	Area (×10⁻² mm²/cm²)		
1	EHEN→BHA	24	16 (66·7)	0·46±0·57[a]	1·29±2·77[a]	6 (25)	0·17±0·33[a]	15·88±44·91[a]	1 (4·2)	0
	EHEN→EQ	27	26 (96·3)[b]	0·93±0·79[b]	5·55±5·12[b]	17 (63·0)[c]	0·52±0·58[c]	23·55±45·18	3 (11·1)	0
2	EHEN	23	12 (52·1)	0·21±0·32	0·88±1·51	5 (21·7)	0·08±0·02	7·67±32·14	0	0
3	BHA	25	0	—	—	0	—	—	0	0
4	EQ	25	0	—	—	0	—	—	0	0

[a] Values are mean ± SD.
[b] Significantly different from group 2 at $p < 0.01$.
[c] Significantly different from group 2 at $p < 0.001$.

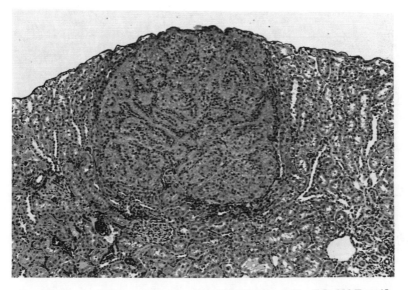

FIG. 8. Renal cell adenoma in a rat given EHEN followed by EQ; H&E; ×40.

ment of preneoplastic and neoplastic lesions in the urinary bladder after pretreatment with N-butyl-N-(4-hydroxybutyl)nitrosamine (BBN) was studied in our laboratory (Fukushima *et al.*, 1983, 1984).

In one experiment, two groups of F344 rats were given drinking water containing 0·05% BBN for 4 weeks, and then powdered diet containing 5·0% (group 1) or 1·0% (group 2) SA for 32 weeks. Group 3 was given only BBN for 4 weeks, whereas group 4 was given drinking water without BBN for 4 weeks, and then powdered diet containing 5·0% SA. The total observation period in this experiment was 36 weeks.

Macroscopically, rats given 0·5% BBN followed by 5·0% SA had a greater incidence of big tumors of the urinary bladder than the controls (Fig. 9). For quantitative analysis, urinary bladder lesions were counted by light microscopy, the total length of the basement membrane was measured with a color video image processor, and the numbers of lesions per 10 cm of basement membrane were calculated (Fukushima *et al.*, 1982).

The histopathological lesions of the urinary bladder observed in rats are summarized in Table 8. As described previously (Fukushima *et al.*, 1982; Ito *et al.*, 1973), the lesions found in the urinary bladder epithelium were

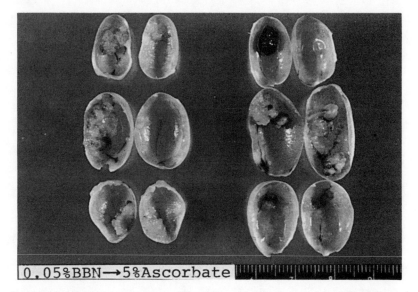

0.05%BBN→5%Ascorbate

FIG. 9. Macroscopic appearance of the urinary bladder in rats given BBN followed by 5·0% SA; big tumors are seen in the urinary bladder.

classified into four types: simple hyperplasia, papillary or nodular hyperplasia (PN hyperplasia, preneoplastic hyperplasia), papilloma and carcinoma (Figs 10–12). On pretreatment with 0·05% BBN followed by 5·0% SA in group 1, the incidence and the number of carcinomas per 10 cm basement membrane were significantly increased. The incidence and the number of PN hyperplasias and papillomas per 10 cm basement membrane were also significantly increased by 5·0% SA. However, 1·0% SA did not significantly increase the occurrence of any bladder lesions in rats pretreated with BBN, although it tended to increase the incidence of PN hyperplasia. There were no remarkable changes in the urinary bladder of rats treated with 5·0% SA alone without BBN. These results showed that SA promotes urinary bladder carcinogenesis in rats initiated with BBN.

Treatment with SA resulted in increases in the contents of AA and its metabolite, dehydroascorbic acid, in the urine (Fukushima *et al.*, 1983). Since these changes might contribute to the induction of carcinoma in the urinary bladder, it was uncertain from these findings whether AA itself has promoting activity.

A second series of experiments with rats was therefore performed. Rats were given drinking water with (groups 1–4) or without (groups 5–7)

TABLE 8
Histological Findings in the Urinary Bladder of Rats Treated with BBN Followed by Test Chemical

Group	Treatment BBN	Treatment Test chemical	Effective no. of rats	Simple hyperplasia Incidence (%)	Papillary or nodular hyperplasia Incidence (%)	No./10 cm of BM[a]	Papilloma Incidence (%)	No./10 cm of BM	Carcinoma Incidence (%)	No./10 cm of BM
Experiment 1										
1	+	5.0% SA	25	25 (100)[c]	25 (100)[c]	7.0 ± 3.0[b,c]	23 (92)[c]	3.1 ± 1.6[b,c]	24 (96)[c]	1.4 ± 0.7[b,c]
2	+	1.0% SA	29	20 (69)	11 (38)	0.6 ± 1.0	12 (41)	0.4 ± 0.6	0 —	0
3	+	—	30	17 (57)	8 (27)	0.3 ± 0.5	12 (40)	0.5 ± 0.5	1 (3)	0.0 ± 0.2
4	−	5.0% SA	20	0	0 —	0	0 —	0	0 —	0
Experiment 2										
1	+	5.0% AA	25	14 (56)	7 (28)	0.3 ± 0.5[b]	10 (40)	0.4 ± 0.5[b]	1 (4)	0.0 ± 0.1[b]
2	+	5.0% SE	23	23 (100)	23 (100)[c]	5.3 ± 4.2[c]	19 (83)[c]	1.4 ± 1.2[c]	15 (65)[c]	0.8 ± 0.7[c]
3	+	0.8% EQ	25	25 (100)	25 (100)[c]	9.4 ± 3.9[c]	17 (68)[c]	1.1 ± 1.0[c]	4 (16)	0.2 ± 0.5
4	+	—	24	14 (58)	8 (33)	0.5 ± 1.0	5 (20)	0.2 ± 0.4	1 (4)	0.0 ± 0.2
5	−	5.0% AA	25	0 (0)	0 (0)	0	0 (0)	0	0 (0)	0
6	−	5.0% SE	25	0 (0)	0 (0)	0	0 (0)	0	0 (0)	0
7	−	0.8% EQ	25	25 (100)	9 (36)	0.4 ± 0.5	9 (0)	0	0 (0)	0

[a] BM = basement membrane.
[b] Mean ± SD.
[c] Significantly different from group 4 at $p < 0.001$.

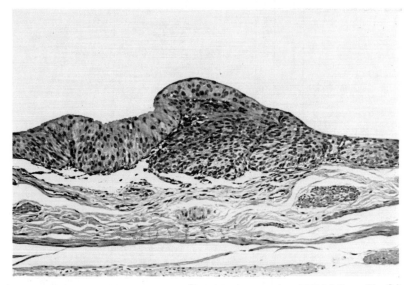

FIG. 10. PN hyperplasia of the urinary bladder in a rat given BBN followed by SA; H&E; ×200.

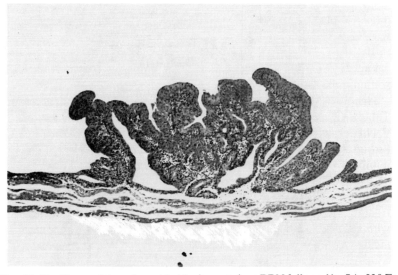

FIG. 11. Papilloma of the urinary bladder in a rat given BBN followed by SA; H&E; ×80.

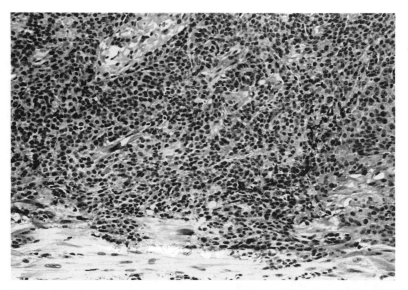

Fig. 12. Transitional cell carcinoma of the urinary bladder in a rat given BBN followed by SA; cancerous tissue invades the muscle layer; H&E; ×200.

0·05% BBN for 4 weeks, and then for 32 weeks they were given powdered basal diet containing 5·0% AA (groups 1 and 5), 5·0% SE (groups 2 and 6) or 0·8% EQ (groups 3 and 7), or pelleted basal diet containing no added chemical (group 4). The total observation period was 36 weeks. (SE is the sodium salt of erythorbic acid, the epimer of AA.)

Histological findings in the urinary bladder of the rats are summarized in Table 8. The incidences and numbers per 10 cm of basement membrane of PN hyperplasia and papilloma were significantly higher in groups given SE (group 2) or EQ (group 3) than in controls (group 4). The incidence and number of carcinomas were increased significantly in group 2 treated with SE, and slightly in group 3 treated with EQ. However, treatment with AA did not increase the incidence of any urinary bladder lesions in rats pretreated with BBN (group 1). In groups given the test chemicals alone without BBN (groups 5, 6 and 7), EQ induced PN hyperplasia at low incidence, but AA and SE had no effect on the mucosa. These results show conclusively that SE and EQ promote urinary bladder carcinogenesis, whereas AA does not. Moreover, EQ might be carcinogenic for the urinary bladder in a long-term carcinogenicity test.

TABLE 9
Histological Findings in the Urinary Bladder in Rats Treated with BBN Followed by BHA or BHT

Group	Treatment BBN	Treatment Test chemical	Effective no. of rats	Simple hyperplasia Incidence (%)	Papillary or nodular hyperplasia Incidence (%)	Papillary or nodular hyperplasia No./10 cm of BM[a,b]	Papilloma Incidence (%)	Papilloma No./10 cm of BM[a]	Carcinoma Incidence (%)	Carcinoma No./10 cm of BM[a]
1	0·05%	2·0% BHA	25	25	25 (100)	4·3 ± 2·7[e]	22 (88·0)[e]	2·0 ± 1·4[e]	19 (76·0)[e]	0·8 ± 0·7[d]
2	0·05%	1·0% BHT	24	24	23 (95·8)	4·0 ± 1·9[e]	17 (70·8)[d]	0·9 ± 0·8[c]	13 (54·2)[c]	0·4 ± 0·6
3	0·05%	—	26	23	24 (92·3)	2·0 ± 0·8	11 (42·3)	0·4 ± 0·6	5 (19·3)	0·2 ± 0·4
4	0·01%	2·0% BHA	25	24	24 (96·0)[c]	3·0 ± 2·3[e]	11 (44·0)	0·7 ± 1·3	5 (20·0)	0·1 ± 0·3
5	0·01%	1·0% BHT	22	21	20 (90·9)[c]	2·0 ± 1·2[d]	3 (13·6)	0·1 ± 0·3	1 (4·5)	0·0 ± 0·0
6	0·01%	—	24	16	15 (62·5)	1·1 ± 1·0	7 (29·2)	0·2 ± 0·5	2 (8·3)	0·1 ± 0·2
7	—	2·0% BHA	25	0	0	0	0	0	0	0
8	—	1·0% BHT	25	0	0	0	0	0	0	0
9	—	—	19	0	0	0	0	0	0	0

[a] Mean ± SD.
[b] BM = basement membrane.
[c] Significantly different from the control at $p < 0.05$.
[d] Significantly different from the control at $p < 0.01$.
[e] Significantly different from the control at $p < 0.001$.

Promoting Activity of BHA and BHT

The promoting effects of BHA and BHT on the development of pre-neoplastic and neoplastic lesions in rats pretreated with BBN were also studied (Imaida et al., 1983). In these studies rats were given drinking water containing 0·05% BBN for 4 weeks and then pellet diet containing 2·0% BHA, basal diet containing 1·0% BHT or basal diet for 32 weeks. Other groups were given drinking water containing 0·01% BBN for 4 weeks and then BHA, BHT or basal diet. All rats were sacrificed at the end of week 36.

The incidences of histopathological lesions of the urinary bladder are shown in Table 9. The incidence and number per 10 cm basement membrane of carcinomas and papillomas were significantly higher in rats given 0·05% BBN followed by BHA than in controls. The incidence of carcinoma and the incidence and number of papillomas were significantly increased in rats given 0·05% BBN followed by BHT. There were also significant increases in the incidences and numbers of PN hyperplasias in rats given 0·01% BBN followed by BHA or BHT, compared with control values. There were no histopathological changes in the urinary bladder of rats given BHA or BHT alone.

Papillomas of the forestomach were observed in rats in all groups treated with BHA, but there was no significant difference between groups with or without prior BBN administration.

These findings show that BHA and BHT promote urinary bladder carcinogenesis.

Effects of Combinations of Four Antioxidants

The promoting activities of BHA, BHT, t-butylhydroquinone (TBHQ) and α-tocopherol (α-TP), and of combinations of pairs of these compounds, on urinary bladder carcinogenesis initiated by BBN in rats were further investigated in our laboratory (Hagiwara et al., 1984).

In these studies 420 F344 rats were divided into 21 groups of 20 rats and tested as shown in Table 10. Rats were given drinking water with or without 0·05% BBN for 4 weeks and then were maintained on diets containing 0·4% BHA plus 0·4% BHT, 0·4% BHA plus 0·4% TBHQ, 0·4% BHA plus 0·4% α-TP, 0·4% BHT plus 0·4% TBHQ, 0·4% BHT plus 0·4% α-TP, 0·4% TBHQ plus 0·4% α-TP, 0·8% BHA, 0·8% BHT, 0·8% TBHQ, 0·8% α-TP, or no chemical. From week 13, all rats treated with 0·8% BHT were given 7 ppm of vitamin K in their drinking water, and the total observation period was 36 weeks.

Quantitative data on histopathological changes of the urinary bladder

TABLE 10

Histological Findings in the Urinary Bladder of Rats Treated with BBN and then Test Chemicals

Group	Treatment		No. of rats examined	PN hyperplasia		Papilloma		Cancer	
	BBN	Test chemical		Incidence No. (%)	Density No./10 cm BM[a]	Incidence No. (%)	Density No./10 cm BM	Incidence No. (%)	Density No./10 cm BM[a]
1-A	+	BHA + BHT	20	17 (85)	$2{\cdot}8 \pm 2{\cdot}1^b$	14 (70)	$1{\cdot}1 \pm 0{\cdot}9$	1 (5)	$0{\cdot}0 \pm 0{\cdot}2$
B	+	BHA + TBHQ	20	19 (95)^b	$5{\cdot}8 \pm 4{\cdot}7^d$	16 (80)	$1{\cdot}8 \pm 1{\cdot}7$	6 (30)	$0{\cdot}3 \pm 0{\cdot}4$
C	+	BHA + α-TP	20	11 (55)	$1{\cdot}4 \pm 2{\cdot}0$	10 (50)	$0{\cdot}7 \pm 1{\cdot}0^b$	1 (5)	$0{\cdot}1 \pm 0{\cdot}2$
D	+	BHT + TBHQ	20	18 (90)	$3{\cdot}6 \pm 2{\cdot}8^c$	15 (75)	$1{\cdot}3 \pm 1{\cdot}0$	3 (15)	$0{\cdot}2 \pm 0{\cdot}7$
E	+	BHT + α-TP	20	18 (90)	$2{\cdot}1 \pm 1{\cdot}6$	9 (45)	$0{\cdot}7 \pm 0{\cdot}8^b$	0 —	—
F	+	TBHQ + α-TP	20	15 (75)	$1{\cdot}6 \pm 1{\cdot}3$	7 (35)	$0{\cdot}4 \pm 0{\cdot}6^c$	1 (5)	$0{\cdot}1 \pm 0{\cdot}2$
G	+	BHA	20	18 (90)	$3{\cdot}6 \pm 3{\cdot}1^c$	15 (75)	$1{\cdot}3 \pm 1{\cdot}1$	3 (15)	$0{\cdot}2 \pm 0{\cdot}5$
H	+	BHT	16	14 (88)	$3{\cdot}3 \pm 2{\cdot}6^b$	11 (69)	$1{\cdot}1 \pm 1{\cdot}1$	4 (25)	$0{\cdot}4 \pm 0{\cdot}8$
I	+	TBHQ	20	18 (90)	$6{\cdot}9 \pm 6{\cdot}5^b$	14 (70)	$3{\cdot}0 \pm 3{\cdot}2$	3 (15)	$0{\cdot}3 \pm 0{\cdot}8$
J	+	α-TP	20	13 (65)	$1{\cdot}3 \pm 1{\cdot}4$	10 (50)	$0{\cdot}8 \pm 1{\cdot}0^b$	0 —	—
2	+	Basal diet	20	14 (70)	$1{\cdot}3 \pm 1{\cdot}6$	15 (75)	$1{\cdot}6 \pm 1{\cdot}2$	2 (10)	$0{\cdot}2 \pm 0{\cdot}5$
3-A	−	BHA + BHT	20	0 —	—	0 —	—	0 —	—
B	−	BHA + TBHQ	20	0 —	—	0 —	—	0 —	—
C	−	BHA + α-TP	20	0 —	—	0 —	—	0 —	—
D	+	BHT + TBHQ	20	0 —	—	0 —	—	0 —	—
E	−	BHT + α-TP	20	0 —	—	0 —	—	0 —	—
F	−	TBHQ + α-TP	20	0 —	—	0 —	—	0 —	—
G	−	BHA	20	0 —	—	0 —	—	0 —	—
H	−	BHT	16	0 —	—	0 —	—	0 —	—
I	−	TBHQ	20	0 —	—	0 —	—	0 —	—
J	−	α-TP	20	0 —	—	0 —	—	0 —	—

[a] BM = basement membrane.

[b,c,d] Significantly different from group 2 at $p < 0{\cdot}05$, $p < 0{\cdot}01$ and $p < 0{\cdot}001$, respectively.

are summarized in Table 10. The incidence of PN hyperplasia was significantly increased only in the group given 0·05% BBN and 0·4% BHA plus 0·4% TBHQ. Quantitative analysis showed that the density of PN hyperplasia (number of lesions per 10 cm basement membrane) was significantly increased in the groups given BBN and BHA plus BHT, BHA plus TBHQ, BHT plus TBHQ, BHA, BHT and TBHQ. There was no significant difference in the incidences of papillomas in control and experimental groups. However, the density of papillomas was significantly decreased in the groups given BHA plus α-TP, BHT plus α-TP, TBHQ plus α-TP and α-TP with BBN. Rats given antioxidant alone or in combination without BBN had no bladder epithelial lesions. No marked histopathological lesions related to treatments were observed in any other organs.

The phenolic antioxidants BHA, BHT and TBHQ, singly or in pairs, were thus found to enhance bladder carcinogenesis in rats initiated by BBN. The promoting effects of BHA and BHT have been demonstrated previously. A significant finding was that α-TP alone, or in combination with BHA or BHT or TBHQ, clearly inhibited BBN-induced urinary bladder carcinogenesis.

EFFECT ON CARCINOGENESIS IN MANY ORGANS

The modifying effects of BHA, BHT and SA after pretreatment with N-methyl-N-nitrosourea (MNU), a wide-spectrum carcinogen inducing tumors in many organs, were studied (Imaida et al., 1984).

Rats were initially treated with 20 mg MNU/kg or vehicle, administered intraperitoneally, twice a week for 4 weeks (Table 11). They were then divided into groups, consisting of 30 rats each, for treatment with 2·0% BHA, 1·0% BHT or 5·0% SA in basal diet from week 4 to 36. Another group of 30 rats was given MNU in the same manner and then placed on basal diet from week 4 to 36. In week 36 the rats were killed. All major organs were carefully examined histologically for the presence of neoplastic lesions.

Neoplastic lesions were found in the stomach (both the forestomach and glandular stomach), urinary bladder, liver, thyroid, lymphatic or hematopoietic tissue, tongue, intestine, nervous system, lung, kidney, ear duct and skin. Statistically significant differences between the incidences in treated and control groups were observed in the forestomach, urinary

TABLE 11

Effects of BHA, BHT and Sodium L-Ascorbate on Forestomach Carcinogenesis in Rats Initiated by MNU

Group	Treatment	Effective no. of rats	Hyperplasia (%)	Papilloma (%)	Carcinoma (%)
1	MNU → 2·0% BHA	25	24 (96)[a]	23 (92)[b]	22 (88)[b]
2	MNU → 1·0% BHT	17	13 (77)	7 (41)	1 (6)
3	MNU → 5·0% SA	29	19 (66)	12 (41)	10 (35)[a]
4	MNU	22	12 (55)	8 (36)	0 —
5	— 2·0% BHA	30	30 (100)	29 (97)	0 —
6	— 1·0% BHT	16	0 —	0 —	0 —
7	— 5·0% SA	30	3 (10)	3 (10)	0 —

[a] Significantly different from group 4 at $p < 0.01$.
[b] Significantly different from group 4 at $p < 0.001$.

bladder and thyroid (Tables 11–13). The incidences of hyperplasia, papilloma and squamous cell carcinomas in the forestomach were significantly higher in animals treated with BHA (Table 11). SA increased the incidence of carcinoma. Atypical cell foci were seen in the fundus and pylorus of the glandular stomach of all MNU-treated animals, but their incidences were not significantly different from those in controls. Animals given BHA, BHT or SA had higher incidences and numbers of PN hyperplasia and papilloma in the urinary bladder than controls (Table 12). The incidences of carcinomas of the urinary bladder were significantly increased in groups given BHT. The numbers of carcinoma were significantly higher in groups given BHA or BHT than in the controls. Although not significant, the incidences and numbers of carcinomas also tended to be higher in groups given SA.

Adenomas and hyperplasias of the lung, and lymphomas and/or leukemia, were observed in all MNU-treated groups but there were no significant differences in incidence in these groups (Table 13). The incidence of adenoma of the thyroid in the MNU+BHT treated group was significantly higher than that in the MNU-treated group, but the incidences of adenocarcinomas in different groups were not significantly different.

The results of these investigations show that BHA, BHT and SA have promoting activities on urinary bladder carcinogenesis in rats initiated with MNU, and that BHA and SA also enhance forestomach carcinogenesis initiated with MNU. BHT may also be a promoter of thyroid tumorigenesis.

DISCUSSION

The carcinogenicity of BHA has been studied by several workers, but none of them found that it was carcinogenic for experimental animals (Allen, 1976; Hodge et al., 1964, 1966; Kohn, 1971). Many investigators have reported that BHA has no mutagenic activity, although it was positive in the rec assay of DNA repair test (Ishidate and Odashima, 1977; Kawachi, 1979). Our recent studies, however, show that BHA is carcinogenic in the forestomach of rats, with dose-dependence (Ito et al., 1983a, 1986). BHT has been reported recently to induce hepatocellular neoplasms in rats (Olsen et al., 1983). Some antioxidants, especially phenolic antioxidants, may inhibit or enhance tumorigenesis in rodents treated concomitantly with carcinogenic agents (Wattenberg, 1976, 1978, 1980; Williams et al., 1983; Witschi, 1981). Apart from BHA or BHT, SA has been shown to

TABLE 12

Effects of BHA, BHT and Sodium L-Ascorbate on Urinary Bladder Carcinogenesis in Rats Treated with MNU

Group	Treatment	Effective no. of rats	Simple hyperplasia Incidence (No. of rats)	Papillary or nodular hyperplasia Incidence (No. of rats)	Papillary or nodular hyperplasia No./10 cm $BM^{a,b}$	Papilloma Incidence (No. of rats)	Papilloma No./10 cm BM^a	Carcinoma Incidence (No. of rats)	Carcinoma No./10 cm BM^a
1	MNU→2·0% BHA	24	24[d]	20[e]	4·7±4·2[e]	10[d]	0·8±1·2[d]	4	0·2±0·4[c]
2	MNU→1·0% BHT	15	14	12[d]	3·3±3·0[d]	9[e]	0·9±1·0[d]	4[c]	0·3±0·4[c]
3	MNU→5·0% sodium L-ascorbate	29	29[d]	17[c]	1·8±3·2[c]	8[c]	0·3±0·4[d]	3	0·1±0·3
4	MNU	21	13	5	0·4±0·8	0	0	0	0
5	— 2·0% BHA	30	0	0	0	0	0	0	0
6	— 1·0% BHT	16	0	0	0	0	0	0	0
7	— 5·0% sodium L-ascorbate	30	0	0	0	0	0	0	0

[a] Values are mean ± SD.
[b] BM = basement membrane.
[c] Significantly different from group 4 at $p < 0·05$.
[d] Significantly different from group 4 at $p < 0·01$.
[e] Significantly different from group 4 at $p < 0·001$.

TABLE 13

Effects of BHA, BHT and Sodium L-Ascorbate on the Lung, Thyroid and Hematopoietic System of Rats Pretreated with MNU

Group	Treatment	Effective no. of rats	Lung Hyperplasia	Lung Adenoma	Thyroid Adenoma	Thyroid Adenocarcinoma	Lymphoma/Leukemia
1	MNU→2·0% BHA	25	14	5	4	0	7
2	MNU→1·0% BHT	17	10	3	11[a]	0	6
3	MNU→5·0% SA	29	23	9	1	2	9
4	MNU	22	16	5	6	1	10
5	— 2·0% BHA	30	0	0	0	0	0
6	— 1·0% BHT	16	0	0	0	0	0
7	— 5·0% SA	30	0	0	0	0	0

[a] Significantly different from group 4 at $p < 0·05$.

inhibit colon carcinogenesis in rats (Reddy *et al.*, 1982) and α-TP oral carcinogenesis in hamsters (Shklar, 1982).

Chemical carcinogenesis is known to occur in two stages in several organs, a first initiation stage and a second promotion stage (Berenblum and Shubik, 1947). In the present studies, administration of antioxidants in the second stage after pretreatment with carcinogens induced modification of the carcinogenic response (MCR) of chemical carcinogenesis. Table 14 summarizes the modifying effects of the antioxidants tested on neoplastic development in six organs: forestomach, glandular stomach, liver, kidney,

TABLE 14
Modifying Effects of Antioxidants on Second Stage of Carcinogenesis in Rats

Organ	BHA	BHT	SA	EQ
Forestomach	↑	↔	↑	NE
Glandular stomach	↔	↔	↔	NE
Liver	↓	↓	↔	↓
Kidney	↔	NE	NE	↑
Urinary bladder	↑	↑	↑	↑
Thyroid	↔	↑	↔	NE

↑, Enhancement; ↓, inhibition; ↔, no effect; NE, not examined.

urinary bladder and thyroid. BHA significantly enhanced tumor development in the forestomach and urinary bladder, but inhibited the development of liver lesions. Similarly, BHT promoted urinary bladder carcinogenesis, but inhibited liver carcinogenesis, and in addition it enhanced the development of MNU-initiated thyroid tumors. BHT is also reported to have 'promoting' effects in lung (Witschi *et al.*, 1977) and liver carcinogenesis in a different system from that used in the present study (Peraino *et al.*, 1977). SA enhanced forestomach and urinary bladder carcinogenesis. EQ enhanced kidney and bladder carcinogenesis, but inhibited liver carcinogenesis.

Clearly then, depending upon the organ, antioxidants modify neoplastic development resulting in either enhancement or inhibition of the appearance of lesions. Several investigators have reported the promoting and inhibitory effects of chemicals *in vivo*, although their studies were usually focused on one or a few main target organs. The fact that a single chemical can exert both a positive or a negative influence is, however, not limited to antioxidants. For example, 4,4'-diaminodiphenylmethane has been shown to inhibit urinary bladder and liver carcinogenesis (Fukushima *et al.*, 1981), and more recently it was found to promote the development of thyroid tumors in rats initiated with *N*-bis-(2-hydroxypropyl)nitrosamine (Hiasa *et al.*, 1984).

Consideration of the literature and information presently available does not allow a clear explanation of the differential modification of the carcinogenic response (MCR) observed with a number of chemicals including antioxidants. Although BHA has been shown to induce hyperplasia in one of its target organs (Nera *et al.*, 1984; Hirose *et al.*, 1985) and BHT induces proliferation of thyroid tissue (Søndergaaed and Olsen, 1982), this is not the only mechanism underlying enhancement of carcinogenesis, as stressed earlier (Weinstein and Troll, 1977), since there was no difference between the thyroid weights of groups treated with BHA and BHT in the present experiment, but only BHT enhanced tumor induction. Possible irritation, as measured by changes in the urine pH and crystalluria, was also not correlated with enhancement of urinary bladder carcinogenesis. This field obviously deserves, and should reward, further investigation.

In conclusion, the studies described in this chapter show that antioxidants, which are widely used as food additives, can modify the neoplastic process in two-stage carcinogenesis when administered at the second stage, although doses of antioxidants employed in the present study are several orders of magnitude (on a molar basis) more effective than antioxidants in inducing the liver microsomal mixed-function oxidases. Since antioxidants exert a wide variety of beneficial or harmful effects in rodents, the extent of exposure of humans to these compounds should be carefully evaluated.

SUMMARY

In two-stage carcinogenesis in rats after appropriate initiation, BHA enhanced carcinogenesis in the forestomach and urinary bladder of rats, but inhibited carcinogenesis in the liver. BHT enhanced the induction of urinary bladder tumors and inhibited that of liver tumors, but had no effect on carcinogenesis in the forestomach. BHT could be a promoter of thyroid carcinogenesis. SA enhanced forestomach and urinary bladder carcinogenesis. EQ enhanced kidney and urinary bladder carcinogenesis, but inhibited liver carcinogenesis. Thus, these antioxidants modify two-stage chemical carcinogenesis in the forestomach, liver, kidney, urinary bladder and thyroid, but show organ-specific differences in effects.

ACKNOWLEDGMENTS

These studies were supported in part by Grants-in-Aid for Cancer Research from the Ministry of Education, Science and Culture and the Ministry of Health and Welfare of Japan, and by grants from the Japan Tobacco and Salt Public Corporation, Aichi Cancer Research Foundation, Meihoku Labour Standards Association, the Society for Promotion of Pathology of Nagoya, and the Experimental Pathological Research Association.

REFERENCES

Allen, J. R. (1976). Long-term antioxidant exposure effects on female primates. *Arch. Environ. Health*, **31**, 47–50.

Ames, S. R., Ludwig, M. I., Swanson, W. J. and Harris, P. L. (1956). Effect of DPPD, methylene blue, BHT, and hydroquinone on reproductive process in the rat. *Proc. Soc. Exp. Biol. Med.*, **93**, 39–42.

Astill, B. D., Mills, J., Fassett, D. W., Roudabush, R. L. and Terhaar, C. J. (1962). Fate of butylated hydroxyanisole in man and dog. *J. Agric. Food Chem.*, **10**, 315–21.

Batzinger, B. P., Ou, S. Y. L. and Bueding, E. (1978). Antimutagenic effects of 2(3)-*tert*-butylhydroxyanisole and of microbial agents. *Cancer Res.*, **38**, 4478–85.

Benson, A. M., Batzinger, R. P., Ou, S.-Y., Bueding, E., Cha, Y.-N. and Talalay, P. (1978). Elevation of hepatic glutathione S-transferase activities and protection against metabolites of benzo[a]pyrene by dietary antioxidants. *Cancer Res.*, **38**, 4486–95.

Benson, A. M., Cha, Y. N., Bueding, E., Heine, H. S. and Talalay, P. (1979). Elevation of extrahepatic glutathione S-transferase and epoxide hydratase activities by 2(3)-*tert*-butyl-4-hydroxyanisole. *Cancer Res.*, **39**, 2971–7.

Berenblum, I. and Shubik, P. A. (1947). A new quantitative approach to the study of the stages of chemical carcinogenesis in the mouse's skin. *Brit. J. Cancer*, **1**, 383–91.

Branen, A. L. (1975). Toxicology and biochemistry of butylated hydroxyanisole and butylated hydroxytoluene. *J. Am. Oil Chem. Soc.*, **52**, 59–63.

Brown, W. D., Johnson, A. R. and O'Halloran, M. W. (1959). The effect of the level of dietary fat on the toxicity of phenolic antioxidants. *Aust. J. Exp. Biol.*, **37**, 533–47.

Cha, Y.-N., Martz, F. and Bueding, E. (1978). Enhancement of liver microsome epoxide hydratase activity in rodents by treatment with 2(3)-*tert*-butyl-4-hydroxyanisole. *Cancer Res.*, **38**, 4496–8.

Clapp, N. K., Boweles, N. D., Satterfield, L. C. and Klima, W. C. (1979). Selective protective effect of butylated hydroxytoluene against 1,2-dimethylhydrazine carcinogenesis in BALB/c mice. *J. Nat. Cancer Inst.*, **63**, 1081–7.

Clegg, D. J. (1965). Absence of teratogenic effect of butylated hydroxyanisole (BHA) and butylated hydroxytoluene (BHT) in rats and mice. *Food Cosmet. Toxicol.*, **3**, 387–403.

Cohen, S. M., Arai, M., Jacobs, J. B. and Friedell, G. H. J. (1979). Promoting effect of saccharin and DL-tryptophan in urinary bladder carcinogenesis. *Cancer Res.*, **39**, 1207–17.

Cook, M. G. and McNamara, P. (1980). Effect of dietary vitamin E on dimethyl-hydrazine-induced colonic tumors in mice. *Cancer Res.*, **40**, 1329–31.

Crampton, R. F., Gray, T. J. B., Grasso, P. and Parke, D. V. (1977). Long-term studies on chemically induced liver enlargement in the rat. I. Sustained induction of microsomal enzymes with absence of liver damage on feeding phenobarbitone or butylated hydroxytoluene. *Toxicology*, **7**, 289–306.

Creaven, P. J., Davies, W. H. and Williams, R. T. (1966). The effect of butylated hydroxytoluene, butylated hydroxyanisole and octyl gallate upon liver weight and biphenyl-4-hydroxylase activity in the rat. *J. Pharm. Pharmacol.*, **18**, 485–9.

Cumming, R. B. and Walton, M. F. (1973). Modification of the acute toxicity of mutagenic and carcinogenic chemicals in the mouse by prefeeding with anti-oxidants. *Food Cosmet. Toxicol.*, **11**, 547–53.

Dacre, J. C. and Denz, F. A. (1956). The metabolism of butylated hydroxyanisole in the rabbit. *Biochem. J.*, **64**, 777–82.

Daniel, J. W. and Gage, J. C. (1965). The absorption and excretion of butylated hydroxytoluene (BHT) in the rat. *Food Cosmet. Toxicol.*, **3**, 405–15.

Daniel, J. W., Green, T. and Phillips, P. J. (1973a). Metabolism of the phenolic antioxidant 3,5-di-*tert*-butyl-4-hydroxyanisole (topanol 354). I. Excretion and tissue distribution in man, rat and dog. *Food Cosmet. Toxicol.*, **11**, 771–9.

Daniel, J. W., Green, T. and Phillips, P. J. (1973b). Metabolism of the phenolic antioxidant 3,5-di-*tert*-butyl-4-hydroxyanisole (topanol 354). II. Biotransform-ation in man, rat and dog. *Food Cosmet. Toxicol.*, **11**, 781–92.

Daniel, J. W., Green, T. and Phillips, P. J. (1973c). Metabolism of the phenolic antioxidant 3,5-di-*tert*-butyl-4-hydroxyanisole (topanol 354). III. The metabolism in rats of the major autoxidation product, 2,6-di-*tert*-butyl-*p*-benzoquinone. *Food Cosmet. Toxicol.*, **11**, 793–6.

Deichmann, W. B., Gables, C., Clemmer, F. J. J., Rakoczy, R. and Bianchine, J. (1955). Toxicity of di-*tert*-butyl-methylphenol. *Arch. Ind. Health*, **11**, 93.

DHEW Publication (1979). *Bioassay of Butylated Hydroxytoluene (BHT) for Possible Carcinogenicity*. No. (NIH) 79-1706.

Epstein, S. S. and Shafner, H. (1968). Chemical mutagens in the human environ-ment. *Nature*, **219**, 385–7.

Fukushima, S., Hirose, M., Hagiwara, A., Hasegawa, R. and Ito, N. (1981). Inhibitory effect of 4,4'-diaminodiphenylmethane on liver, kidney and bladder carcinogenesis in rats ingesting N-ethyl-N-hydroxyethylnitrosamine or N-butyl-N-(4-hydroxybutyl)nitrosamine. *Carcinogenesis*, **2**, 1033–7.

Fukushima, S., Murasaki, G., Hirose, M., Nakanishi, K., Hasegawa, R. and Ito, N. (1982). Histopathological analysis of preneoplastic changes during N-butyl-N-(4-hydroxybutyl)nitrosamine induced urinary bladder carcinogenesis in rats. *Acta Pathol. Japan*, **32**, 243–50.

Fukushima, S., Imaida, K., Sakata, T., Okumura, T., Shibata, M. and Ito, N. (1983). Promoting effects of sodium L-ascorbate on two-stage urinary bladder carcinogenesis in rats. *Cancer Res.*, **43**, 4454–7.

Fukushima, S., Kurata, Y., Shibata, M., Ikawa, E. and Ito, N. (1984). Promotion by ascorbic acid, sodium erythorbate, and ethoxyquin of neoplastic lesions in rats initiated with N-butyl-N-(4-hydroxybutyl)nitrosamine. *Cancer Lett.*, **23**, 29–37.

Hagiwara, A., Miyata, Y., Ogiso, T., Fukushima, S. and Ito, N. (1984). Promoting or inhibiting effects of four antioxidants in rat urinary bladder carcinogenesis initiated by BBN. *Proc. Jap. Cancer Assoc.*, **43**, 47.

Hansen, E. and Meyer, O. (1978). A study of the teratogenicity of butylated hydroxyanisole on rabbits. *Toxicology*, **10**, 195–201.

Hathway, D. E. (1966). Metabolic fate in animals of hindered phenolic antioxidants in relation to their safety evaluation and antioxidant function. *Adv. Food Res.*, **15**, 1–56.

Hiasa, Y., Ohshima, M., Kitahori, Y., Konishi, N., Fujita, T. and Yuasa, T. (1983). β-Cyclodextrin: promoting effect on the development of renal tubular cell tumors in rats treated with N-ethyl-N-hydroxyethylnitrosamine. *J. Nat. Cancer Inst.*, **69**, 963–7.

Hiasa, Y., Kitahori, Y., Enoki, N., Konishi, M. and Shinoyama, T. (1984). 4,4′-Diaminodiphenylmethane: promoting effect of development of thyroid tumors in rats treated with N-bis(2-hydroxypropyl)nitrosamine. *J. Nat. Cancer Inst.*, **72**, 471–6.

Hicks, R. M., Wakefield, J. and Chowaniec, J. (1975). Evaluation of a new model to detect bladder carcinogens or co-carcinogens: results obtained with saccharin, cyclamate and cyclophosphamide. *Chem. Biol. Interact.*, **11**, 225–33.

Hirose, M., Shibata, M., Hagiwara, A., Imaida, K. and Ito, N. (1981). Chronic toxicity of butylated hydroxytoluene in Wistar rats. *Food Cosmet. Toxicol.*, **19**, 147–51.

Hirose, M., Masuda, A., Kurata, Y., Ikawa, E., Mera, Y. and Ito, N. (1985). Histological and autoradiographical studies on the forestomach of hamsters treated with 2-*tert*-butylated hydroxyanisole, 3-*tert*-butylated hydroxyanisole, crude butylated hydroxyanisole or butylated hydroxytoluene. *J. Nat. Cancer Inst.*, **76**, 143–9.

Hodge, H. C., Fassett, D. W., Mayard, E. A., Downs, W. L. and Coye, R. D. (1964). Chronic feeding studies of butylated hydroxyanisole in dogs. *Toxicol. Appl. Pharmacol.*, **6**, 512–9.

Hodge, H. C., Maynard, E. A., Down, W. L., Ashton, J. K. and Selerno, L. L. (1966). Tests on mice for evaluating carcinogenicity. *Toxicol. Appl. Pharmacol.*, **9**, 583–96.

Holder, G. M., Ryan, A. J., Watson, T. R. and Wiebe, L. I. (1970). The metabolism of butylated hydroxytoluene (3,5-di-t-butyl-4-hydroxytoluene) in man. *J. Pharm. Pharmacol.*, **22**, 375–6.

Imaida, K., Fukushima, S., Shirai, T., Ohtani, M., Nakanishi, K. and Ito, N. (1983). Promoting activities of butylated hydroxytoluene on 2-stage urinary bladder carcinogenesis and the inhibition of γ-glutamyl transpeptidase-positive foci development in the liver of rats. *Carcinogenesis*, **4**, 895–9.

Imaida, K., Fukushima, S., Shirai, T., Masui, T., Ogiso, T. and Ito, N. (1984). Promoting activities of butylated hydroxyanisole, butylated hydroxytoluene and sodium L-ascorbate on forestomach and urinary bladder carcinogenesis initiated with methylnitrosourea in F344 male rats. *Gann*, **75**, 769–75.

Ishidate, M. and Odashima, S. (1977). Chromosome tests with 134 compounds on Chinese hamster cells *in vitro*. A screening for 14 chemical carcinogens. *Mutat. Res.*, **48**, 337–54.

Ito, N., Matayoshi, K., Arai, M., Yoshioka, Y., Kamamoto, Y., Makiura, S. and Sugihara, S. (1973). Effects of various factors on induction of urinary bladder tumors in animals by N-butyl-N-(4-hydroxybutyl)nitrosamine. *Gann*, **64**, 151–9.

Ito, N., Tsuda, H., Hasegawa, R. and Imaida, K. (1982). Sequential observation of pathomorphologic alterations in preneoplastic lesions during the promoting stage of hepatocarcinogenesis and the development of short-term test system for hepatopromoters and hepatocarcinogens. *Toxicol. Pathol.*, **10**, 37–49.

Ito, N., Fukushima, S., Hagiwara, A., Shibata, M. and Ogiso, T. (1983*a*). Carcinogenicity of butylated hydroxyanisole in F344 rats. *J. Nat. Cancer Inst.*, **70**, 343–52.

Ito, N., Fukushima, S., Imaida, K., Sakata, T. and Masui, T. (1983*b*). Induction of papilloma in the forestomach of hamsters by butylated hydroxyanisole. *Gann*, **74**, 459–61.

Ito, N., Fukushima, S., Shirai, T. and Nakanishi, K. (1983*c*). Effects of promoters on N-butyl-N-(4-hydroxybutyl)nitrosamine-induced urinary bladder carcinogenesis in the rat. *Environ. Health Perspect.*, **50**, 61–9.

Ito, N., Tsuda, H., Hasegawa, R. and Imaida, K. (1983*d*). Comparison of the promoting effects of various agents in induction of preneoplastic lesions in rat liver. *Environ. Health Perspect.*, **50**, 131–8.

Ito, N., Fukushima, S., Tamano, S., Hirose, M. and Hagiwara, A. (1986). Dose-response of induction of forestomach carcinogenesis in F344 rats by butylated hydroxyanisole. *J. Nat. Cancer Inst.*, **77**, 1261–5.

Johnson, A. R. (1965). A re-examination of the possible teratogenic effects of butylated hydroxytoluene (BHT) and its effect on the reproductive capacity of the mouse. *Food Cosmet. Toxicol.*, **3**, 371–5.

Joner, P. R. (1977). Butylhydroxyanisole (BHA), butylhydroxytoluene (BHT) and ethoxyquin (EMQ) tested for mutagenicity. *Acta Vet. Scand.*, **18**, 187–93.

Kahe, R. and Wulff, U. (1979). Induction of rat hepatic epoxide hydratase by dietary antioxidants *Toxicol. Appl. Pharmacol.*, **47**, 217–27.

Kawachi (1979). Ministry of Health and Welfare of Japan. *Annual Report of Cancer Research*, Nat. Cancer Center, Tokyo, pp. 1111–20 (in Japanese).

King, M. M., Bailey, D. M., Gibson, D. D., Pitha, J. V. and McCay, P. B. (1979). Incidence and growth of mammary tumors induced by 7,12-dimethyl-benz(a)anthracene as related to the dietary content of fat and antioxidant. *J. Nat. Cancer Inst.*, **63**, 657–63.

King, M. M., McCay, P. B. and Kosanke, S. D. (1981). Comparison of the effect of butylated hydroxytoluene on N-nitroso methylurea and 7,12-dimethyl-benz[a]anthracene-induced mammary tumors. *Cancer Lett.*, **14**, 219–26.

Kitahara, A., Satoh, K., Nishimura, K., Ishikawa, T., Ruike, K., Sato, K., Tsuda, H. and Ito, N. (1984). Changes in molecular forms of rat hepatic glutathione S-transferase during chemical hepatocarcinogenesis. *Cancer Res.*, **44**, 2698–703.

Kohn, R. R. (1971). Effect of antioxidants on life-span of C57BL mice. *J. Gerontol.*, **26**, 378–80.

Ladomery, L. G., Ryan, A. J. and Wright, S. E. (1967). The excretion of [^{14}C] butylated hydroxytoluene in the rat. *J. Pharm. Pharmacol.*, **19**, 383–7.

Lam, L. K. T. and Wattenberg, L. W. (1979). Effects of butylated hydroxyanisole on the metabolism of benzo[a]pyrene by mouse liver microsomes. *J. Nat. Cancer Inst.*, **58**, 413–7.

Maeura, Y., Weisburger, J. H. and Williams, G. M. (1984). Dose-dependent reduction of N-2-fluorenylacetamide-induced liver cancer and enhancement of bladder cancer in rats by butylated hydroxytoluene. *Cancer Res.*, **44**, 1604–10.

Martin, A. D. and Gilbert, D. (1968). Enzyme changes accompanying liver enlargement in rats treated with 3-*tert*-butyl-4-hydroxyanisole. *Biochem. J.*, **106**, 321–9.

Matsuo, M., Mihara, K., Okuno, M., Ohdawa, H. and Miyamoto, J. (1984). Comparative metabolism of 3,5-di-*tert*-butyl-4-hydroxytoluene (BHT) in mice and rats. *Food Chem. Toxicol.*, **22**, 345–54.

Miller, E. C., Miller, J. A., Brown, R. R. and MacDonald, J. (1958). On the protective action of certain polycyclic aromatic hydrocarbons against carcinogenesis by aminoazo dyes and 2-acetylaminofluorene. *Cancer Res.*, **18**, 469–77.

Minegishi, K., Watanabe, M. and Yamaha, T. (1981). Distribution of butylated hydroxyanisole and its conjugates in the tissues of rats. *Chem. Pharm. Bull.*, **29**, 1377–81.

Nera, E. A., Lok, E., Iverson, F., Ormsby, E., Karpinski, K. F. and Clayson, D. B. (1984). Short-term pathological and proliferative effects of butylated hydroxyanisole and other phenolic antioxidants in the forestomach of Fischer 344 rats. *Toxicology*, **32**, 197–213.

Olsen, P., Bille, N. and Meyer, O. (1983). Hepatocellular neoplasms in rats induced by butylated hydroxytoluene (BHT). *Acta Pharmacol. Toxicol.*, **53**, 433–4.

Peraino, C., Fry, R. J. and Staffeldt, E. (1971). Reduction and enhancement by phenobarbital of hepatocarcinogenesis induced in the rat by 2-acetylaminofluorene. *Cancer Res.*, **31**, 1506–12.

Peraino, C., Fry, R. J. M., Staffeldt, E. and Christopher, J. P. (1977). Enhancing effects of phenobarbitone and butylated hydroxytoluene on 2-acetylaminofluorene-induced hepatic tumorigenesis in the rat. *Food Cosmet. Toxicol.*, **15**, 93.

Reddy, B. S., Hirota, N. and Katayama, S. (1982). Effect of dietary sodium ascorbate on 1,2-dimethylhydrazine- or methylnitrosourea-induced colon carcinogenesis in rats. *Carcinogenesis*, **3**, 1097.

Reddy, B. S., Maeura, Y. and Weisburger, J. H. (1983). Effect of various levels of dietary butylated hydroxyanisole on methylazoxymethanol acetate-induced colon carcinogenesis in CF1 mice. *J. Nat. Cancer Inst.*, **71**, 1299–305.

Richardson, H. L., Stier, A. R. and Borsoo-Nachtenbel, E. (1952). Liver tumor inhibition and adrenal histologic responses in rats to which 3'-methyl-4-dimethylaminoazobenzene and 20-methylcholanthrene were simultaneously administered. *Cancer Res.*, **12**, 356–61.

Shirai, T., Hagiwara, A., Kurata, Y., Shibata, M., Fukushima, S. and Ito, N. (1982). Lack of carcinogenicity of butylated hydroxytoluene on long-term administration to B6C3F₁ mice. *Food Chem. Toxicol.*, **20**, 861–5.

Shirai, T., Fukushima, S., Ohshima, M., Masuda, A. and Ito, N. (1984). Effects of butylated hydroxyanisole, butylated hydroxytoluene, and NaCl on gastric carcinogenesis initiated with N-methyl-N'-nitro-N-nitrosoguanidine in F344 rats. *J. Nat. Cancer Inst.*, **72**, 1189–98.

Shirai, T., Ikawa, E., Hirose, M., Thamavit, W. and Ito, N. (1985). Modification by five antioxidants of 1,2-dimethylhydrazine-initiated colon carcinogenesis in F344 rats. *Carcinogenesis*, **6**, 637–9.

Shklar, G. (1982). Oral mucosal carcinogenesis in hamsters: inhibition by vitamin E. *J. Nat. Cancer Inst.*, **68**, 791.

Søndergaaed, D. and Olsen, P. (1982). The effect of butylated hydroxytoluene

(BHT) on the rat thyroid. *Toxicol. Lett.*, **10**, 239–44.

Sparnins, V. L., Venegas, P. L. and Wattenberg, L. W. (1982). Glutathione S-transferase activity: enhancement by compounds inhibiting chemical carcinogenesis and by dietary constituents. *J. Nat. Cancer Inst.*, **68**, 493–6.

Speier, J. L. and Wattenberg, L. W. (1975). Alterations in microsomal metabolism of benzo[a]pyrene in mice fed butylated hydroxyanisole. *J. Nat. Cancer Inst.*, **55**, 469–72.

Takahashi, O. and Hiraga, K. (1978). Dose-response study of hemorrhagic death by dietary butylated hydroxytoluene (BHT) in male rats. *Toxicol. Appl. Pharmacol.*, **43**, 399–406.

Takahashi, M., Kokubo, T., Furukawa, F., Kurokawa, Y., Tatematsu, M. and Hayashi, Y. (1983). Effect of high salt diet on rat gastric carcinogenesis induced by N-methyl-N'-nitro-N-nitrosoguanidine. *Gann*, **74**, 28–34.

Takahashi, M., Kokubo, T., Furukawa, F., Kurokawa, Y. and Hayashi, Y. (1984). Effects of sodium chloride, saccharin, phenobarbital and aspirin on gastric carcinogenesis in rats after initiation with N-methyl-N'-nitro-N-nitrosoguanidine. *Gann*, **75**, 494–501.

Tatematsu, M., Takahashi, M., Fukushima, S., Hananouchi, M. and Shirai, T. (1975). Effects in rat of sodium chloride on experimental gastric cancer induced by N-methyl-N'-nitro-N-nitrosoguanidine or 4-nitroquinoline-1-oxide. *J. Nat. Cancer Inst.*, **55**, 101–6.

Telford, I. R., Woodruff, C. S. and Linford, R. H. (1962). Fetal resorption in the rat as influenced by certain antioxidants. *Am. J. Anat.*, **110**, 29–36.

Thamavit, W., Tatematsu, M., Ogiso, T., Mera, Y., Tsuda, H. and Ito, N. (1985). Dose-dependent effects of butylated hydroxyanisole, butylated hydroxytoluene and ethoxyquin in induction of foci of rat liver cells containing the placental form of glutathione S-transferase. *Cancer Lett.*, **27**, 295–303.

Toth, B. and Patil, K. (1983). Enhancing effect of vitamin E on murine intestinal tumorigenesis by 1,2-dimethylhydrazine dihydrochloride. *J. Nat. Cancer Inst.*, **70**, 1107–11.

Tsuda, H., Fukushima, S., Imaida, K., Kurata, Y. and Ito, N. (1983). Organ-specific promoting effect of phenobarbital and saccharin in induction of thyroid, liver, and urinary bladder tumors in rats after initiation with N-nitrosomethylurea. *Cancer Res.*, **43**, 3292–6.

Tsuda, H., Sakata, T., Masui, T., Imaida, K. and Ito, N. (1984). Modifying effects of butylated hydroxyanisole, ethoxyquin and acetaminophen on induction of neoplastic lesions in rat liver and kidney initiated by N-ethyl-N-hydroxyethylnitrosamine. *Carcinogenesis*, **5**, 525–31.

Ulland, B. M., Weisburger, J. H., Yamamoto, R. S. and Weisburger, E. K. (1973). Antioxidants and carcinogenesis: butylated hydroxytoluene, but not diphenyl-*p*-phenylenediamine, inhibits cancer induction by N-2-fluorenylacetamide and by N-hydroxy-N-fluorenylacetamide in rats. *Food Cosmet. Toxicol.*, **11**, 199–207.

Vorhees, C. V., Butcher, R. E., Brunner, R. L. Wootten, V. and Sabotka, T. J. (1981). Developmental neurobehavioral toxicity of butylated hydroxyanisole (BHA) in rats. *Neurobehav. Toxicol. Teratol.*, **3**, 321–9.

Wattenberg, L. W. (1976). Inhibition of chemical carcinogenesis by antioxidants and some additional compounds. In: *Fundamentals in Cancer Prevention*, P. N.

Magee, S. Takayama, T. Sugimura and T. Matsushima (Eds), Univ. Tokyo Press, Tokyo, p. 153.

Wattenberg, L. W. (1978). Inhibitors of chemical carcinogenesis. *Adv. Cancer Res.*, **26**, 197.

Wattenberg, L. W. (1980). Inhibitors of chemical carcinogens. *J. Environ. Pathol. Toxicol.*, **3**, 35–52.

Weinstein, I. B. and Troll, W. (1977). National cancer institute workshop on tumor promotion and cofactors in carcinogenesis. *Cancer Res.*, **37**, 3461–3.

Weisburger, E. K., Evarts, R. P. and Wenk, M. L. (1977). Inhibitory effect of butylated hydroxytoluene (BHT) on intestinal carcinogenesis in rats by azoxymethane. *Food Cosmet. Toxicol.*, **15**, 139–41.

Williams, G. M., Maeura, Y. and Weisburger, J. H. (1983). Simultaneous inhibition of liver carcinogenicity and enhancement of bladder carcinogenicity of N-2-fluorenylacetamide by butylated hydroxytoluene. *Cancer Lett.*, **19**, 55–60.

Witschi, H. (1981). Enhancement of tumor formation in mouse lung by dietary butylated hydroxytoluene. *Toxicology*, **21**, 95–104.

Witschi, H. P., Williamson, D. and Lock, S. (1977). Enhancement of urethan tumorigenesis in mouse lung by butylated hydroxytoluene. *J. Nat. Cancer Inst.*, **58**, 301.

Chapter 9

FOOD IRRADIATION

P. S. ELIAS

*Federal Research Centre for Nutrition, Karlsruhe, Federal Republic of
Germany*

HISTORICAL INTRODUCTION

Foods may be preserved by a variety of physical, chemical or biological
methods, with the ultimate goal of preventing undesirable tissue changes
and extending shelf life. The final objective is the preservation of quality

295

against undesirable microbial, physical, chemical and biochemical action. Until the early 1950s widely used traditional methods were available for these purposes, e.g. heat treatment by cooking or pasteurisation and heat sterilisation by canning. Removal of heat by cold storage or deep freezing and chemical treatment by the addition of preservatives were suitable alternatives. Biological fermentation processes represented another commonly used technology for preserving food.

Minck (1896) discovered the bactericidal action of X-rays but research on the biological effects of ionising radiation was hampered largely by the low radiation energies then available from existing installations. In 1943 the first report appeared on the successful preservation of hamburgers by irradiation (Goldblith, 1966). The efforts to find a peaceful use for atomic energy later led to proposals for employing the ionising energy of γ-rays emanating from radioactive isotopes, of X-rays or of accelerated electrons for the preservation of foodstuffs.

The physical principle on which food irradiation is based is essentially the absorption of energy quanta of electromagnetic radiation by the treated food. The radiation employed is either the radiation continuously emitted by the isotopes ^{60}Co and ^{137}Cs during their radioactive decay or the radiation emitted discontinuously by X-ray sources or linear electron accelerators. The common technological results of the action of this high energy radiation are:

(i)   the reduction or elimination of the damage and health hazards consequent upon microbial and parasitic contamination of food;
(ii)   the delaying of germination or ripening of certain foods of plant origin;
(iii) the disinfestation of important crops to be stored over considerable periods of time.

It should be noted that irradiation can in no circumstances improve the nature and quality possessed by the food at the time it undergoes this treatment. It does however improve its hygienic status and consequently permits a longer shelf life. Deception of the discerning consumer is therefore not likely.

PHYSICAL ASPECTS OF IRRADIATION

The electromagnetic radiation suitable for treating foodstuffs has a wavelength between 10^3 and 10^{-1} nm. The corresponding radiation energies lie between 10^2 and 10^6 eV. This is illustrated in Fig. 1.

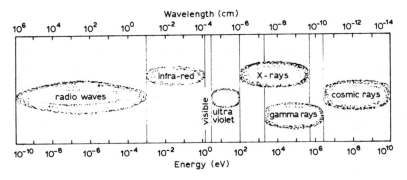

FIG. 1. Electromagnetic spectrum (from Langerak, 1982).

$1\,eV = 1\cdot6 \times 10^{-12}\,erg = 1\cdot6 \times 10^{-19}\,J;$ $1\,MeV = 10^6\,eV = 1\cdot6 \times 10^{-13}\,J;$
$1\,erg = 10^{-7}\,J;\ 1\,J = 6\cdot25 \times 10^{18}\,eV$

The energy of the photons, which arise in the case of γ-rays within the atomic nucleus and in the case of X-rays outside it, as well as the energy of the accelerated electrons is measured in electron volts (1 eV is the energy absorbed by an electron when accelerated through an electric field potential of 1 volt). The radiation dose, the amount of incident radiation energy absorbed by the irradiated matter, is measured in grays or rads (1 Gy is the absorption of 1 J per kg irradiated matter). It should be noted that, because the action of γ-rays or X-rays is due to the fast electrons they produce on entering matter, the irradiation effects are in fact the result of fast electrons for both γ-radiation and accelerated electrons. Table 1 gives some typical energy values for the radiation treatment used in food preservation compared to other preservation processes.

TABLE 1
Energy Equivalents (kJ kg^{-1}) Used in Food Preservation (after Brynjolfsson, 1980)

Radurisation (2·5 kGy)	20
Radappertisation (30 kGy)	160
Heat sterilisation	920
Freezing chicken	7 550
Storage at −25°C for 3·5 weeks	5 150
Storage at 0°C for 10 days	390

$1\,Gy = 100\,rad;\ 1\,rad = 10^{-2}\,J\,kg^{-1} = 6\cdot25 \times 10^{16}\,eV\,kg^{-1} = 6\cdot25 \times 10^{10}\,MeV\,kg^{-1};$
$1\,Gy = 1\,J\,kg^{-1} = 6\cdot25 \times 10^{12}\,MeV\,kg^{-1};\ 1\,kGy = 1\,kJ\,kg^{-1} = 1\,J\,g^{-1}$

The energy of the photonic quanta or of the moving electrons must be sufficiently high to exceed the ionisation energy of atoms or molecules in the food to be irradiated. There must also be an upper limit to that radiation energy so that it does not exceed the values which would induce nuclear reactions and consequently radioactivity by creating radioactive isotopes in the treated food. The upper limit for inducing nuclear reactions lies for almost all atoms in the range 13–16 MeV. To prevent this it is therefore conventional to restrict electron beams to 10 MeV and γ- and X-rays to 5 MeV.

TECHNOLOGICAL ASPECTS OF FOOD IRRADIATION

The application of food irradiation may be considered under three headings: high doses above 10 kGy for sterilisation; medium doses of 1–10 kGy to reduce the microbial load and prolong shelf life; low doses of less than 1 kGy for disinfestation and inhibition of sprouting. Table 2 lists the various areas of application.

Post-harvest losses of foodstuffs due to insect and parasite infestation, microbial spoilage, premature sprouting or maturation are reckoned to amount to 25–40% of the total world food production. Prevention or reduction of these losses and the prolongation of shelf life by irradiation of foods would therefore represent an immense potential contribution to ensuring an adequate food supply in developing countries. The radiation sterilisation of meat, vegetables and fish products is commercially of little interest at present because of the high costs of processing. It is used however for special situations, e.g. to supply food for patients after organ transplantation, for those suffering from severe immune deficiencies, for astronauts etc. The need for applying high radiation doses necessitates special technological procedures and a thorough evaluation of the nutritional and toxicological aspects of the treated foods. These fields of application are therefore still restricted to pilot investigations.

Applications of Low Dose Irradiation

Low doses of radiation, i.e. between 30 Gy and 1 kGy, are used predominantly for the prevention of sprouting of potatoes and onions. The technique makes use of the irreversible inhibition of cell division by doses of 30–200 Gy. The treatment was permitted as early as 1958 in the USSR. It is applied at any time post-harvest before storing varieties of potatoes which are destined for further processing. The usual radiation dose is 0·05–0·15 kGy. Potatoes damaged during harvesting or transport can be

TABLE 2
Approximate Radiation Doses (kGy) Required in Food Irradiation (modified from McLaughlin, 1982)

Sprouting inhibition:	potatoes, onions	0·03–0·12
Insect disinfestation:	cereals, flour, fresh and dried fruits	0·2–0·8
Destruction of parasites:	trichinae, tapeworms	0·1–0·3
Pasteurisation:	fruit, vegetables, poultry, fish, meat	0·5–10
Elimination of pathogens:	poultry, eggs, frozen meat	3·0–10
Reducing bacterial load:	spices, starches, enzyme preparations	8·0–20
Sterilisation:	poultry, meat, meat products, shrimps	25–60

irradiated only after the wounds have healed. Excessive doses cause increased contamination and spoilage by microbial invasion at the site of damage. Only the best quality should therefore be treated and at the same time handled as little as possible. For these purposes γ- or X-rays are needed because internal sprouting has to be prevented. Irradiation has the advantage over chemical anti-sprouting treatment of being irreversible and leaving no residues.

Onions need somewhat smaller doses. Irradiation is again preferable to chemical treatment but needs penetrating γ- or X-rays applied immediately after harvest to reach the quiescent germinal centre. Subsequent cold storage prevents the browning of the interior. Irradiated onions may be stored for up to 7 months.

Low doses are particularly suitable for the disinfestation of cereals and cereal products in tropical and subtropical climates. When stored in silos it is also possible to use insecticides but products packed in plastic containers can only be protected against destruction by larvae through irradiation with doses of 0·03–0·05 kGy. This radiation dose also kills insect eggs. Rice and pulses require doses up to 1 kGy for disinfestation without sustaining any significant losses of nutritional value, quality and organoleptic properties. However, irradiation does not provide protection against reinfestation with insects and pests; that requires storage under the best possible conditions.

Subtropical fruits like citrus, papaya and mango are often carriers of important insect pests. When irradiated with doses of 0·3–0·5 kGy these implanted pests and their eggs are killed, so that no further development occurs during storage. Somewhat higher doses may be used for prolonging the shelf life through the reduction of the microbial load. Irradiation is also an effective alternative for the treatment of citrus fruit against attack by the Mediterranean fruitfly (*Ceratitis capitata*) in view of the hazardous nature of the presently used carcinogenic fumigant ethylene dibromide. Dried fruits, e.g. dates, an important foodstuff in subtropical countries, can be disinfested with doses up to 1 kGy.

Parasitic worms, the larvae of trichinae and toxoplasma may be eliminated by deep-freezing or by irradiation with doses of 0·5–1 kGy. Disinfestation of dried fish may be carried out in tropical countries with doses up to 1 kGy.

Applications of Intermediate Dose Irradiation

Doses in this range, i.e. 1–10 kGy, reduce the microbial load and eliminate such non-spore-forming pathogens as Salmonella, Yersinia, Campylobacter, *Staphylococcus aureus* and *Clostridium perfringens*. This prolongs the shelf life. Combination with heat treatment may occasionally yield synergistic effects.

Up to 90% of deep-frozen poultry may be contaminated with Salmonella as a result of intensive rearing and mass slaughtering (Kampelmacher, 1984). Salmonellosis is a common food poisoning disease and is occasionally fatal in elderly patients. Salmonella can be effectively eliminated from packaged poultry by irradiation with doses of 3·5–7·5 kGy, the treatment reducing at the same time the total bacterial load by a factor of 10^3. The same applies to deep-frozen frog legs which are almost always contaminated with Salmonella and need 4 kGy for pasteurisation.

Doses between 7·5 and 15 kGy kill *Clostridium botulinum* in cured meat and ham products and thus permit a reduction in nitrite addition to bacon from 120 mg to 20–40 mg kg^{-1}, to ham and corned beef from 156 mg to 50 mg kg^{-1} and in certain types of sausage from 156 mg to 75 mg kg^{-1}. Nitrite is liable to react with biogenic amines to form *N*-nitrosamines, many of which are known to be carcinogenic. The possibility of reducing the addition of nitrite in curing meat without any concomitant rise in the hazard from botulinum toxin production is a major contribution to the safety of cured foods.

Fresh fruit and vegetables are generally sensitive to irradiation and yield products of inferior quality and poor taste with only slightly longer shelf life. However, strawberries, fresh figs, bananas, papayas and mangoes are suitable for this treatment. Using doses of 2·5–4·0 kGy will prolong the shelf life of strawberries by delaying mould development by 3–7 days depending on the conditions of storage. Appropriate dose selection in the range 1–3 kGy can achieve a delay in post-harvest maturation of certain fruits such as apples, pears and tomatoes. More important is the application of this treatment to tropical and subtropical fruits. Bananas are irradiated on an industrial scale in South Africa, while other countries prefer storage in a controlled atmosphere. Mangoes given a combination treatment of 5 min dipping into water at 55°C followed by irradiation with 7·5 kGy may be stored for up to 4 weeks at 10°C. This treatment controls at the same time the infestation with the mango weevil and with fruitfly eggs. Doses of 0·5 kGy suffice to kill the eggs of the oriental fruitfly, so that treated mangoes could meet the quarantine regulations of many countries.

Cultivated mushrooms can be treated with 1–2·5 kGy to prevent further growth and opening of the head, thereby delaying the development of lamellae and spores. This treatment can prolong shelf life to 6–9 days.

Spoilage of fish and seafood occurs as the result of microbial activity immediately after being caught. Irradiation, in combination with storage on ice, of filleted fish prolongs shelf life and reduces the microbial load. Doses of the order of 1·5–2·5 kGy are needed for this purpose. Only prepacked fish and fish fillets are suitable for this form of preservation. The treatment is particularly suitable for deep-frozen shrimps which are frequently highly contaminated with pathogens.

Irradiation of dry products, such as spices, dried herbs, dried vegetables and enzymes, is an excellent alternative to fumigation with the toxic and carcinogenic gases ethylene oxide and methyl bromide against the common contaminating spore-formers and thermophilic bacteria. If dried contaminated products are incorporated into other foods, e.g. meat, semi-conserved goods or cheese, they tend to reduce quality and storage life through the added spoilage organisms. Reduction in the bacterial load and elimination of pathogenic microorganisms without the toxic residues of chlorohydrins and bromides arising from fumigation is a useful contribution to public health. Radiation doses of 7·5–10 kGy are able to reduce the initial bacterial count, which may be as high as 10^8 organisms g^{-1}, to 10^4 g^{-1} and to eliminate enterobacteria. Heat treatment is not satisfactory because of the heat sensitivity of the flavouring substances in these foodstuffs, while alcohol vapour treatment cannot be applied to powdered material and causes loss of flavours by alcohol extraction.

Irradiation with doses up to 10 kGy changes the permeability of plant cells. This has been utilised to increase the extractability of cane sugar and beet sugar (Han *et al.*, 1983). Similar effects on yield have been obtained by irradiation in the production of juice from fruit and vegetables. Irradiated dried soups have a reduced cooking time (Paul *et al.*, 1969). However, none of these uses are economically feasible.

Applications of High Dose Irradiation
Irradiation can be used as alternative to canning for foods with high protein content such as meat, poultry and fish, which require to be stored for long periods. The process may also be applied for the sterilisation of precooked foods packed in individual portions which cannot be stored by deep-freezing or chilling. The radiation dose required to reduce the number of *Clostridium botulinum* by 10^{12} (the 12D dose) lies in the range 25–45 kGy for most products. At these dosage levels protein-rich products develop adverse organoleptic properties unless the treatment is carried out at temperatures of −40°C. In addition, the proteolytic enzymes in these products require inactivation through initial heating to an internal temperature of 70–75°C. The foods to be irradiated must also be vacuum

packed to exclude oxidative reactions and recontamination with micro-organisms and insect pests. The storage life of radiation-sterilised food is about 2 years at ambient temperatures up to 20°C. For the production of sterilised, precooked, individually packed meal portions a radiation dose of up to 60 kGy is needed (Grünewald, 1984).

Disadvantages of Irradiation

Too high radiation doses adversely affect the colour and texture of foodstuffs. Some of the flavouring characteristics are also sensitive to irradiation, resulting in the development of off-flavours especially in foods with a high content of proteins and fat. In these circumstances it is feasible to use irradiation in combination with other methods of preservation, e.g. moderate cooling, mild heat treatment or irradiation under vacuum. A combination of mild heat treatment and irradiation is an effective anti-mould treatment for mangoes and papayas and may even be synergistic as may be seen from Fig. 2. This would allow the use of lower heat and lower radiation doses on these rather delicate products.

Irradiation Facilities

The process of food irradiation can only be carried out in specially constructed facilities and under strict observance of radiological protection and safety measures. The Recommended International Code of Practice for the Operation of Radiation Facilities Used for the Treatment of Foods (Codex Alim. Comm., 1984) contains useful instructions which aim at easing the international acceptance of irradiated foods treated in facilities known to follow this code of practice. Moreover, the development of modern high-energy electron accelerators and of X-ray machines as well as radioactive sources with a high irradiation capacity has now provided the means for the commercial application of this processing technique (Herrnhut, 1985). Facilities suitable for irradiating foodstuffs may be of three types (Grünewald, 1984; Fraser, 1983).

Gamma Cells

The radiation sources are either ^{60}Co or ^{137}Cs. ^{60}Co is formed through neutron bombardment of ^{59}Co; ^{137}Cs is a byproduct of nuclear reactor operation. ^{60}Co has a specific activity of 370×10^{10} Bq (100 Ci g^{-1}) and a half-life of 5·27 years, hence every year 25% of the source must be replaced by new isotopic material. The energies of the γ-radiation produced by ^{60}Co are 1·17 and 1·33 MeV. One ton of uranium yields

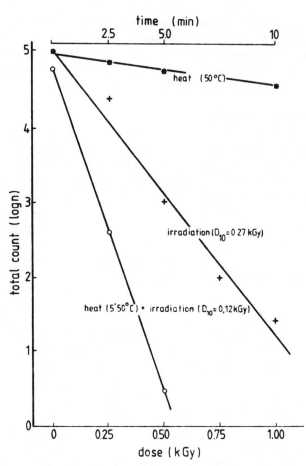

FIG. 2. Effect of heat (50°C), irradiation and a combination of both on a D_{10} value of *Penicillium expansum* spores (from Langerak, 1982).

2·88 kg Cs, of which the ^{137}Cs component delivers radioactivity amounting to $3·8 \times 10^{13}$ Bq (1 kCi).* ^{137}Cs has a half-life of 30 years and its γ-rays have an energy of 0·66 MeV. At present ^{60}Co is more easily available and used preferentially in irradiators. To deliver a radiation energy of 1 kilowatt requires about 70 kCi of ^{60}Co or 280 kCi of ^{137}Cs. This amount of energy

*curie (Ci) measures the radioactivity equivalent to $3·7 \times 10^{10}$ atomic nuclear disintegrations per second; 1 becquerel (Bq) is the radioactivity produced by 1 nuclear transformation per second.

suffices theoretically to irradiate 3.6 kGy t h^{-1}, although in practice the efficiency of utilising this energy is less than 30%. The total energy output of all the industrial irradiating plants existing in Europe corresponds to about 20×10^6 Ci (Kaylor *et al.*, 1980).

The lay-out of a γ-irradiation facility is relatively simple. The source isotopes are encapsulated in zirconium/stainless steel rods in the case of ^{60}Co and in stainless steel tubes in the case of ^{137}CsCl$_2$ cylinders. An automatic transport system surrounds the radiation source, which is kept under about 33 feet of water at rest. In this way no contact between the food and the radioactive material is possible. The penetration power of the radiation is measured by the distance travelled at which half its energy is absorbed by the irradiated goods (half-value section thickness). The pathway of the transport system is designed so that all sides of the goods are uniformly irradiated. Goods are transported by a pneumatic system, stacked either in a container or on a pallet. The duration of irradiation amounts to 15 h for sterilisation in a high capacity facility, assuming an energy utilisation efficiency of 30%. A pallet type plant handles about 3.2 t per throughput. A Japanese facility for irradiating potatoes, which has existed since 1973, handles about 350 t of potatoes per day during a period of 3 months, i.e. a total of 30000 t per year, with an operating efficiency of 20%. As irradiation lowers the capacity of potatoes to heal wounds sustained during harvesting, the Japanese plant has been specially designed to avoid handling of the goods as far as possible. Potatoes are therefore packaged in special containers holding 1.5 t for irradiation and subsequent storage. The goods travel around the source at a distance of 4 m. This of course raises the price but potatoes are not a staple food item in Japan. The utility of such an irradiation facility therefore depends on the market situation. Facilities are illustrated in Figs 3–5.

Linear Electron Accelerators
Modern installations have a range of electrical tension from 0.5 to 5.0 MeV and radiation energy outputs of 20–200 kW. They employ high-tension generators and indirect acceleration of electrons by microwaves to enable the generation of pulsed electron beams up to 10 MeV with a beam power spread of 25–75 kW. Electrons with this energy can penetrate about 3.8 cm of matter. A 50 kW beam can treat theoretically 18 t h^{-1} with a dose of 10 kGy. In practice only 25–40% of this output is achieved. A 6 MeV 300 kW facility corresponds to a ^{60}Co source of 20 MCi. If such an accelerator is used to generate bremsstrahlung from a metal target, the hard X-rays produced have a broad energy spectrum and can penetrate

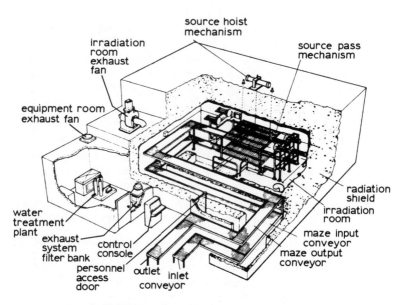

FIG. 3. JS 8500 irradiator (from Leemhorst, 1982).

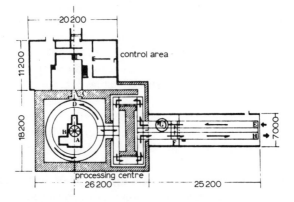

FIG. 4. Shihoro Agricultural Cooperative Association potato irradiator (plane view):
(A) source; (B) waterpool; (C) window; (D) irradiation conveyor; (E) entrance;
(F) line transfer; (G) turntable; (H) exit line (from Matsuyama and Umeda, 1983).

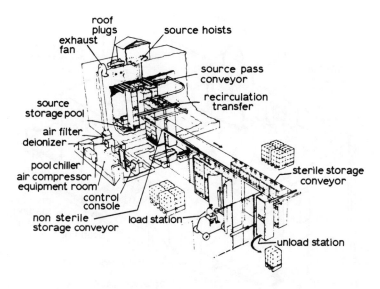

FIG. 5. JS 9000 pallet irradiator (from Leemhorst, 1982).

30 cm. This would be equivalent to the radiation from 317 Ci of [60]Co. However, this is not an efficient utilisation of the output capacity of an accelerator, because only a few % of the beam energy is converted to X-rays.

Linear accelerators have the advantage of a very high dose rate application, well beyond that of an isotope source. This shortens the duration of irradiation sufficiently to permit the installation of an accelerator as part of a continuous production line, but has the disadvantage of a possible adiabatic (no heat removal) temperature rise in the irradiated product. An absorbed radiation dose of 25 kGy can result adiabatically in a temperature rise of from 6 (water) to 54 (steel) K depending on the nature of the material being irradiated. 10 kGy would raise the temperature of water, an abundant component of most foods, by 2·4°C. Figure 6 illustrates such a facility.

X-ray Generating Machines
Machine sources generating X-rays with energies of 5–10 MeV are a very recent development. No commercial installation using X-rays is as yet available.

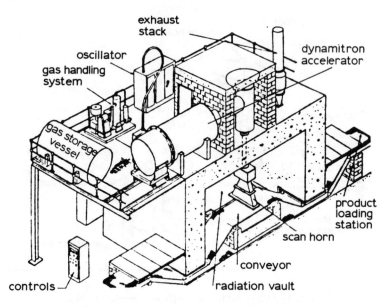

FIG. 6. Dynamitron electron accelerating facility (from Cleland *et al.*, 1980).

Dosimetry

When foodstuffs are being irradiated it is of fundamental importance to supervise the applied radiation dose strictly. Different foods require different accurately measured doses to avoid any significant reduction in quality. The radiation dose is defined as that fraction of the total radiation energy delivered into a unit volume which is absorbed by the mass contained in the volume; it is measured in J kg^{-1}.

Procedures for measuring radiation doses are given in the code of practice elaborated by the Codex Alimentarius Commission (1984). They depend essentially on the strategic placement of calibrated dosimeters within the bulk of the food to be irradiated. This permits statistical control of the parameters, such as minimum and maximum dose, necessary to establish the average radiation doses applied. These dosimeters use either iron sulphate or iron–copper sulphate solutions, polymer films or other systems, depending on the dose range to be measured.

In practice the overall average dose applied is calculated from the dose distribution curve in the total product volume. If the positions of the smallest and largest applied dose are known, it is possible to estimate the average value of the average minimum (D_{min}) and average maximum (D_{max}) absorbed doses by the formula $\frac{1}{2}(D_{max} + D_{min})$. It should be noted that a small fraction (2·5%) of the irradiated food will always receive a dose about 50% higher than the overall average dose, because a uniform dose distribution is not possible due to the geometry of the product and source arrangement (Codex Alim. Comm., 1984).

ECONOMIC ASPECTS OF FOOD IRRADIATION

In calculating the costs of food irradiation a number of factors must be allowed for which are difficult to estimate precisely. In theory a centralised service irradiation facility involves the added expenditure of loading and transporting the food to and from the facility. Irradiation of finished packaged goods at the end of the production line is a cheaper approach but technically difficult to achieve. For small quantities it is more economical to use centralised facilities.

The capital cost of a 200 kW facility which could handle about 50000 tons annually would amount to about US $ 10^7 for a ^{60}Co or ^{137}Cs installation (at 1980 prices) while 5 or 10 MeV linear accelerator installations would cost between US $ 1·8 and $2·5 \times 10^6$. Expressed as costs in US cents kg^{-1}, including depreciation, the corresponding figures would be (at 1980 prices) 7·12 for ^{60}Co, 5·25 for ^{137}Cs and 1·65–2·03 for 5–10 MeV facilities. Any additional procedures such as cooling, freezing or enzyme inactivation would escalate the cost considerably. The expenditure on low or medium dose irradiation in one's own facility would amount to US c 1·4 kg^{-1} for sprout inhibition, 5·4 for radicidation of poultry and 10·8 for decontamination of spices (Brynjolfsson, 1980).

The estimated capital cost of a facility for disinfestation of citrus fruits with a throughput of 900 t/day at a dose of about 0·25 kGy would be about US $ $3·2 \times 10^6$, the total annual running costs about US $ 670000, equivalent to an additional 0·21 c kg^{-1} to the price of the fruit. Similar capital estimates for an electron accelerator installation of the 3–6 MeV range are US $ $2·4 \times 10^6$, and the annual running costs including amortisation for about 6000 operational hours come to US $ $0·5$–$0·9 \times 10^6$. A 5 kGy electron irradiation treatment would thus cost about US c 0·7 kg^{-1} or as X-ray treatment US c 1·5 kg^{-1}. Potato irradiation might thus come to US $ 4–12 t^{-1}. The Japanese facility involves costs of US $ 7–10 t^{-1} (Brynjolfsson, 1980).

METHODS FOR IDENTIFICATION OF IRRADIATED FOODS

The fact that radiation-specific products have not been found in all irradiated foods is of help in assessing the safety of the process. However, it makes it difficult to demonstrate analytically for inspection purposes that food on sale or in transit has been irradiated. Methods exist to show differences between irradiated and non-irradiated foods but their reliability has not been demonstrated in practice and no quantitative estimates can be made of the radiation dose received by individual foods. Several physical measurements may be used to detect irradiation (Bögl and Heide, 1984).

Because of their short life only a few foods are suitable for electron spin resonance (ESR) measurements. Free radicals react quickly with water, so ESR signals are detectable only in dry foods for any length of time. However, energy absorption from processes such as grinding also gives rise to ESR signals, so ESR measurements cannot be regarded as unique evidence of irradiation. The rapid decay of radicals at ambient temperature and in contact with water militates against the use of this technique in food control.

Comparison of the fall in conductance over a 3 min period has been found to be unreliable. Impedance measurements are a reliable and practical technique for identifying irradiated potatoes and estimating the irradiation dose.

The luminescence effect of radiation treatment differs from spice to spice and can be measured against a control sample. Irradiation treatment can be identified for about 2–3 weeks. However, the thermoluminescence intensities have a rather broad range. Nevertheless irradiation can be identified in some materials many months later.

Chemical measurements can also be useful (Bögl and Heide, 1984). Certain irradiated substances, when subsequently in contact with water, emit a short light pulse (chemiluminescence) which can be reinforced by adding a photosensitiser. In the case of spices, irradiation with 10 kGy can be identified for up to 3 weeks. Several other chemical methods such as identification of volatile hydrocarbons, measurement of carbonyl compounds and isoelectric focussing of proteins have been tried but none has achieved practical use.

Biological measurements can be used for identifying irradiation treatment (Bögl and Heide, 1984). For example, changes in the microflora could be useful, if a particularly radiation-sensitive common organism normally present on the food were to be absent. Thus strawberries with low enterobacteriaceae and Pseudomonas counts but high yeast contamination are likely to have been irradiated. Irradiated fish would show pre-dominantly Moraxella-type organisms and absence of radiosensitive spoilage organisms. In the case of onions the inhibition of germination in 95% of treated bulbs would be evidence of irradiation.

ENVIRONMENTAL CONSIDERATIONS

The following environmental concerns apply to food irradiation. If ^{137}Cs sources are used, a waste product from the nuclear industry would be utilised under strict control. Any ^{60}Co would have to be intentionally produced for irradiation purposes and would increase the total load of radioactive isotopes in the environment. However, strict control of these sources would ensure their safe operation. For this purpose nuclear regulatory controls already exist in most countries. Inspection of the facilities by health authorities would add further safeguards. The environmental impact of isotope sources is therefore small, and that of electron accelerators is minimal. Adequate control for assuring good manu-facturing practice in accordance with the Codex Alimentarius Commission provisions relating to irradiated food would ensure that the process is used only where it serves a food hygiene purpose and not as a substitute for good food manufacturing practices (Brynjolfsson, 1985).

CHEMICAL CHANGES DUE TO IRRADIATION

Absorption of energy quanta from the photons of the incident radiation results in energy-induced changes in the atomic and molecular structure of irradiated matter. The energy of the photons of the radiation used for treating foodstuffs is sufficiently high to liberate electrons from the constituent atoms and molecules, i.e. to induce ionisation. The absorption of radiation energy leads as the primary process to the formation of ionised molecules or free radicals which are chemically very reactive. Primary radical formation is independent of temperature and these intermediates have only a short life. Free radicals then undergo secondary reactions which eventually lead to the formation of stable radiochemical compounds of a constitution determined by the molecular composition and structure of the irradiated matter. These secondary reactions are dependent on temperature, on the presence of oxygen and on other variables. The overall irradiation damage to a molecule is approximately proportional to its molecular weight. For example, a radiation dose destroying sufficient

DNA molecules (i.e. bacteria) to reduce a *Clostridium botulinum* population by 10^{-12} would cause changes in frozen or dry macronutrients of the order of 0·14% of proteins, 0·3% of carbohydrates and 0·4% of lipids (Brynjolfsson, 1980).

The chemical effects of irradiation are expressed quantitatively as *G*-values. The *G*-value is defined as the number of molecules changed by the absorbed radiation for every 100 eV of absorbed energy. For the radiation doses normally applied in food processing, *G*-values lie between 1 and 3. Thus, for a *G*-value of 3 and 10 Gy ($= 1$ krad) absorbed dose, $3\cdot1 \times 10^{-6}$ mol kg^{-1} of substance will be changed. For a dose of *D* krad the radiochemical products generated will amount to $D \times G \times 10^{-3}$ mmol kg^{-1} of substance.

It is possible to determine *G*-values by irradiating solutions of individual compounds or simple mixtures and analysing for the presence of breakdown products. A knowledge of the *G*-values of the components of a foodstuff can be used to calculate the *G*-value of the whole irradiated foodstuff because the individual components yield the same radiochemical products whether irradiated in isolation or as part of the complex food. For appropriately irradiated foods a *G*-value of 1 is generally applicable. A dose of 10 kGy ($= 1$ Mrad) would therefore produce 300 mg kg^{-1} radiochemical products, assuming a *G*-value of 1 and an average molecular weight of 300 for the irradiated substance. Most of the compounds identified after irradiation also occur in unirradiated but otherwise processed food, leaving about 10% unique radiolytic products not normally found in food (Takeguchi, 1983). Low and medium dose applications cause nearly negligible chemical changes in the target food material.

Reactive free radicals have also been identified in dry cereals after milling or in fats under the action of light. The radicals commonly produced by irradiation are OH, H, O_2, e_{aq} as well as H_2, H_2O_2, and H_3O^+. In dry foods mainly organic radicals are formed. The nature of the radiochemical products differs depending on whether the food component is irradiated in isolation or as part of the complex food (Elias and Cohen, 1977; Urbain, 1978). Isolated fatty acids yield CO_2, H_2, CO, C_{n-1}-alkanes and C_n-aldehydes. Saturated fatty acids undergo C–C chain scission preferably next to the carbonyl bond whereas unsaturated fatty acids form hydroperoxides. Triglycerides split off free fatty acid radicals and C_{n-1}-hydrocarbons, the latter being mostly alkanes and alkenes, and alcohols and carbonyl compounds are also formed. Carbonyl compounds form mainly in the presence of oxygen (Nawar, 1977).

Isolated amino acids and peptides release NH_3, ketoacids and α,α-

diamino acids on irradiation. Peptide chains are deaminated, the main chain undergoing scission to form both backbone radicals and side-chain radicals. Proteins are reductively deaminated and decarboxylated and disulphide bridges are reduced. Hydrogen bonds are frequently disrupted and the molecular conformation is altered by unfolding. The aromatic and sulphur-containing amino acid residues form short-lived intermediate radicals. Alanine may release ethylamine and propionic acid, glycine liberates methylamine and acetic acid (Urbain, 1977).

Globular proteins aggregate and unfold while fibrous proteins degrade. Protein solutions are less sensitive to irradiation if they also contain carbohydrates and lipids. Deep-frozen and dry proteins are also radiation-resistant, hence irradiated enzymes lose little activity. Radiation-induced free radicals in protein-rich foods disappear quickly at normal temperature but can remain for up to 8 months in dried food.

Irradiation of different meats produces S-containing compounds, while irradiated meat fat releases alkanes, alkenes and some carbonyl compounds. The nature of the radiochemical compounds is independent of the type of irradiated meat. Most of the volatiles identified in irradiated meat are innocuous and also found in heated meat. Benzene has been detected in ppb quantities at the highest radiation doses used but it also occurs naturally in meat, fish, vegetables, nuts, eggs and bevereges (Van Straten, 1977). Enzymes in food are relatively protected and would need very large radiation doses for inactivation.

Isolated monosaccharides are oxidised and fragmented when irradiated, mainly carbonyls being released. Carbohydrate solutions containing amino acids or proteins form far fewer radiochemical products than pure solutions. Irradiated polysaccharides like starch and cellulose form glucose, maltose, dextrins, malonaldehyde, formaldehyde, acetaldehyde, glyceraldehyde, formic acid and hydrogen peroxide (see Table 3). Chain length is reduced by 30% through depolymerisation (Diehl, 1983).

Irradiation of fruit and fruit juice leads mostly to radical formation from the water component and these radicals then react with the fruit sugars (Dauphin and St. Lèbe, 1977; Diehl et al., 1978; Adam, 1983).

Vitamins have differing sensitivities towards irradiation. Vitamins E, B_1, C and K are the most sensitive, and are rapidly destroyed. Doses over 10 kGy degrade vitamin C and B_1 to the same extent as occurs on cooking, whereas vitamins B_2, B_6, B_{12}, A and D are more resistant (Tobback, 1977; Diehl, 1979).

Irradiation of dilute aqueous solutions of DNA yields mostly damaged purine and pyrimidine bases (Wilmer and Schubert, 1981).

In general it is found that food irradiation with appropriate doses

TABLE 3

Major Radiolytic Products (mg/kg/Mrad) of Maize Starch Irradiated in the Presence of Air, at a Moisture Content of 12–13% (from Dauphin and St. Lèbe, 1977)

Formic acid	100
Glycolaldehyde	9
Malonaldehyde	2
Acetaldehyde	40 (up to 800 krad)
Maltose	9·8
Hydrogen peroxide	6·6 (100–400 krad)
Glucose	5·8
Glyceraldehyde and/or dihydroxyacetone	4·5
Acetone	2·1 (above 2 Mrad)

produces no greater damage than heat treatment. Moreover, the reactions occurring in irradiated food, though smaller in number, are similar to those taking place in heat-treated food. Actual analyses of the compounds generated in food and of the reaction products in model systems, as well as consideration of the theoretically estimated concentrations, show that the products of irradiation and their concentrations could be predicted from the radiation dose, the temperature and the composition of the food (Merritt and Taub, 1983). Most of the changes in irradiated food result in products commonly found in food or generated from it during processing and digestion.

TOXICOLOGICAL ASPECTS OF FOOD IRRADIATION

Because the chemical and toxicological effects of irradiation arise through the action of fast electrons, there is no difference from the toxicological point of view between a foodstuff treated by γ-rays and the same foodstuff treated by accelerated electrons. Only dose rate effects will differ between these two types of treatment. The wholesomeness of irradiated food and of irradiated isolated food components has been studied in a large number of *in vivo* and *in vitro* investigations by private, national and international organisations during the last 37 years. Numerous studies exist also on identified radiation chemical products. Some 20 out of 60 different foods have been extensively tested in animal feeding studies, including lifespan and multigeneration studies in laboratory animals. Almost all these studies showed no adverse toxicological effects as a result of feeding irradiated foodstuffs. Indeed, as early as 1965 the Surgeon General of the US Army declared, on the basis of extensive studies conducted in the US between 1948 and 1965, that foods irradiated up to absorbed doses of 5·6 kGy with a ^{60}Co source of γ-radiation or with electrons with energies up to 10 MeV had been found to be wholesome, i.e. safe and nutritionally adequate (USA, 1965). At the international level, the 1980 Joint FAO/IAEA/WHO Expert Committee on Wholesomeness of Irradiated Food (JECFI) reviewed the extensive data collected up to that time and concluded that the irradiation of any food commodity up to an overall average dose of 10 kGy presented no toxicological hazard; hence toxicological testing of foods so treated was no longer required. Furthermore, such processing introduced no special nutritional or microbiological problems (JECFI, 1981).

In designing animal feeding studies with irradiated foods, certain methodological difficulties were encountered. For example, in studies with irradiated meats in laboratory rodents, which are essentially herbivores, the amount of meat which could be incorporated in the diet was limited because of deleterious effects on the renal system. Similar considerations did not apply in the case of irradiated plant proteins. Problems also arose over the extent to which irradiated foods could be incorporated in the diet without disturbing the nutritional balance. The selection of the control diet presented difficulties in some cases. Strictly speaking, controls should be fed the unpreserved food, which is not feasible in long-term studies on easily spoiled foodstuffs. In the case of meat products one could also argue that heat treatment might destroy some natural toxicant in the meat and therefore heat-treated meat should represent the control feed. On the other hand, heat treatment might possibly produce minute amounts of toxic substances and therefore frozen meat should serve as control.

Radiochemical Products

A few studies are available on identified radiochemical products. Some 26 of these substances were selected among those detected and quantified in beef fat irradiated at 60 kGy. The compounds investigated were essentially straight-chain alkanes and 1-alkenes, from C_5 to C_{17}, in the proportions found after irradiation. The yield of the 26 radiochemical products was about 22 mg per 100 g of irradiated beef fat and the average human daily intake was estimated at 0·77 mg kg^{-1} b.w. The mixed compounds were administered to female mice in a three-generation reproduction study at levels of 0·55%, 1·8% and 5·5% of the diet. Additional groups of mice were fed 9, 8, 3 or 2 radiochemical products at concentrations varying from

0·76% to 2·1% in the diet. The combined 26 products reduced survival and body weight gain of F_3 pups of both sexes at weaning. Small necrotic hepatic foci increased dose-relatedly in the test groups compared to controls. At 1·8% of the diet only male F_3 pups showed a reduced body weight. Haematocrit values showed inconsistent decreases. No data on urinalysis or clinical chemistry were obtained. Histopathology of 9 major organs showed only the hepatic lesions. The combined C_{13}, C_{14} and C_{17} 1-alkenes, when fed at 3·82% of the diet, were toxic for the reproductive function; infertility, increased pup mortality and absent litters were observed in the second generation (Mafarachisi, 1974).

Oral acute, 3-weeks subacute and 6-months subacute studies were carried out in rats with a mixture of 9 radiochemical products identified in aqueous extracts of starch irradiated with 3 kGy. The doses used in the subacute studies were 0·015, 0·072, 0·1, 0·3 and 0·63 g kg^{-1} b.w. in drinking water; in the 6-months study 0·072, 0·1 and 0·3 g kg^{-1} b.w. were used. Fluid consumption was reduced at the 0·3 and 0·63 g kg^{-1} b.w. level but no haematological or clinico-chemical abnormalities were found. Only in the 3-week study was epithelial hyperplasia of the forestomach seen at 0·63 g kg^{-1} b.w. (Truhaut and St. Lèbe, 1978).

Carbohydrates

A few positive findings require however closer discussion. Aqueous solutions of glucose and other monosaccharides are cytotoxic and mutagenic to mammalian and non-mammalian cells if tested *in vitro* immediately after treatment with doses up to 20 kGy (Rao, 1978). On the other hand, anhydrous glucose irradiated up to 50 kGy was not mutagenic for Drosophila and caused no dominant lethal mutations in mice (Varma *et al.*, 1982*a,b*). Irradiated sucrose solutions were mutagenic *in vitro* for *Salmonella typhimurium* but not when used in a host-mediated assay in mice (Aiyar and Rao, 1977). Fructose, glucose, sucrose, maltose and ribose solutions irradiated with doses of 10–25 kGy were mutagenic only for *S. typhimurium* T100 in oxygenated solutions, using the preincubation procedure, but little activity was found in the absence of oxygen (Rao, 1978).

The mutagenic compounds identified in irradiated sugars were glyoxal, D-erythrohexo-2,3-diulose and D-arabinohexo-2-ulose. Despite the findings obtained with isolated fruit sugars no mutagenic activity was detected in irradiated fruit juices or in the supernatant of the pulp of irradiated whole fruit at doses up to 20 kGy (Niemand *et al.*, 1983). In fact addition of supernatant decreased the mutagenic activity of D-arabinohexo-2-ulose. High-dose irradiation of pineapple, citrus and apple juice induced chromosome breaking activity when tested against onion root cells. Doses of 10 kGy caused very little radiolysis of glucose in apple juice. Irradiation of solutions of 2-deoxy-D-ribose and ribose, the sugar moieties of DNA and RNA respectively, induced mutagenic activity against *S. typhimurium* TA100 and TA98. Irradiated solutions of nucleic acid bases, using doses of 10 kGy, were non-mutagenic but irradiated nucleosides were mutagenic for TA100 (Wilmer *et al.*, 1981). These data indicate that the sugar moiety is the main target yielding mutagenic radicals and then only in fresh solutions at high radiation doses. The mutagenic activity depended on the quantity of carbonyl compounds produced, and could be reduced or removed entirely by heating. No *in vivo* mutagenic activity was found, possibly because of rapid biotransformation of radicals to non-genotoxic substances.

Fruit and Vegetables
Very extensive and comprehensive data are available on four different fruits (mangoes, dates, strawberries, papayas). They show that mangoes, dates and papayas, irradiated up to 1 kGy, as well as strawberries, irradiated up to 3 kGy, caused no adverse health effects in life-span feeding studies (WHO, 1977, 1981). Less comprehensive feeding studies were made on oranges, apples, bananas, apricots and peaches irradiated with doses from 0·3 to 3 kGy, none of which showed any adverse toxicological effects (Zaitsev, 1980).

Onions irradiated up to 0·15 kGy were extensively tested in long-term reproduction and genotoxicity studies. At levels of 2% in the diet of laboratory rodents no adverse effects were noted but higher levels were not tolerated because of haemolysis and anaemia due to naturally occurring toxic constituents (WHO, 1977, 1981). Mushrooms irradiated at 3 kGy caused no adverse effects on reproduction and embryogenesis when fed to rats but other tests were less adequate and high dietary levels were not well tolerated by rats and dogs (WHO, 1977). Other irradiated vegetables like lettuce, celery, carrots and cauliflower have only been tested in bacterial systems (Van Kooij *et al.*, 1978).

Cereals, Pulses and Other Plant Foods
Wheat, rice and maize have been submitted to extensive toxicological investigations including short-term, long-term, teratogenicity and mutagenicity studies. None of these showed any effects on test animals as a consequence of eating wheat irradiated up to 1 kGy and stored after irradiation (WHO, 1977, 1981).

A few of the large number of feeding studies and mutagenicity studies carried out with wheat, rice and maize yielded contradictory results. Two Russian studies (Kamaldinova, 1970; Shillinger and Osipova, 1970) showed detrimental effects in rats given food irradiated with γ-rays at doses of 8 and 6 kGy. Careful review established poor design for both studies. The study by Kamaldinova used a substandard basic diet. The changes in fat metabolism were ascribed to alterations in tributyrinase activity but liver enzyme activities in the parent test group, F_1 test group and F_1 control group were identical and slightly lower in parent controls. No statistically significant data were presented. The Shillinger and Osipova study used diets with Ca/P imbalance and test diets were mistreated after irradiation by improper storage. The conclusions were not supported by the data presented. Indeed a further six Russian papers between 1972 and 1981 confirmed the safety of irradiated foods (Zaitsev and Osipova, 1981; Zaitsev and Maganova, 1981).

The administration of freshly irradiated wheat to a small number of malnourished children, monkeys and rats led to an apparent increase in polyploidy demonstrated in cytogenetic tests. No polyploidy was seen when wheat was ingested that had been stored for 3 months after irradiation (Bhaskaram and Sadasivan, 1975; Vijayalaxmi, 1975, 1978a). The data reported by Bhaskaram and Sadasivan were meagre and failed to take into account large statistical variations, the design was poor and the results failed to support the conclusions of a mutagenic potential present in irradiated wheat. The 1·5% polyploidy observed in 5 children given irradiated wheat are within the normal range and the 0% incidence in 5 controls is an improbable result. Other studies in laboratory animals were unable to confirm these effects (Reddi et al., 1977; Murthy, 1981a, b). Rats fed for 15 weeks some 70% freshly irradiated wheat in their diet showed some reduction in the responsiveness of their immune system to antigen challenge but not sufficient to impair their ability to overcome artificially induced infections (Vijayalaxmi, 1978b).

Cooked irradiated potatoes produced no adverse effects in feeding tests or in mutagenicity tests (WHO, 1977). However, alcoholic extracts of freshly irradiated raw potatoes were reported to cause in vitro mutagenic effects and, in some feeding tests, chromosomal damage and dominant lethal mutations (WHO, 1977). Again it was not possible to confirm these observations when the experiments were repeated (WHO, 1977).

These positive toxicological findings with freshly irradiated foodstuffs, using high radiation doses and without subsequent storage, are probably the result of the presence of short-lived radiochemical products. Similar effects were not observed when technologically relevant doses had been employed. It may be concluded therefore that in practice these toxic products are either not formed or occur in biologically insignificant amounts or are inactived by reaction with other food components.

Long-term feeding studies with irradiated rice are available in the rat, mouse and dog. Multigeneration reproduction studies and genotoxicity tests were also carried out (WHO, 1977, 1981). On maize only a three-generation reproduction study in mice has been performed. These investigations show that no adverse effects were associated with the ingestion by several animal species of rice and maize irradiated up to 1 kGy. Pulses were administered to laboratory animals in their diet only over comparatively short periods. When high levels of both irradiated and non-irradiated beans were fed, growth rates were reduced. Mutagenicity studies with beans irradiated at 1 kGy were negative for a number of different genetic end points (WHO, 1981).

Spices and Condiments

Onion powder and spice mixtures containing mainly paprika and pepper irradiated up to 15 kGy have been examined in long-term feeding studies as well as in reproduction, teratology and mutagenicity tests. Apart from reduced food intake, reduced body weight and increased liver weight, noted at feeding levels above 10% in the diet with treated and untreated material, no significant toxic effects occurred after the ingestion of irradiated spices (Barna, 1973, 1976; WHO, 1981). Cocoa beans irradiated up to 5 kGy and untreated beans depressed the growth and reduced the food intake of rats at high dietary levels. Foetal development and survival of pups were adversely affected. These effects are related to the high theobromine content of the diet and could be reproduced by administering theobromine. No genotoxic properties were found in irradiated cocoa beans (WHO, 1981).

Fish, Fish Products and Shellfish

Foodstuffs containing polyunsaturated fatty acids turn rancid in presence of oxygen through the formation of hydroperoxides and carbonyl compounds such as malonaldehyde. Irradiation causes the same effects. The free radicals and active oxygen destroy the polyunsaturated fatty acids present in the membranes of mitochondria, lysosomes and the endoplasmic reticulum, thereby causing toxic damage. Thus feeding irradiated herring oils reduces mixed function oxidase activity and alters the spectrum of fatty acids in the endoplasmic reticulum of the rat liver but also raises the activity of P_{450} and P_{448}. These changes are too small to affect the metabolic transformation of xenobiotics (Wills, 1981).

The possible formation of toxic substances has been examined in several fish species. Most of the investigations were carried out in cod, haddock and mackerel, irradiated up to 2 kGy, and fish paste irradiated at 4·5 kGy. Most investigations used mixtures of cod and haddock, irradiated at 1·75 kGy, boiled and then incorporated at 45% of the diet of mice and rats. Subchronic and long-term studies as well as multigeneration reproduction and teratogenicity investigations were performed. Except for an inconsistent and non-reproducible rise in serum alkaline phosphatase in a few of the feeding tests on rats, which could not be confirmed in mice and dogs, no adverse health effects were noted. Several genotoxicity tests on cod irradiated up to 6 kGy remained negative (WHO,1977, 1981).

Only a few wholesomeness studies have been carried out on crustaceans. A subacute feeding study with shrimp irradiated up to 3 kGy and fed at 28% in the diet of rats revealed no toxic effects (Aravindakshan et al., 1973). A four-generation reproduction study on dehydrated shrimp irradiated at 2·5 kGy also showed no adverse findings (van Logten et al., 1972), while a 2-year feeding study in dogs confirmed similarly the absence of toxic effects in a non-rodent species (Fegley and Edmonds, 1968). Mackerel irradiated up to 2 kGy was also examined in subchronic, long-term, multigeneration and mutagenicity studies without yielding any result giving rise to concern over adverse health effects (Chaubey et al., 1979; Anukarahanonta et al., 1980).

Meat and Poultry

The irradiation of freshly slaughtered chicken contributes considerably to the prevention of the spread of salmonellosis as Salmonella is frequently carried by poultry. Hence it seemed particularly important to examine thoroughly the safety to health of irradiated chicken in life-span feeding studies in rats and mice, in a multigeneration reproduction study in rats, in several subchronic feeding studies in dogs and rodents and in mutagenicity studies. Chicken meat irradiated with 7 kGy doses gave no adverse effect in all these investigations (WHO, 1977, 1981). Similar feeding tests in rats and dogs with chicken meat irradiated with 28 and 56 kGy also remained negative. A further extensive feeding study in mice using chicken meat irradiated with 58 kGy by either γ-rays or accelerated electrons was conducted for the US Army Medical R&D Command between 1979 and 1983. The study used two control groups fed either enzyme-inactivated meat stored frozen or meat made shelf-stable by heat sterilisation and two test groups fed either electron-irradiated or γ-irradiated meat. The average radiation dose was 58 kGy at −25°C. After irradiation the meat was stored at 24°C. No serious detrimental effects were noted as a result of irradation except for an apparent increase in testicular interstitial (Leydig) cell tumours in the test groups compared to the controls fed frozen untreated meat. The reproductive performance through three generations showed, as the only adverse effect, a comparatively decreased fertility in the control group fed heat sterilised meat; all other parameters of reproductive function, such as the number of offspring born, the number of stillbirths and the survival of pups, remained unaffected. A subsequent review of the histological slides failed to confirm any statistically significant increase in the incidence of testicular tumours. Moreover, these tumours had occurred only unilaterally, there was no associated hyperplasia of the interstitial cells in the testes and no evidence of progression from hyperplasia to neoplasia. There was no demonstrable testicular atrophy or necrosis as a contributory factor. None of the tumours was frankly malignant. Because cystic vascular interstitial cell tumours mimic other testicular tumours the historical control data were probably unreliable. Hence it was possible to conclude that feeding of irradiated chicken meat did not cause cancer (USA, 1985).

Several different kinds of mutagenicity studies were carried out on the same irradiated, heat-treated and deep-frozen chicken meat. Only in tests using Drosophila was it noted that fewer progeny developed from all groups fed chicken meat and even fewer in the group fed ^{60}Co-irradiated meat. Mutagenic changes were not observed. No satisfactory explanation could be found for this reproductive effect (Brynjolfsson, 1985).

Beef and beef products, pork, ham, bacon and mixed offal were tested in feeding studies in rats and dogs. Meat was usually fed to rodents at 35% of their diet and to dogs at the same rate or at 200 g/day. The meat was either raw or cooked and had been treated with 6–8 kGy or with 28 or 56 kGy. The cured meats were irradiated variously at 20, 50 or 74 kGy at −10°C to −30°C. Feeding studies extended from a few weeks to 2 years and included multigeneration reproduction, dominant lethal tests, studies in Drosophila and cytogenetic tests. No significant deleterious effects were noted in any study (Read *et al.*, 1959; Shillinger *et al.*, 1965; Ke-Wen and Dao-Jing, 1983; van Logten *et al.*, 1983).

Human Observations

Irradiation-sterilised food has been used over many years by patients suffering from immunological deficiencies either as a result of cytotoxic drug treatment or following organ transplantation. These foods are treated by doses of 25 kGy or more. Irradiated food has also been used in diets for astronauts. No general conclusions regarding safety can be drawn from these applications but it should be noted that no overt adverse effects have been reported.

Irradiated Animal Feeds

Irradiated commercial diets for laboratory and farm animals have been used in breeding colonies for laboratory animals and in animal husbandry. Radiation doses of 15–25 kGy were used for sterilisation. Reproduction of rats and mice over many generations was no different from that in controls fed autoclaved diets. No toxic effects were seen except for an unexplained 15–20% reduction in lymphocytes in male rats.

NUTRITIONAL CONSIDERATIONS

There is good evidence that irradiation of foodstuffs does not materially alter their nutritional value. Feeding trials set up to raise large numbers of laboratory rodents have shown normal growth and development of the animals when irradiated laboratory feed was used. When doses above 15 kGy were applied, vitamin supplementation became necessary; doses of 1 kGy caused no significant loss of nutrients in animal feeds.

In irradiation of fresh foods destruction of vitamins is nutritionally the most important change. The most sensitive water-soluble vitamin is ascorbic acid. Low doses cause losses comparable to those occurring during cold storage. When higher doses are used, the losses compare to those following cooking. The most sensitive fat-soluble vitamins are E and K (Diehl, 1979; Tobback, 1977).

Loss of vitamin B_1 and of polyunsaturated fatty acids is the most significant effect of irradiation. Being both temperature and dose dependent it is possible to reduce these losses by irradiating at low temperatures, e.g. $-30°C$ to $-40°C$, and by excluding oxygen by packaging in vacuum or under a nitrogen atmosphere. Digestibility of meat and its biological value are generally little affected. Irradiation in the presence of oxygen favours lipid oxidation and formation of carbonyls which then react with proteins and amino acids to yield a lower net protein utilisation.

Irradiation of fruit, vegetables and tubers reduces vitamin C and carotene to a nutritionally significant degree. Loss of vitamin E can be partly prevented by excluding oxygen during irradiation and storage.

Considerable losses of vitamins B_1 and C also occur on cooking and storage. Some amino acids and vitamin A are more sensitive to autoclaving than to irradiation.

MICROBIOLOGICAL CONSIDERATIONS

Irradiation damages living organisms mainly at sites of the genetic system through alterations of macromolecular cellular components such as DNA, RNA and other macroproteins. Because the molecular weight of DNA is about 10^6 times that of an amino acid, fatty acid or monosaccharide, and because the number of chemical changes in a molecule after irradiation is roughly proportional to its molecular weight, the sensitivity of DNA to radiation damage is about 10^6 times that of the basic food constituents. Bacteria are therefore much more sensitive to radiation because they consist largely of DNA. Bacterial spores however are radiation-resistant.

Irradiation reduces or eliminates the spoilage microflora as well as pathogens occurring in the food chain. The killing of bacteria is independent of the total count and always affects a constant fraction in similar time intervals. It therefore proceeds at a logarithmic rate so that the logarithm of the number of surviving organisms is linearly related to the irradiation dose. The heat sensitivity of bacteria parallels their radiation sensitivity. Both processes therefore achieve the same end result by reduction of the microbial load. Radiation resistance depends not only on the radiation dose but also on the temperature and the medium (Grecz *et al.*, 1981). Vegetative forms are 2–3 times more resistant in a dry or frozen system than in water. Similarly resistance to irradiation in a vacuum or in a nitrogen atmosphere is higher than in oxygen. Sensitivity of microorganisms to radiation is generally expressed as the number of Gy killing 90% of bacteria (D_{10} value). Radiation-resistant bacteria such as *Micrococcus radiodurans* have a D_{20} value of 5 kGy but are generally non-pathogenic and do not cause spoilage of food. Table 4 gives some D_{10} values for a number of microorganisms and Fig. 7 relates survival to radiation dose.

Fungi and moulds are more sensitive to radiation than yeasts. Resistant species are unknown. Viruses are resistant to radiation. Food irradiation alone cannot therefore guarantee the microbiological safety of food so treated. On the other hand, irradiated organisms, having lost genes important for plain survival, are more sensitive to heat treatment, drying and other processes. Increased pathogenicity has not been observed so far.

Increased production of mycotoxins has been observed only under very special circumstances. Two Indian studies showed that irradiated wheat, maize, sorghum, pearl millet, potatoes and onions produced more aflatoxins than non-irradiated foods (Priyadarshini and Tulepule, 1976, 1979). As the samples were heat-sterilised before infection with fungi the natural antifungal components were destroyed. These observations are

TABLE 4
D_{10} Values (kGy) for Some Microorganisms (modified from Langerak, 1982)

Pseudomonas spp.	0·10–0·20
E. coli (aerobic)	0·12–0·35
Salmonella spp.	0·20–0·50
Streptococcus faecalis	0·50–1·00
Penicillium, Aspergillus (spores)	0·50–0·70
Clostridium botulinum	1·50–2·50
Micrococcus radiodurans	5·00

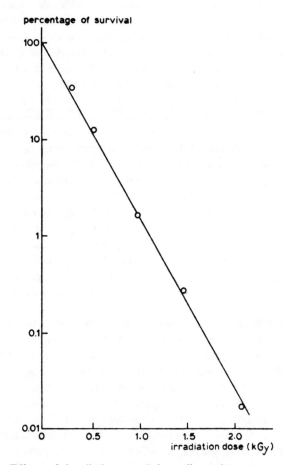

FIG. 7. Effect of irradiation on *Salmonella typhimurium* in ground beef: $7D_{10} = 3·85$ kGy (after Simard *et al.*, 1973).

therefore irrelevant for the irradiation of raw agricultural commodities. Related studies showed that irradiation of cultures of *Aspergillus flavus* and *Aspergillus parasiticus* could produce organisms generating more toxin than the non-irradiated culture, but growth conditions in practice would curtail the development of mutants because of their greater sensitivity (Schindler *et al.*, 1980). Single irradiation treatment causes temporary damage in surviving microorganisms but so far no toxin-producing or pathogenic mutants have been discovered.

Increased radiation resistance has been demonstrated under experimental but never under practical working conditions. Moreover these mutants lose their resistance if not irradiated constantly and they possess a weaker growth potential and lower virulence.

Most processes using heating, drying, freezing or chemical preservation will generate mutants or favour by selection pressure some naturally produced mutants. However, these mutants are usually less competitive (Cliver, 1977; Maxcy, 1977). The natural exposure of bacteria to background radiation in our environment, or heat and chemicals, produces many more mutations than the radiation doses used for food processing. The use of sub-sterilising doses may selectively destroy some organisms and thus favour some strains by removing the natural competition. This process is not restricted to food irradiation and occurs also with pasteurisation (Brynjolfsson, 1985).

Because of the natural radiation resistance of some microorganisms, irradiation at low doses cannot solve by itself all problems related to the microbiological safety of foods. Some problems require combination treatment for their solution. However, irradiation creates another barrier to the transmission of pathogens through food, especially Gram-negative organisms, leaving survivors which are usually more sensitive to heat, drying and other technological treatments of food. The problems due to suppression of spoilage organisms are not likely to be greater than those encountered with other methods of partial preservation, e.g. pasteurisation and salting.

LEGAL ASPECTS OF FOOD IRRADIATION

At present about 23 countries have given permission for the irradiation of about 40 different foods. Most of the clearances are restricted to experimental batches or products for test marketing. The sale of 12 irradiated foods is freely permitted in different countries. It is likely, in future, that foods irradiated according to the conditions contained in the International Standard developed by the Codex Alimentarius Commission, an organisation representing 122 member countries, may become items of international trade. The Cedex Standard for these products prescribes a maximum overall average dose of 10 kGy absorbed radiation energy. Irradiated foodstuffs should in addition be appropriately labelled to inform the consumer and to prevent unnecessary re-irradiation (Codex Alim. Comm., 1984). In accordance with the General Agreement on Tariffs and Trade (GATT) these Codex Standards should be accepted also by the member countries of GATT, unless there is a good reason for not doing so.

In the Netherlands and South Africa a symbol as well as a text are prescribed in the labelling provisions for irradiated foods. In the USA the irradiation of foods up to 1 kGy is permitted generally. Herbs and spices and certain dried products can be irradiated up to 30 kGy, provided they amount to no more than 0·01% of the daily food intake (i.e. 200 mg/day). In the FRG and the UK the sale of irradiated foods is not yet permitted, while in other EEC members the sale of certain specific irradiated foods is permitted. In the Netherlands full clearance for sale has been granted for irradiated chicken and onions, and provisional clearance for spices, frozen frog legs, rice, rye bread, frozen cooked shrimps, frozen fish, egg powder and dried vegetables. A whole series of other irradiated foods have been permitted for test marketing. In France full clearance has been given for the decontamination of spices and certain dried vegetables including powdered onions and garlic. Provisional approval was granted 9 years ago for the irradiation of onions, garlic and shallots to inhibit sprouting. A general survey of irradiated food products for human consumption in different countries has been published recently (van Kooij, 1985) (see Appendix).

The main hurdle to be overcome by commercialisation of the process is acceptance of marketed irradiated foods by the consumer. Much resistance both from the food industry and from the consumer has to be overcome. Proper information and education of the public as well as careful consideration of the form in which irradiated foods should be labelled without arousing unwarranted fears and prejudices in the purchaser will determine future developments. There is also the potential obstacle from political exploitation of the understandable fears and disquiet of the public related to anything connected with atomic or nuclear power. The other danger to be avoided is to make claims for advantages of food irradiation which cannot be fully supported or which are clearly exaggerated (Grünewald, 1984).

REFERENCES

Adam, S. (1983). Recent developments in radiation chemistry of carbohydrates. In: *Recent Advances in Food Irradiation*, P. S. Elias and A. J. Cohen (Eds), Elsevier, Amsterdam, pp. 149–70.

Aiyar, A. S. and Rao, V. S. (1977). Studies on mutagenicity of irradiated sugar solutions in *Salmonella typhimurium. Mutat. Res.*, **48**, 17–27.

Anukarahanonta, T. *et al.* (1980). Wholesomeness study of irradiated salted and dried mackerel in rats. Unpublished report to IAEA.

Aravindakshan, M., Vakil, U. K. and Sreenivasan, A. (1973). *Nutritional and Wholesomeness Studies with Dehydroirradiated Shrimp*. Report No. 455, Bhabha Atomic Research Centre, Bombay, India.

Barna, J. (1973). Toxicity studies of radiation- and heat-treated paprika powder in animal feeding experiments. Central Food Res. Inst., Budapest, Hungary.

Barna, J. (1976). Final report on preliminary studies relating to investigation of the wholesomeness of irradiated spices. Central Food Res. Inst., Budapest, Hungary.

Bhaskaram, C. and Sadasivan, G. (1976). Effects of feeding irradiated wheat to malnourished children. *Int. J. Radiat. Biol.*, **27**, 93; and *Am. J. Clin. Nutr.* (1975), **28**, 130–35.

Bögl, W. and Heide, L. (1984). Nachweis der Gewürzbestrahlung. *Fleischwirtsch.*, **64**(9), 1120–6.

Brynjolfsson, A. (1980). Food irradiation in the United States. In: *Proc. 26th European Meeting of Meat Research Workers*, Amer. Meat Sci. Assoc., Chicago, Vol. 1, pp. 172–7.

Brynjolfsson, A. (1985). Wholesomeness of irradiated foods: a review. *J. Food Safety*, **7**, 107–26.

Chaubey, R. C., Kavi, B. R., Chauhan, P. S., Sundaram, K. and Barna, J. (1979). Cytogenetic studies with irradiated ground paprika as evaluated by the micronucleus test in mice. *Acta Alim.*, **8**(2), 197–201.

Cleland, M. R., Farrell, J. P. and Morganstern, K. H. (1980). The use of high energy electrons and X-rays for the preservation of meat and other food products. In: *Proc. 26th European Meeting of Meat Research Workers*, Amer. Meat Sci. Assoc., Chicago, Vol. 1, pp.255–7.

Cliver, D. O. (1977). Unlikelihood of mutagenic effects of irradiation on viruses. *Wholesomeness of Irradiated Food*, WHO Tech. Rep. Ser., No. 604, Annex 2, 43–4, WHO, Geneva.

Codex Alimentarius Commission (1984), Codex general standard for irradiated foods and recommended international code of practice for the operation of radiation facilities used for the treatment of foods. *Codex Alim.*, Vol. XV, FAO, Rome.

Dauphin, J. F. and St. Lèbe, L. R. (1977). Radiation chemistry of carbohydrates. In: *Radiation Chemistry of Major Food Components*, P. S. Elias and A. J. Cohen (Eds), Elsevier, Amsterdam, pp.131–85.

Diehl, J. F. (1979). Verminderung von strahleninduzierten Vitamin E und -B$_1$-Verlusten durch Bestrahlung von Lebensmitteln bei tiefen Temperaturen und durch Ausschluss von Luftsauerstoff. *Z. Lebensm. Unter. Forsch.*, **169**, 276–82.

Diehl, J. F. (1983). Radiolytic effects in foods. In: *Preservation of Food by Ionizing*

Radiation, E. S. Josephson and M. S. Peterson (Eds), CRC Press, Boca Raton, USA, Vol. I, pp.279–357.

Diehl, J. F., Adam, S., Delincee, H. and Jakubick, V. (1978). Radiolysis of carbohydrates and of carbohydrate-containing foodstuffs. *J. Agric. Food Chem.*, **26**, 15–20.

Elias, P. S. and Cohen, A. J. (Eds) (1977). *Radiation Chemistry of Major Food Components*, Elsevier, Amsterdam, The Netherlands.

Fegley, H. C. and Edmonds, S. R. (1968). *Long-term Feeding Experiments on Radiation Pasteurized Foods*. Final Report, NYO-3573-1-Unclass.

Fraser, F. M. (1983). Gamma radiation processing equipment and associated energy requirements in food irradiation. In: *Preservation of Food by Ionizing Radiation*, E. S. Josephson and M. S. Peterson (Eds), CRC Press, Boca Raton, USA, Vol. III, pp.253–7.

Goldblith, S. A. (1966). Historical development of food irradiation. In: *Food Irradiation* (Proc. Int. Symp. Food Irradiation). STI/PUB 127, IAEA, Vienna, pp.3–21.

Grecz, N., Bruszew, G. and Amin, I. (1981). In: *Combination Processes in Food Irradiation*, IAEA, Vienna, pp.3–20.

Grünewald, Th. (1984). In: *Isotopes and Radiation in Agricultural Sciences*, M. F. l'Annunziata and J. O. Legg (Eds), Academic Press, New York, Vol. 2, pp.271–301.

Han, Y. W., Catalano, E. A. and Ciegler, A. (1983), Chemical and physical properties of sugar cane bagasse irradiated with gamma rays. *J. Agric. Food Chem.*, **31**(1), 34–8.

Herrnhut, H. (1985). Anwendungsorientierte Lebensmittelbestrahlungsanlagen, deren Wirtschaftlichkeit und Energieverbrauch. *Mitt. Gebiete Lebensm. Hyg.*, **76**, 28–33.

JECFI (1981). *Wholesomeness of Irradiated Food* (Report of a Joint FAO/IAEA/WHO Expert Committee), WHO Tech. Rep. Ser. No. 659, WHO, Geneva.

Kamaldinova, Z. M. (1970). Effect of culinary pretreated gamma-irradiated beef on the organism of rats. *Voprosy Pitaniya*, **29**(2), 73–7.

Kampelmacher, E. H.' (1984). Irradiation of food: a new technology for preserving and ensuring the hygiene of foods. *Fleischwirtsch.*, **64**(3), 322–7.

Kaylor, J. D., Slavin, J. W., Ronsivalli, L. J. and Lane, J. P. (1980). A prototype seafood irradiator. In: *Proc. 26th European Meeting of Meat Research Workers*, Amer. Meat Sci. Assoc., Chicago, USA, Vol. I, pp.217–20.

Ke-Wen, Cheng and Dao-Jing, Zhang (1983). Wholesomeness studies on gamma-irradiated rice. *Radiat. Phys. Chem.*, **22**(3), 792.

Langerak, D. Is. (1982). Irradiation of foodstuffs: technological aspects and possibilities. In: *Food Irradiation Now*, M. Nijhoff/Dr. W. Junk Publ., The Hague, pp.40–59.

Leemhorst, J. G. (1982). Industrial application of food irradiation. In: *Food Irradiation Now*, M. Nijhoff/Dr. W. Junk Publ., The Hague, pp. 60–8.

Mafarachisi, B. A. (1974). Growth, fertility and tissue studies of mice fed radiolytic products arising from gamma-irradiated beef fat. PhD. Thesis, Univ. Massachusetts.

Matsuyama, A. and Umeda, K. (1983). Sprout inhibition in tubers and bulbs. In:

Preservation of Food by Ionizing Radiation, E. S. Josephson and M. S. Peterson (Eds), CRC Press, Boca Raton, USA, Vol. III, p.197.

Maxcy, R. B. (1977). Comparative viability of unirradiated and gamma-irradiated bacterial cells. *J. Food Sci.*, **42**, 1056–9.

McLaughlin, W. L. (1982). Trends in radiation dosimetry. *Int. J. Appl. Radiat. Isot.*, **33**, 953–1310.

Merritt, C., Jr. and Taub, I. A. (1983). Commonality and predictability of radiolytic products in irradiated meats. In: *Recent Advances in Food Irradiation*, P. S. Elias and A. J. Cohen (Eds), Elsevier Biomedical Press, Amsterdam, pp. 27–57.

Minck, F. (1896). Zur Frage über die Einwirkung der Röntgenschen Strahlen auf Bakterien und ihre eventuelle therapeutische Verwendbarkeit. *Münch. Med. Wochenschr.*, **5**, 101; **9**, 202.

Murthy, P. B. K. (1981a), SCE in monkeys fed irradiated wheat. *Food Cosmet. Toxicol.*, **12**, 523.

Murthy, P. B. K. (1981b). Sister-chromatid exchanges in mice given irradiated wheat. *Toxicology*, **20**, 247–9.

Nawar, W. W. (1977). Radiation chemistry of lipids. In: *Radiation Chemistry of Major Food Components*, P. S. Elias and A. J. Cohen (Eds), Elsevier, Amsterdam, pp. 21–61.

Niemand, J. G., den Drijver, L., Pretorius, C. J., Holzapfel, C. W. and Van der Linde, J. (1983). Study of the mutagenicity of irradiated sugar solutions: implication for the radiation preservation of sub-tropical fruits. *J. Agric. Food Chem.*, **31**, 1016–20.

Paul, N., Grünewald, Th. and Kuprianoff, J. (1969). Über die Möglichkeiten einer Behandlung von Trockensuppen mit ionisierenden Strahlen. *Deutsch. Lebensm. Rundschau*, **65**(9), 279–81.

Priyadarshini, E. and Tulepule, P. G. (1976). Aflatoxin production in irradiated food. *Food Cosmet. Toxicol.*, **14**, 293–5.

Priyadarshini, E. and Tulepule, P. G. (1979). Effect of graded doses of gamma-irradiation on aflatoxin production by *Aspergillus parasiticus* in wheat. *Food Cosmet. Toxicol.*, **19**, 505–7.

Rao, V. S. (1978). Biochemical studies on the toxicity of irradiated sugar solutions in microorganisms. Ph.D. Thesis, Univ. Bombay.

Read, M. S., Trabosh, H. M., Worth, W. S., Kraybill, H. F. and Witt, N. F. (1959). Short-term rat feeding studies with gamma-irradiated food products. II. Beef and pork stored at elevated temperature. *Toxicol. Appl. Pharmacol.*, **1**, 417–23.

Reddi, O. S., Reddy, P. P., Ebenezer, D. N. and Naidu, N. V. (1977). Lack of genetic and cytogenetic effects in mice fed on irradiated wheat. *Int. J. Radiat. Biol.*, **31**, 589–601.

Schindler, A. F., Abadie, A. N. and Simpson, R. E. (1980). Enhanced aflatoxin production by *Aspergillus flavus* and *Aspergillus parasiticus* after gamma-irradiation of the spore inoculum. *J. Food Protect.*, **43**, 7–9.

Shillinger, Yu. I. and Osipova, I. N. (1970). The effect of gamma-irradiated fresh fish on the organism of white rats. *Voprosy Pitaniya*, **32**(6), 45–50.

Shillinger, Yu. I., Kachkova, V. O. and Maganova, N. B. (1965). Influence produced on the canine organism by meat food products gamma-irradiated in radio-pasteurization doses. *Voprosy Pitaniya*, **24**(1), 19.

Simard, C., Lachance, R. A. and Moreau, R. R. (1973). Traitement des viandes par irradiation. *Can. Inst. Food Sci. Technol. J.*, **6**, 250.

Takeguchi, C. A. (1983). Regulatory and toxicological aspects of food irradiation. *J. Food Safety*, **5**, 213–7.

Tobback, P. P. (1977). Radiation chemistry of vitamins. In: *Radiation Chemistry of Major Food Components*, P. S. Elias and A. J. Cohen (Eds), Elsevier, Amsterdam, pp.187–220.

Truhaut, R. and St. Lèbe, L. (1978). Différentes voies d'approche pour l'évaluation toxicologique de l'amidon irradié. In: *Food Preservation by Irradiation*, Vol. II (STI/PUB/470), IAEA, Vienna.

Urbain, W. M. (1977). Radiation chemistry of proteins. In: *Radiation Chemistry of Major Food Components*, P. S. Elias and A. J. Cohen (Eds), Elsevier, Amsterdam, pp.63–130.

Urbain, W. M. (1978). Food irradiation. *Adv. Food Res.*, **24**, 155–227.

USA (1965). *Statement on the Wholesomeness of Irradiated Foods by the Surgeon General of the Army.* Hearings Subcommittee on Research, Development and Radiation. 89th Congress, 9–10 June. US Government Printing Office, Washington, DC, pp.105–6.

USA (1985). *Chronic Toxicity, Oncogenicity and Multigeneration Reproduction Study Using CD-1 Mice to Evaluate Frozen, Thermally Sterilized, Cobalt-60 Irradiated and 10 MeV Electron Irradiated Chicken Meat.* Nat. Tech. Inf. Serv., Order No: PB-84-187012.

Van Kooij, J. G. (1985). Updated list of clearances for irradiated foods in member states. *IAEA Food Irrad. Newslett.*, **9**(2), 29–39.

Van Kooij, J. G., Leveling, H. B. and Schubert, J. (1978). Application of the Ames mutagenicity test to food processed by physical preservation methods. In: *Food Preservation by Irradiation*, Proc. Int. Symp. Food Preservation by Irradiation, IAEA, Vienna, Vol. 2, pp.63–71.

van Logten, M. J., den Tonkelaar, E. M., van Esch, G. J. and Kroes, R. (1972). The wholesomeness of irradiated shrimps. *Food Cosmet. Toxicol.*, **10**(6), 781.

van Logten, M. J., de Vries, T., van der Heyden, C. A., van Leeuwen, E. Y. R., Garbis-Berkvens, M. J. M. and Strik, J. J. T. W. A. (1983). Report 61740001, N. I. Public Health, Netherlands.

Van Straten, S. (1977). *Volatile Compounds in Food*, 4th edn, CIVO-TNO, Zeist, The Netherlands.

Varma, M. B., Rao, K. P., Nadan, S. D. and Rao, M. S. (1982*a*). Mutagenic effects of irradiated glucose in Drosophila melanogaster. *Food Chem. Toxicol.*, **20**, 947–9.

Varma, M. B., Nadan, D. S., Rao, K. P. and Rao, M.S. (1982*b*). Non-induction of dominant lethal mutations in mice fed irradiated glucose. *Int. J. Radiat. Biol.*, **42**, 559–63.

Vijayalaxmi, C. (1975). Cytogenetic studies in rats fed irradiated wheat. *Int. J. Radiat. Biol.*, **27**, 283.

Vijayalaxmi, C. (1978*a*). Cytogenetic studies in monkeys fed irradiated wheat. *Toxicology*, **9**, 181–4.

Vijayalaxmi, C. (1978*b*). Immune response in rats given irradiated wheat. *Brit. J. Nutr.*, **40**, 535–41.

WHO (1977). *Wholesomeness of Irradiated Food.* WHO/FOOD ADD/77.45, WHO, Geneva.

WHO (1981). *Wholesomeness of Irradiated Food.* EHE/81.24, WHO, Geneva.

Wills, E. D. (1981). *Studies of Irradiated Food with Special Reference to Its Lipid Peroxide Content and Carcinogenic Potential.* IFIP Tech. Rep. Ser. No. 55, Karlsruhe, FRG.

Wilmer, J. and Schubert, J. (1981). Mutagenicity of irradiated solutions of nucleic acid bases and nucleosides in *Salmonella typhimurium. Mutat. Res.*, **88**, 337–42.

Wilmer, J., Schubert, J. and Leveling, H. (1981). Mutagenicity of gamma-irradiated oxygenated and deoxygenated solutions of 2-deoxy-D-ribose and D-ribose in *Salmonella typhimurium. Mutat. Res.*, **90**, 385–97.

Zaitsev, A. (1980). USSR submission to WHO.

Zaitsev, A. N. and Maganova, N. B. (1981). Effect of the diet including gamma-irradiated fish on embryogenesis and chromosomes of rats. *Voprosy Pitaniya*, **40**(6), 61–3.

Zaitsev, A. N. and Osipova, I. N. (1981). Study on mutagenic properties of irradiated fresh fish in chronic experiments. *Voprosy Pitaniya*, **40**, 53–6.

APPENDIX
Irradiated Food Products Cleared for Human Consumption in Different Countries (August 1985)

Country (Organisation)	Product	Purpose	Clearance	Dose permitted (kGy)	Approval date
Argentina	potatoes	sprout inhibition	provisional	up to 0·15	14 December 1978
	onions	sprout inhibition	test marketing	0·05 average	June 1984
	garlic	sprout inhibition	test marketing	0·05 average	June 1984
Australia	frozen shrimps	decontamination	provisional	6 or 8	11 September/ 16 October 1978
Bangladesh	chicken	shelf-life extension/ decontamination	unconditional	up to 7	28 December 1983
	papaya	insect disinfestation/ control of ripening	unconditional	up to 1	28 December 1983
	potatoes	sprout inhibition	unconditional	up to 0·15	28 December 1983
	wheat and ground wheat products	insect disinfestation	unconditional	up to 1	28 December 1983
	fish	shelf-life extension/ decontamination/ insect disinfestation	unconditional	up to 2·2	28 December 1983
	onions	sprout inhibition	unconditional	up to 0·15	28 December 1983
	rice	insect disinfestation	unconditional	up to 1	28 December 1983
	frog legs	decontamination	provisional		
	shrimp	shelf-life extension/ decontamination	provisional		
	mangoes	shelf-life extension/ insect disinfestation/ control of ripening	unconditional	up to 1	28 December 1983
	pulses	insect disinfestation	unconditional	up to 1	28 December 1983
	spices	decontamination/ insect disinfestation	unconditional	up to 10	28 December 1983

Country (Organisation)	Product	Purpose	Clearance	Dose permitted (kGy)	Approval date
Belgium	potatoes	sprout inhibition	provisional	up to 0·15	16 July 1980
	strawberries	shelf-life extension	provisional	up to 3	16 July 1980
	onions	sprout inhibition	provisional	up to 0·15	16 October 1980
	garlic	sprout inhibition	provisional	up to 0·15	16 October 1980
	shallots	sprout inhibition	provisional	up to 0·15	16 October 1980
	black/white pepper	decontamination	provisional	up to 10	16 October 1980
	paprika powder	decontamination	provisional	up to 10	16 October 1980
	gum arabic	decontamination	provisional	up to 9	29 September 1983
	spices (78 different products)	decontamination	provisional	up to 10	29 September 1983
	(semi)-dried vegetables (7 different products)	decontamination	provisional	up to 10	29 September 1983
Brazil	rice	insect disinfestation	unconditional	up to 1	7 March 1985
	potatoes	sprout inhibition	unconditional	up to 0·15	7 March 1985
	onions	sprout inhibition	unconditional	up to 0·15	7 March 1985
	beans	insect disinfestation	unconditional	up to 1	7 March 1985
	maize	insect disinfestation	unconditional	up to 0·5	7 March 1985
	wheat	insect disinfestation	unconditional	up to 1	7 March 1985
	wheat flour	insect disinfestation	unconditional	up to 1	7 March 1985
	spices (13 different products)	decontamination/ insect disinfestation	unconditional	up to 10	7 March 1985
	papaya	insect disinfestation/ control of ripening	unconditional	up to 1	7 March 1985
	strawberries	shelf-life extension	unconditional	up to 3	7 March 1985
	fish and fish products (fillets, salted, smoked, dried, dehydrated)	shelf-life extension/ decontamination/ insect disinfestation	unconditional	up to 2·2	8 March 1985
	poultry	shelf-life extension/ decontamination	unconditional	up to 7	8 March 1985

(continued)

APPENDIX—contd.

Country (Organisation)	Product	Purpose	Clearance	Dose permitted (kGy)	Approval date
Bulgaria	potatoes	sprout inhibition	experimental batches	0·1	30 April 1972
	onions	sprout inhibition	experimental batches	0·1	30 April 1972
	garlic	sprout inhibition	experimental batches	0·1	30 April 1972
	grain	insect disinfestation	experimental batches	0·3	30 April 1972
	dry food concentrates	insect disinfestation	experimental batches	1	30 April 1972
	dried fruits	insect disinfestation	experimental batches	1	30 April 1972
	fresh fruits (tomatoes, peaches, apricots, cherries, raspberries, grapes)	shelf-life extension	experimental batches	2·5	30 April 1972
Canada	potatoes	sprout inhibition	unconditional	up to 0·1	9 November 1960
	onions	sprout inhibition	unconditional	up to 0·15	14 June 1963
	wheat, flour, wholewheat flour	insect disinfestation	unconditional	up to 0·15	25 March 1965
				up to 0·75	25 February 1969
	poultry	decontamination	test marketing	up to 7	20 June 1973
	cod and haddock fillets	shelf-life extension	test marketing	up to 1·5	2 October 1973
	spices and certain dried vegetables, seasonings	decontamination	unconditional	up to 10	September 1984
Chile	potatoes	sprout inhibition	experimental batches, test marketing	up to 0·15	31 October 1974
			unconditional		29 December 1982
	papaya	insect disinfestation	unconditional	up to 1	29 December 1982
	wheat and ground wheat products	insect disinfestation	unconditional	up to 1	29 December 1982

Country (Organisation)	Product	Purpose	Clearance	Dose permitted (kGy)	Approval date
	strawberries	shelf-life extension	unconditional	up to 3	29 December 1982
	chicken	decontamination	unconditional	up to 7	29 December 1982
	onions	sprout inhibition	unconditional	up to 0·15	29 December 1982
	rice	insect disinfestation	unconditional	up to 1	29 December 1982
	teleost fish and fish products	shelf-life extension decontamination insect disinfestation	unconditional	up to 2·2	29 December 1982
	cocoa beans	decontamination/ insect disinfestation	unconditional	up to 5	29 December 1982
	dates	insect disinfestation	unconditional	up to 1	29 December 1982
	mangoes	shelf-life extension/ insect disinfestation/ control of ripening	unconditional	up to 1	29 December 1982
	pulses	insect disinfestation	unconditional	up to 1	29 December 1982
	spices and condiments	decontamination/ insect disinfestation	unconditional	up to 10	29 December 1982
China	potatoes	sprout inhibition	unconditional	up to 0·20	30 November 1984
	onions	sprout inhibition	unconditional	up to 0·15	30 November 1984
	garlic	sprout inhibition	unconditional	up to 0·10	30 November 1984
	peanuts	insect disinfestation	unconditional	up to 0·40	30 November 1984
	grain	insect disinfestation	unconditional	up to 0·45	30 November 1984
	mushrooms	growth inhibition	unconditional	up to 1	30 November 1984
	sausage	decontamination	unconditional	up to 8	30 November 1984
Czechoslovakia	potatoes	sprout inhibition	experimental batches	up to 0·1	26 November 1976
	onions	sprout inhibition	experimental batches	up to 0·08	26 November 1976
	mushrooms	growth inhibition	experimental	up to 2	26 November 1976

(continued)

APPENDIX—contd.

Country (Organisation)	Product	Purpose	Clearance	Dose permitted (kGy)	Approval date
Denmark	potatoes	sprout inhibition	unconditional	up to 0·15	27 February 1970
France	potatoes	sprout inhibition	provisional	0·075–0·15	8 November 1972
	onions	sprout inhibition	provisional	0·075–0·15	9 August 1977
	garlic	sprout inhibition	provisional	0·075–0·15	9 August 1977
	shallots	sprout inhibition	provisional	0·075–0·15	9 August 1977
	spices and aromatic substances (72 products inclusive powdered onion and garlic)	decontamination	unconditional	up to 11	10 February 1983
	gum arabic	decontamination	unconditional	up to 9	16 June 1985
	muesli-like cereal	decontamination	unconditional	up to 10	16 June 1985
	dehydrated vegetables	decontamination	unconditional	up to 10	16 June 1985
	mechanically deboned poultry meat	decontamination	unconditional	up to 5	16 February 1985
Federal Republic of Germany	deep frozen meals	sterilization	hospital patients/ test marketing		
	potatoes	sprout inhibition	test marketing		1981
German Democratic Republic	onions	sprout inhibition	test marketing	50	30 January 1984
	onions	sprout inhibition	unconditional	20	7 June 1983
	enzyme solutions	decontamination	unconditional	10	29 December 1982
	spices	decontamination	provisional	up to 10	
Hungary	potatoes	sprout inhibition	test marketing	0·1	23 December 1969
	potatoes	sprout inhibition	test marketing	0·15 max.	10 January 1972
	potatoes	sprout inhibition	test marketing	0·15 max.	5 March 1973
	onions	sprout inhibition	test marketing		5 March 1973
	strawberries	shelf-life extension	test marketing		5 March 1973

Country (Organisation)	Product	Purpose	Clearance	Dose permitted (kGy)	Approval date
Hungary	mixed spices (black pepper, cumin, paprika, dried garlic: for use in sausages)	decontamination	experimental batches	5	2 April 1974
	onions	sprout inhibition	test marketing	0·06	6 August 1975
	onions	sprout inhibition	experimental batches	0·06	6 September 1976
	mixed dry ingredients for canned hashed meat	decontamination	experimental batches	5	20 November 1976
	potatoes	sprout inhibition	test marketing	0·10	4 May 1980
	onions	sprout inhibition	experimental batches	0·05	15 September 1980
	onions (for dehydrated flakes processing)	sprout inhibition	test marketing	0·05	18 November 1980
	mushrooms (Agaricus)	growth inhibition	test marketing	2·5	20 June 1981
	strawberries	shelf-life extension	test marketing	2·5	20 June 1981
	potatoes	sprout inhibition	test marketing	0·1	13 October 1981
	potatoes	sprout inhibition	test marketing	0·10	2 December 1981
	spices for sausage production	decontamination	test marketing	5	4 January 1982
	strawberries	shelf-life extension	test marketing	2·5	15 April 1982
	mushrooms (Agaricus)	growth inhibition	test marketing	2·5	15 April 1982
	mushrooms (Pleurotus)	growth inhibition	test marketing	3	15 April 1982
	grapes	shelf-life extension	test marketing	2·5	15 April 1982
	cherries	shelf-life extension	test marketing	2·5	15 April 1982

(continued)

APPENDIX—contd.

Country (Organisation)	Product	Purpose	Clearance	Dose permitted (kGy)	Approval date
Hungary	sour cherries	shelf-life extension	test marketing	2·5	15 April 1982
	red currant	shelf-life extension	test marketing	2·5	15 April 1982
	onions	sprout inhibition	unconditional	0·05 ± 0·02	23 June 1982
	spices for sausage	decontamination	test marketing	5	28 June 1982
	pears	shelf-life extension	test marketing	2·5	7 December 1982
	pears	shelf-life extension	test marketing	1·0 + CaCl$_2$ treatment	24 January 1983
	spices	decontamination	test marketing	5	1983
	potatoes (for processing into potato flakes)	sprout inhibition	test marketing	0·1	28 January 1983
	frozen chicken	decontamination	test marketing	4	3 October 1983
Israel	potatoes	sprout inhibition	unconditional	0·15 max.	5 July 1967
	onions	sprout inhibition	unconditional	0·10 max.	25 July 1968
	poultry and poultry sections	shelf-life extension/ decontamination	unconditional	7 max.	23 April 1982
	onions	sprout inhibition	unconditional	0·15	6 March 1985
	garlic	sprout inhibition	unconditional	0·15	6 March 1985
	shallots	sprout inhibition	unconditional	0·15	6 March 1985
	spices (36 different products)	decontamination	unconditional	10	6 March 1985
Italy	potatoes	sprout inhibition	unconditional	0·075–0·15	30 August 1973
	onions	sprout inhibition	unconditional	0·075–0·15	30 August 1973
	garlic	sprout inhibition	unconditional	0·075–0·15	30 August 1973
Japan	potatoes	sprout inhibition	unconditional	0·15 max.	30 August 1972

Country (Organisation)	Product	Purpose	Clearance	Dose permitted (kGy)	Approval date
Netherlands	asparagus	shelf-life extension/ growth inhibition	experimental batches	2 max.	7 May 1969
	cocoa beans	insect disinfestation	experimental batches	0·7 max.	7 May 1969
	strawberries	shelf-life extension	experimental batches	2·5 max.	7 May 1969
	mushrooms	growth inhibition	unconditional	2·5 max.	23 October 1969
	deep-frozen meals	sterilization	hospital patients	25 min.	27 November 1969
	potatoes	sprout inhibition	unconditional	0·15 max.	23 March 1970
	shrimps	shelf-life extension	experimental batches	0·5–1	13 November 1970
	onions	sprout inhibition	experimental batches	0·15	5 February 1971
	spices and condiments	decontamination	experimental batches	8–10	13 September 1971
	poultry, eviscerated (in plastic bags)	shelf-life extension	experimental batches	3 max.	31 December 1971
	chicken	shelf-life extension/ decontamination	unconditional	3 max.	10 May 1976
	fresh, tinned and liquid foodstuffs	sterilization	hospital patients	25 min.	8 March 1972
	spices	decontamination	provisional	10	4 October 1974
	powdered batter mix	decontamination	test marketing	1·5	4 October 1974
	vegetable filling	decontamination	test marketing	0·75	4 October 1974
	endive (prepared, cut)	shelf-life extension	test marketing	1	14 January 1975
	onions	sprout inhibition	unconditional	0·05 max.	9 June 1975
	spices	decontamination	provisional	10	26 June 1975
	peeled potatoes	shelf-life extension	test marketing	0·5	12 May 1976
	chicken	shelf-life extension/ decontamination	unconditional	3 max.	10 May 1976
	shrimps	shelf-life extension	test marketing	1	15 June 1976
	fillets of haddock, coal-fish, whiting	shelf-life extension	test marketing	1	6 September 1976

(continued)

APPENDIX—contd.

Country (Organisation)	Product	Purpose	Clearance	Dose permitted (kGy)	Approval date
Netherlands	fillet of cod and plaice	shelf-life extension	test marketing	1	7 September 1976
	fresh vegetables (prepared, cut, soupgreens)	shelf-life extension	test marketing	1	6 September 1977
	spices	decontamination	provisional	10	4 April 1978
	frozen frog legs	decontamination	provisional	5	25 September 1978
	rice and ground rice products	insect disinfestation	provisional	1	13 March 1979
	rye bread	shelf-life extension	provisional	5 max.	12 February 1980
	spices	decontamination	provisional	7 max.	15 April 1980
	frozen shrimp	decontamination	provisional	7 max.	9 May 1980
	malt	decontamination	provisional	10 max.	8 February 1983
	boiled and cooled shrimp	shelf-life extension	provisional	1 max.	8 February 1983
	frozen shrimp	decontamination	provisional	7 max.	8 February 1983
	frozen fish	decontamination	provisional	6 max.	24 August 1983
	egg powder	decontamination	provisional	6 max.	25 August 1983
	dry blood protein	decontamination	provisional	7 max.	25 August 1983
	dehydrated vegetables	decontamination	provisional	10 max.	27 October 1983
	refrigerated snacks of minced meat	shelf-life extension	test marketing	2	12 July 1984
New Zealand	herbs and spices (one batch)	decontamination	provisional	8	March 1985
Norway	spices	decontamination	unconditional	up to 10	
Philippines	potatoes	sprout inhibition	provisional	0·15 max.	13 September 1972
	onions	sprout inhibition	provisional	0·07	1981
	garlic	sprout inhibition	provisional	0·07	1981

Country (Organisation)	Product	Purpose	Clearance	Dose permitted (kGy)	Approval date
Poland	potatoes	sprout inhibition	provisional	up to 0·15	1982
	onions	sprout inhibition	provisional		March 1983
South Africa	potatoes	sprout inhibition	unconditional	0·12–0·24	19 January 1977
	dried bananas	insect disinfestation	provisional	0·5 max.	28 July 1977
	avocadoes	insect disinfestation	provisional	0·1 max.	28 July 1977
	onions	sprout inhibition	unconditional	0·05–0·15	25 August 1978
	garlic	sprout inhibition	unconditional	0·1–0·20	25 August 1978
	chicken	shelf-life extension/ decontamination	unconditional	2–7	25 August 1978
	papaya	shelf-life extension	unconditional	0·5–1·5	25 August 1978
	mangoes	shelf-life extension	unconditional	0·5–1·5	25 August 1978
	strawberries	shelf-life extension	unconditional	1–4	25 August 1978
	bananas	shelf-life extension	unconditional		1982
	litchis	shelf-life extension	unconditional		1982
	pickled mangoes (achar)	shelf-life extension	unconditional		1982
	avocadoes	shelf-life extension	unconditional		1982
	frozen fruit juices	shelf-life extension	unconditional		
	green beans		unconditional		
	tomatoes	control of ripening	unconditional		
	brinjals		unconditional		
	soya pickle products		unconditional		
	ginger		unconditional		
	vegetable paste		unconditional		
	bananas (dried)	insect disinfestation	unconditional		
	almonds	insect disinfestation	unconditional		
	cheese powder	insect disinfestation	unconditional		

(continued)

APPENDIX—contd.

Country (Organisation)	Product	Purpose	Clearance	Dose permitted (kGy)	Approval date
South Africa	yeast powder		unconditional		
	herbal tea		unconditional		
	various spices		unconditional		
	various dehydrated vegetables		unconditional		
Spain	potatoes	sprout inhibition	unconditional	0·05–0·15	4 November 1969
	onions	sprout inhibition	unconditional	0·08 max.	1971
Thailand	onions	sprout inhibition	unconditional	0·1 max.	20 March 1973
Union of Soviet Socialist Republics	potatoes	sprout inhibition	unconditional	0·1 max.	14 March 1958
	potatoes	sprout inhibition	unconditional	0·3 (1 MeV electrons)	17 July 1973
	grain	insect disinfestation	unconditional	0·3	1959
	fresh fruit and vegetables	shelf-life extension	experimental batches	2–4	11 July 1964
	semi-prepared raw beef, pork and rabbit products (in plastic bags)	shelf-life extension	experimental batches	6–8	11 July 1964
	dried fruits	insect disinfestation	unconditional	1	15 February 1966
	dry food concentrates (buckwheat mush, gruel, rice pudding)	insect disinfestation	unconditional	0·7	6 June 1966
	poultry, eviscerated (in plastic bags)	shelf-life extension	experimental batches	6	4 July 1966
	culinary prepared meat products (fried meat, entrecote) (in plastic bags)	shelf-life extension	test marketing	8	1 February 1967

Country (Organisation)	Product	Purpose	Clearance	Dose permitted (kGy)	Approval date
United Kingdom	onions	sprout inhibition	test marketing	0·06	25 February 1967
	onions	sprout inhibition	unconditional	0·06	17 July 1973
	any food for consumption by patients who require a sterile diet as an essential factor in their treatment	sterilization	hospital patients		1 December 1969
United States of America	wheat and wheat flour	insect disinfestation	unconditional	0·2–0·5	21 August 1963
	white potatoes	shelf-life extension	unconditional	0·05–0·1	30 June 1964
	white potatoes	shelf-life extension	unconditional	0·05–0·15	1 November 1965
	spices and dry vegetable seasonings (38 commodities)	decontamination/ insect disinfestation	unconditional	30 max.	5 July 1983
	dry or dehydrated enzyme preparations (including immobilized enzyme preparations)	control of insects and/or micro-organisms	unconditional	10 max.	10 June 1985
	pork carcasses or fresh, non-heat processed cuts of pork carcasses	control of Trichinella spiralis	unconditional	0·3 min.–1·0 max.	22 July 1985
Uruguay	potatoes	sprout inhibition	unconditional		23 June 1970

(continued)

APPENDIX—contd.

Country (Organisation)	Product	Purpose	Clearance	Dose permitted (kGy)	Approval date
Yugoslavia	cereals	insect disinfestation	unconditional	up to 10	17 December 1984
	legumes	insect disinfestation	unconditional	up to 10	17 December 1984
	onions	sprout inhibition	unconditional	up to 10	17 December 1984
	garlic	sprout inhibition	unconditional	up to 10	17 December 1984
	potatoes	sprout inhibition	unconditional	up to 10	17 December 1984
	dehydrated fruits and vegetables	sprout inhibition	unconditional	up to 10	17 December 1984
	dried mushrooms	decontamination	unconditional	up to 10	17 December 1984
	egg powder	decontamination	unconditional	up to 10	17 December 1984
	herbal teas, tea extracts	decontamination	unconditional	up to 10	17 December 1984
	fresh poultry	shelf-life extension/ decontamination	unconditional	up to 10	17 December 1984
FAO/IAEA/WHO Expert Committee, 1969	potatoes	sprout inhibition	provisional	0·15 max.	12 April 1969
	wheat and ground wheat products	insect disinfestation	provisional	0·75 max.	12 April 1969

Country (Organisation)	Product	Purpose	Clearance	Dose permitted (kGy)	Approval date
FAO/IAEA/WHO Expert Committee 1976	potatoes	sprout inhibition	unconditional	0·03–0·15	7 September 1976
	onions	sprout inhibition	provisional	0·02–0·15	7 September 1976
	papaya	insect disinfestation	unconditional	0·5–1	7 September 1976
	strawberries	shelf-life extension	unconditional	1–3	7 September 1976
	wheat and ground wheat products	insect disinfestation	unconditional	0·15–1	7 September 1976
	rice	insect disinfestation	provisional	0·1–1	7 September 1976
	chicken	shelf-life extension/ decontamination	unconditional	2–7	7 September 1976
	cod and redfish	shelf-life extension/ decontamination	provisional	2–2·2	7 September 1976
FAO/IAEA/WHO Expert Committee, 1980	any food product	sprout inhibition/ shelf-life extension/ decontamination/ insect disinfestation/ control of ripening/ growth inhibition	unconditional	up to 10	3 November 1980

Chapter 10

FOOD INTOLERANCE

Klara Miller

British Industrial Biological Research Association, Carshalton, Surrey, UK

INTRODUCTION

Intolerance to certain foods or food components is a long-recognized phenomenon, and there is clear evidence that a number of mechanisms may be responsible for eliciting the symptoms ascribed to food intolerance. The most commonly described reactions are urticaria, angio-oedema and asthma, and gastrointestinal symptoms such as vomiting and diarrhoea. Although anaphylactic reactions can occur they are infrequent. In children, enuresis, irritability and hyperactivity have also been reported after ingestion of certain foods or chemical additives such as azo-dyes and preservatives. In adults, early reactions tend to be described in more detail and include swelling of the lips and tingling of the mouth and throat. Other symptoms are sometimes so vague as to be almost impossible to define, for example, nausea, abdominal distension, joint pains, irritability and headaches. In addition, clinical descriptions and the terms used for classification of untoward reactions vary widely, and the vocabulary used by

347

scientists and immunologists is not the same as the one used by clinicians or the one used by the general public.

In this chapter food intolerance is taken to mean a reproducible, unpleasant (i.e. adverse) reaction to a specific food or food ingredient as defined by the joint report of the Royal College of Physicians and the British Nutrition Foundation (1984). The term 'food allergy' is used only when there is proof that an immunological component is involved, and the term 'idiosyncratic reactions' describes abnormal but non-immune responses in certain individuals. Lactase deficiency in the gut, resulting in lactose intolerance, is an example of an idiosyncratic response; fat intolerance in biliary tract disease is another. Urticaria due to strawberries or vomiting and diarrhoea on eating shellfish are examples of intolerance due to non-immunological mechanisms which may arise from a variety of causes. These include pharmacological effects, the release of histamine from mast cells and circulating basophils without the involvement of reaginic antibody, and certain inflammatory bowel conditions. Diagnosis is rendered still more difficult in that symptoms may be the same for each category (Table 1); furthermore, the complexity of the Western diet often prevents identification of the offending substance.

Immunologically mediated responses can be demonstrated only in a minority of cases. Ideally the diagnosis of allergy should rest on the demonstration of specific cytophilic antibodies such as IgE or lymphocytes sensitized to the causative substance, but in practice this is difficult without

TABLE 1
Symptoms Commonly Associated with Food Intolerance

Local (GI tract)
Swelling of lips
Nausea
Vomiting
Diarrhoea
Constipation
Systemic
Headache
Urticaria
Angio-oedema
Eczema
Asthma

the correct purified antigen. Although allergens have been isolated from cow's milk, egg white, tomato, crab, cod fish, soya beans and peanuts, among others, the range of foods reported to have caused adverse reactions is very wide. Virtually all foods have the potential to elicit specific immune responses involving antibodies or cells. The diagnosis of food allergy therefore often rests upon clinical documentation of symptoms that recur after only a small amount of the substance has been ingested, and where the response is unrelated to any physiological effect of the food additive.

The possibility that an allergic reaction to a food will occur in an individual, however, is much less than a non-allergic reaction. This is because in the majority of individuals a gut-associated immunological regulatory system exists to ensure that specific and prolonged tolerance to ingested compounds will occur. However, in individuals predisposed to allergic diseases the tolerance response is either not effective or does not occur. This failure to achieve tolerance is currently believed to be one of the major underlying causes of dietary allergies.

PROTECTIVE MECHANISMS OF THE GASTROINTESTINAL TRACT

Because the gut is designed to absorb nutriments and has a vast surface area that is in contact with the outside world, it requires special protection against the onslaughts of pathogenic bacteria, viruses and toxins. Accordingly, the gut is richly endowed with lymphoreticular tissue able to generate immune effector mechanism as well as to 'sample' antigenic material. The protection afforded to the gut by this gut-associated lymphoid tissue (GALT) is by no means absolute and, even in communities with sophisticated sanitary arrangements and medical supervision, illnesses caused by enteric infections are not uncommon. In undeveloped communities, especially where the population is high, such infections cause continual morbidity and even mortality. The young of both man and animals are particularly at risk as GALT is poorly developed at birth, and the adaptation (in an immunological sense) to pathogenic and commensal bacterial flora necessarily takes time. During the process of adaptation GALT will occasionally over-react and produce antibodies and sensitized lymphocytes directed at normal dietary constituents, so an allergic state may develop.

From an anatomical standpoint the gut wall is protected by its mucous coating, by the tight junctions between epithelial cells and the lympho-reticular tissue (GALT) beneath them. GALT is distributed throughout the whole length of the gut, extending into the villi and surrounding the crypts. It is made up of diffuse lymphoid tissue in the *lamina propria* of the intestine, the Peyer's patches (aggregates of lymphoid follicles that are distributed along the length of the intestine) and the mesenteric lymph nodes (Brandtzaeg *et al.*, 1987).

The cells of the *lamina propria* consist of macrophages, lymphocytes and granulocytes (mainly eosinophils and mast cells). The macrophages appear inconspicuous but modern techniques have demonstrated the *laminae* to be amply supplied with dendritic macrophages (Mayrhofer *et al.*, 1983), which are especially important in the presentation of antigens to competent B and T lymphocytes. Lymphoid cells are made up of small lymphocytes, immunoblasts (small lymphocytes that have transformed into large lymphoid blast cells as a result of appropriate stimuli) and very large numbers of actively antibody-secreting plasma cells. This is because GALT is subject, even in health, to continual antigenic stimulation and because lymph-borne immunoblasts 'home' back to the *lamina propria* almost as soon as they reach the blood (Gowans and Knight, 1964; Hall and Smith, 1970). These immunoblasts, which have become disseminated throughout the gut, develop into mature plasma cells which, during a life span of only a few days (Mattioli and Tomasi, 1973), secrete the immuno-globulins which protect the gut. Most of the cells secrete immunoglobulin A (IgA), the principal antibody of external secretions, but significant numbers produce IgM, IgG and IgE as well (Durkin and Waksman, 1979). IgE-bearing cells increase significantly during infection with metazoan parasites as do mucosal T mast cells (Wakelin and Giences, 1987).

Peyer's patches can be found in the anti-mesenteric wall of the intestine. They are easily identified as the overlying epithelium has lost its villous pattern and become a flat membrane composed of columnar epithelial cells. Some of the membrane ('M') cells have a phagocytic function and appear to sample the contents of the gut and pass small amounts of material to the underlying lymphoid tissue (Owen and Jones, 1974; Owen, 1977). Much of this lymphoid tissue is arranged in follicles similar to the germinal centres found in lymph nodes, but the Peyer's patches contain very few antibody-forming plasma cells.

The mesenteric lymph nodes receive and filter the lymph that is formed in the wall of the intestine and conveyed to them by afferent lymphatics. As they lie downstream of both the diffuse lymphoid tissue and the Peyer's patches, small lymphocytes, immunoblasts and macrophages are conveyed

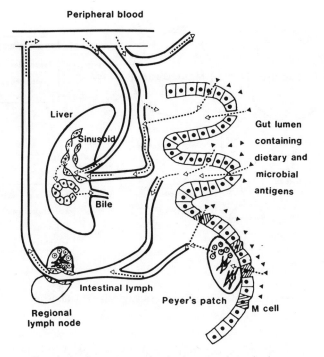

FIG. 1. Antigen penetration in the gastrointestinal tract.

in significant numbers to the mesenteric nodes (Hall *et al.*, 1977). Furthermore, macromolecular material, whether from dietary components or intestinal micro-organisms, that has penetrated the epithelium depends absolutely for its transport on the lymphatic system (Fig. 1). Only in the case of injury or pathology could macromolecules enter the blood capillaries, although of course small molecules such as haptens can be absorbed directly into the portal blood and conveyed, initially, to the liver.

Dietary compounds could also gain access to the body via villus uptake (Lee, 1971) or following uptake and transport through gut enterocytes. Although such a process would be very inefficient it could, because of the large number of enterocytes, be sufficient to carry immunologically significant amounts of protein across the gut. It is believed that this process is particularly susceptible to steric hindrance by secreted antibody, and there is experimental evidence that secretory antibody specific for a given antigen will inhibit significantly its uptake by the gut. This steric hindrance by IgA antibodies is probably their most important function as many

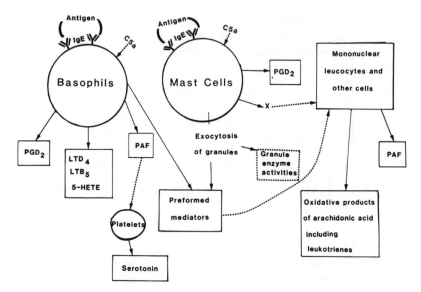

FIG. 2. Role of mediators in allergic-like reactions.

enteropathogenic micro-organisms can only succeed in infecting their potential victim by first attaching themselves to specific receptors on the surfaces of the enterocytes or other mucosal epithelia. There is also evidence that mucosal IgA plays a role in controlling the populations of indigenous flora and that antibodies of appropriate specificity may be able to prevent the acquisition of dangerous characteristics by bacteria through inhibiting the transfer of plasmids (Porter *et al.*, 1978). Mucosal immunity thus appears most effective against organisms which can survive and multiply in the gut or which can bind to epithelial cells, thus remaining long enough to come into contact with the secretory immune system.

Although the amounts of IgE produced in the *laminae* are very low, the ability of even small amounts to bind to and 'sensitize' mast cells has extremely important consequences (Fig. 2). Mast cells in the mucosa reside primarily in the *lamina propria*, although they are occasionally found within the epithelial layer. Small amounts of antigen which succeed in crossing the mucosa cause sensitized mast cells to degranulate immediately. Histamine released from the granules acts on local blood vessels to increase their permeability, and other preformed mediators such as proteases are believed to destabilize the intracellular junctions between enterocytes. Degranulation also generates secondary mediators including prostaglandins and leukotrienes. They possess pro-inflammatory activities and can modulate permeability, cause muscle constriction, and attract and activate both neutrophils and macrophages. These IgE 'triggering' effects may induce a general 'leakyness' in the gut, favouring the absorption of successively larger amounts of food and other components. In this way, hypersensitivity to a particular dietary constituent may lead to the ingress of unrelated antigens and the establishment of allergy to a progressively expanding repertoire of ingested antigenic material.

Perhaps the most significant thing about allergic reactions to food constituents is that they are comparatively rare. In spite of the quantity of protein ingested every day, to say nothing of polysaccharide and bacterial antigens, few individuals suffer overt allergic reactions. This is because dietary antigens are thought to stimulate a local, protective immunity in the gut (IgA-mediated immune exclusion) while, at the same time, they induce an immunologically specific, systemic unresponsiveness (oral tolerance) (Tomasi, 1980; Challacombe and Tomasi, 1980). Orally presented antigens are known to stimulate both specific effector and suppressor cells. The T and B lymphocytes in the GALT, however, are thought to be shielded from the effects of suppression by a resident population of contra suppressor cells which inhibit the suppressors. When T and B effector cells migrate out of the gut, however, they are no longer shielded from suppression and so are unable to initiate potentially damaging allergic reactions. The subject is complicated and more fundamental research is required to understand the regulation of the complex mechanisms involved in the development of oral tolerance. All that can be stated at present is that orally administered antigens may induce allergy, or they may induce tolerance, or they may have no detectable effect at all.

ALLERGIC REACTIONS

Although allergic reactions to food components may not occur often, one group of individuals, namely young children and infants, are particularly at risk of developing allergic reactions. Not only is the gut epithelium in infants immature in terms of limiting antigen absorption, but infants depend at first upon maternal immunoglobulins for much of their immunity. When weaning occurs the infant is deprived of antibodies in the gut until the independent intrinsic activity of GALT can fully take over.

This period of sub-optimal defence often coincides with drastic changes in the composition of the diet, and it is believed that it is during this time that dietary allergies are likely to arise. Clinical and laboratory observations emphasize that allergen avoidance in infancy is important also because of the risk that patterns of response may be established in genetically susceptible infants which will lead to persistent allergic disorders.

Genetic factors are known to predispose individuals to a number of diseases, and this may also hold true for certain food intolerance syndromes. There are, for example, suggestive links between the HLA haplotype A1/B8 and atopic eczema (Soothill *et al.*, 1976) and between HLA B8/DW3 and gluten sensitivity (Dansset and Svejgaard, 1977).

No genetic markers exist for predicting dietary intolerance, however, and genetic factors can only come into play following the appropriate environmental stimulus. Predisposition to food intolerance is no doubt a real phenomenon, as demonstrated, for example, in one study where a family history of allergy was found in 70% of babies with cow's milk intolerance (Jacobsson and Lindberg, 1979).

Atopic subjects also appear to have a greater potential for developing allergic reactions to food components. In a large clinical study of children with allergy to fish, characterized by asthma and urticaria, the majority of children were found to have multiple allergies and were also hypersensitive to inhaled allergens such as house dust, pollen and fungi (Aas, 1966). Several later studies have also demonstrated that at least 10% of children under the age of 6 with asthma, rhinitis and atopic dermatitis showed clinical symptoms after challenge with food.

In some older atopic individuals food provokes or leads to an aggravation of atopic symptoms in 1–3% of this population (Gonzalez de la Reguera *et al.*, 1971). Food allergy *per se* may occur in both atopic and non-atopic individuals, and may be due to a very wide range of ingested substances. Reactions are not necessarily induced by the same food in adults as in children, again demonstrating the complex nature of food reactions. The most common proven allergies in adults are to egg, nuts and fish, where over 70% of cases have been shown to have evidence of IgE-mediated reactions (Lessof *et al.*, 1980). Intolerance to milk and dairy products, on the other hand, although they provoke similar reactions, appears to be due to cytophilic antibodies in only about 30% of cases, although other immunological mechanisms may be involved. Other foods commonly involved include wheat, corn, coffee, tea and citrus fruit. Of these, coffee, tea and citrus fruit are not foods associated with a classical allergic reaction and, in general, although food allergy is by no means rare, food intolerance due to non-immunological causes is far more common and attracts far more attention from the point of view of diagnosis.

INTOLERANCE DUE TO NON-IMMUNOLOGICAL MECHANISMS

As mentioned earlier, symptoms resembling allergic reactions but not elicited by immunological phenomena are said to occur far more frequently than defined food allergies. A proportion of these may be due to contamination by toxic products of microbes or algae (see Chapter 1). For example, seafoods which contain toxic algal contaminants such as saxitoxin, found in mussels, cockles, clams and scallops (Popkiss *et al.*, 1979), can give rise to severe symptoms minutes after ingestion. Such acute chemical intoxications are well recognized, however, and not generally confused with allergic-type mechanisms, and do not fall within the scope of this chapter.

A variety of foods contain vasoactive amines and other pharmacological agents capable of inducing a wide range of symptoms that affect the gastrointestinal tract and the central nervous system. The ingestion of stimulants such as caffeine and theobromine (discussed in detail in Chapter 11) can be associated with stimulation of the central nervous system, headaches and abdominal pain. The majority of intolerant reactions, however, are caused by foods which cause an increase in the level of circulating histamine to which some individuals are particularly sensitive. The offending food could contain histamine, contain a histamine-releasing agent, or enhance the production of histamine by gut microorganisms (Table 2).

Histamine-rich foods include fish (in particular tuna and mackerel), yeast extracts such as Marmite and, in particular, fermented foods such as cheese and wine. Conversion of histidine to histamine by bacterial decarboxylases occurs naturally during the ripening of cheeses (Rice *et al.*, 1976), and in some cases histamine levels can be as high as 260 mg/100 g of cheese. Lower levels of histamine are also naturally present in many foods including avocados, bananas, plums, pineapples and oranges. Other foods such as egg white, shellfish, strawberries and chocolate contain histamine-releasing agents which cause the release of histamine from mast cells and circulating basophils without the involvement of IgE antibody. Alcohol too is a potent histamine releaser, and injudicious use of alcohol at meal time could thus destabilize the intracellular junctions between gut enterocytes, causing ingress of potentially allergenic food components.

TABLE 2
Some Foods Implicated in Non-immunological Mechanisms

Histamine-rich foods
Cheese
Beer
Tuna fish
Mackerel
Histamine-releasing foods
Strawberries
Chocolate
Salicylate-containing foods
Grapes
Bananas
Tea
Rhubarb
Peas
Pickles
Benzoate-containing foods
Cranberries
Blueberries
Red wine

Another vasoactive amine, tyramine, has been found in high concentrations in fermented cheeses such as Stilton, Blue and Roquefort, as well as in pickled fish. In contrast to the action of histamine, tyramine also elevates blood pressure as it releases noradrenaline from tissue stores, which in turn causes the blood pressure to rise (Rice *et al.*, 1976). It is for this reason that patients on drugs used in the treatment of depression which inhibit the monoamine oxidases that rapidly destroy tyramine in the body are routinely advised to avoid foods high in tyramine (Smith and Durack, 1978).

In the majority of susceptible individuals symptoms produced by the various mechanisms described above mimic the allergic phenomena mediated by histamine and other mediators released as a consequence of antigen–antibody reactions (Fig. 3). The terms 'pseudo-allergy' or 'false food-allergy' have therefore been proposed for this condition (Moneret-Vautrin, 1983). General symptoms include flushing, oedema and urticaria. Localized abdominal symptoms include abdominal pain, flatulence,

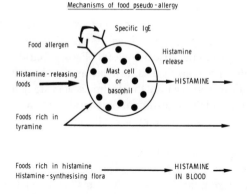

FIG. 3. Role of histamine in allergic and pseudo-allergic reactions.

constipation and diarrhoea. In contrast to true food allergy, the response is initiated by a relatively large quantity of one category of food and is generally associated with a functional impairment of the digestive mucosa.

Other investigators have demonstrated an association between increased levels of prostaglandins and abdominal symptoms after ingestion of specific food (Buisseret *et al.*, 1978), suggesting that in some cases of food intolerance local inflammatory mediators would be released from the gut and disseminated in the blood stream. Mussels, milk and peanuts have been identified as the causative agents in individual cases. If prostaglandins and other mediators transmit their effects to distant organs they might also be responsible for the headaches and other symptoms described in some groups of people. It is claimed that pseudo-allergy is much more common than true food allergy, but firm comparative clinical studies are not available to substantiate this point.

GASTROINTESTINAL DISEASES

Some gastrointestinal conditions which are associated with allergic symptoms or reactions relate to inborn errors of enzyme metabolism such as lactase deficiency. The intestinal enzyme lactase is necessary for the metabolism of lactose found in cow's milk. A lack of this enzyme results in fermentation of lactose to lactic acid and an osmotic effect in the bowel, with resultant symptoms of malabsorption and diarrhoea (Levin *et al.*, 1970). A further complication is that chronic bowel problems and acute infectious diarrhoea in otherwise healthy individuals can cause secondary lactase deficiency to develop as the gut mucosa is denuded (Gray, 1983). These individuals may also have difficulty with digestion of other carbohydrates found in foods because of general oligosaccharidase deficiency. In most individuals there is also a decline in lactase levels after childhood, and in some population groups where the decline is very steep the prevalence of lactase deficiency is high. Ingestion of only moderate amounts of milk may thus result in symptoms resembling allergic reactions in susceptible individuals.

A number of inflammatory bowel diseases, such as coeliac disease and Crohn's disease, although not classical food allergies, are thought to involve allergic or immunological mechanisms (Table 3). Coeliac disease is

TABLE 3
Gastrointestinal Diseases Associated with Food Intolerance

Inborn errors of metabolism
Lactase deficiency
Secretory IgA deficiency

Cow's milk protein intolerance (CMPI)

Inflammatory bowel diseases
Coelic disease
Crohn's disease

caused by hypersensitivity to gluten although the mechanism is unknown. Initially it was considered to be due to a peptidase deficiency which, by allowing toxic gliadin metabolites to accumulate, caused internal damage (Frazer *et al.*, 1959). No such enzyme deficiency has been discovered, however, and interest has therefore focused on the immune pathogenesis of the disease. Patients with coeliac disease have been shown to have increased numbers of intraepithelial lymphocytes (Ferguson and Murray, 1971), particularly T cells, as well as elevated serum levels of IgA (Asquith *et al.*, 1969). Patients with untreated coeliac disease have higher titres of antibodies to d-gliadin than healthy controls (O'Farrelly *et al.*, 1983), suggesting a local cellular hypersensitivity to gluten which induces mucosal tissue damage. It is also possible that a specific immune response gene, linked to HLA-B8 and/or DR3 (Simpson *et al.*, 1981) facilitates the specific immune response to gluten seen in coeliac disease.

Virtually all infants fed cow's milk develop milk antibodies but in the majority there are no clinical consequences (May *et al.*, 1982). As many as 1–3% of the children, however, do develop cow's milk protein intolerance (CMPI) (Bahna and Gandhi, 1983), usually within the first 6 months of life, and symptoms usually disappear by 1–2 years. The development of CMPI often follows gastrointestinal infection. In the acute syndrome, vomiting after cow's milk ingestion is the usual manifestation. Infants in which the sensitivity causes reversible small intestine abnormalities (enteropathy) have malabsorption, with diarrhoea, vomiting, weight loss and failure to thrive (Kuitunen *et al.*, 1975). Many infants also develop urticaria, eczema and other reactions which provide evidence for an immunological basis to these symptoms. It is believed that on a milk-free diet the systemic immune response abates and, with increasing maturity of the local immune system, the vulnerability to intestinal infection and mucosal permeability diminish. This would explain the transient nature of CMPI. It is of interest in this respect that infants with CMPI possess similar HLA antigens to the general population (Verkasalu *et al.*, 1983).

Some adults also show intolerance to milk and dairy products and, although some form of delayed immunological reaction cannot be excluded, the majority of patients do not have positive skin or radio-allergosorbent tests for IgE antibody (Lessof *et al.*, 1980). It has been suggested that foods (including milk) which contain linoleic acid may provide a substrate for prostaglandin synthesis and could therefore provoke adverse effects (through increased levels of prostanoids) in subjects who lack the enzyme which converts linoleic to γ-linolenic acid.

The pathogenesis of inflammatory bowel disease, i.e. Crohn's disease and ulcerative colitis, is also not known. A number of mechanisms have been suggested, including autoimmunity, toxic environmental factors, genetic susceptibility, infection and diet. A marked increase in immunological reactivity in the gastrointestinal tract is evident in inflammatory bowel disease, but whether this activity causes the disease or it is a secondary phenomenon perpetuating the inflammatory process has yet to be resolved (Mike and Asquith, 1987). Specific food intolerance has, however, been identified in a number of Crohn's patients (Hunter *et al.*, 1983) and in one clinical trial 20 of 33 patients with active Crohn's disease were identified as having specific food intolerance (Alun Jones *et al.*, 1984). The commonest foods implicated were dairy products, wheats and other cereals. In addition, one recent clinical study found a high sensitization to mould allergens which contaminate food (Tschaikowski, 1984). The findings of these recent studies need to be confirmed by others but they could be of great importance in elucidating other conditions where intolerance to ingested material is thought to be a causative factor in the development of the disease.

FOOD ADDITIVES

A steadily increasing number of reports associate ingestion of chemicals used to colour or preserve foods with symptoms characteristic of food intolerance (Table 4). Tartrazine (FD&C yellow No. 5; E102) is the colour most frequently implicated in food intolerance reports, although some allowance must be made for the selective usage of the colours as well as for the frequency of testing for responses to other synthetic colours in clinical trials (Miller, 1982).

Tartrazine

Tartrazine is added to many pharmaceutical products as well as to foods and soft drinks, and very many reports on adverse reactions appear confined to pharmaceutical preparations. The first report of intolerance to

TABLE 4
Additives Associated with Food Intolerance

Natural colours
Annatto

Synthetic colours
Tartrazine
Ponceau 4R
Amaranth
Sunset Yellow FCF

Flavours
Balsam of Peru

Preservatives
Benzoate derivatives
(Sulphur dioxide)

Antioxidants
Butylated hydroxytoluene
Butylated hydroxyanisole

tartrazine appeared in 1959 and described three patients, each of whom reacted to a corticosteroid product containing tartrazine (Lockey, 1959). One of the patients had a history of intolerance to acetylsalicylic acid and another to drugs of coal-tar origin, suggesting that some degree of cross-reactivity could have occurred.

The possibility of multiple reactivity to a number of chemicals was strengthened by reports that aspirin-sensitive patients who reacted to tartrazine also reacted adversely to 4-hydroxybenzoic acid (Juhlin *et al.*, 1972). In another investigation 52 patients with recurrent urticaria or angio-oedema, together with 33 control subjects (Michaelsson and Juhlin, 1973), were tested with various other azo dyes and food preservatives in addition to tartrazine; the dyes included Amaranth, Sunset Yellow and Ponceau 4R. Whilst no definite pattern for the reaction to the different azo colours was seen, 27 patients reacted to some azo dyes at dosages similar to those applied for tartrzine. Several other investigators have also reported that patients reacted to different azo dyes during provocation tests (Green, 1974; Thunel and Granholt, 1975). Furthermore, between 10% and 40% of aspirin-sensitive patients, depending on the test protocol followed (Settipane *et al.*, 1976; Stenius and Lemola, 1976), responded to tartrazine with reactions ranging from severe asthma to urticaria and mild rhinitis. In adults the great majority of cases of reported tartrazine intolerance have occurred in subjects who are also sensitive to aspirin (Genton *et al.*, 1985). A similar pattern appears likely to occur in children. In one investigation on asthmatic children, 1 in 3 of the 32 children studied reacted to aspirin and 1 in 5 to tartrazine and/or benzoates (Syvanen and Beckman, 1978).

A major breakthrough in the understanding of the mechanisms involved in ASA intolerance came with the discovery that aspirin inhibits prosta-glandin synthesizing enzymes (Vane, 1971) which are activated during destabilization of mast and basophil membranes. In addition to the release of histamine and other preformed mediators described earlier, degranula-tion also results in the generation of secondary mediators through arachidonic acid metabolism. This metabolism is highly complex but, after the release of arachidonic acid from membrane phospholipids via calcium-dependent phospholipases, biologically active compounds such as the prostaglandins are synthesized via the cyclo-oxygenase pathways and leukotrienes via 5-lipo-oxygenase pathways. These mediators possess varied regulatory and pro-inflammatory activities and can modulate vascular permeability, cause muscle constriction, and attract and activate neutrophils and other phagocytes.

Aspirin and other non-steroidal anti-inflammatory agents have been convincingly shown to inhibit the prostaglandin synthetase system in cells or tissues in man and in almost all laboratory species (Vane, 1971; Szczeklik et al., 1975). Furthermore, studies where plasma concentrations of prostaglandin have been measured during the onset of clinical reactions to aspirin have shown significantly reduced concentrations of prostaglandin F_2 though not of prostaglandin E_2 (Asad et al., 1983) suggesting an aspirin-induced alteration in the balance between the various prostanoid metabolites rather than a total inhibition of cyclo-oxygenase pathways. It is conceivable that selected cyclo-oxygenase inhibition may result in a diversion of substrates toward the production of lipo-oxygenase products such as for example SRS-A (slow reacting substance of anaphylaxis), a mixture of leukotrienes which are likely to be important mediators of smooth muscle contraction in asthma. The recent finding that blood prostaglandin levels may be abnormal in aspirin-intolerant individuals (Asad et al., 1984) also implies an inherent defect of prostaglandin metabolism which could be triggered by both pharmacological and allergic reactions. This may well be the underlying mechanism in aspirin sensitivity, as the effect of aspirin on arachidonic acid metabolism would theoretically be the same for every individual.

On the other hand, aspirin has been shown to cause an improvement in asthma (Szczeklik and Nizankowska, 1983), and this again supports the hypothesis that the balance between arachidonic acid metabolites may differ in normal and aspirin-intolerant individuals. The familial nature of some cases of both aspirin and tartrazine intolerance (Lockey et al., 1973; Turton et al., 1979) underlines the need for future research into possible inborn or acquired errors of metabolism which might be involved in adverse reactions to some chemicals.

It must be emphasized that, although a substantial proportion of aspirin-sensitive individuals do react to tartrazine, no effects of tartrazine on the inhibition of prostaglandin pathways have been observed (Gerber et al., 1979; Vargraftig et al., 1980). On reflection, this is not really an unexpected finding. Firstly, if tartrazine was to inhibit cyclo-oxygenase pathways in a manner analogous to aspirin, intolerance to both compounds ought to have occurred much more commonly than the highest reported level of 40% cross-reactivity. Secondly, many reports of tartrazine intolerance involve patients on corticosteroid therapy. Anti-inflammatory steroidal drugs inhibit phospholipase activity and thus prevent the liberation of archidonic acid from cell membranes, thereby blocking the production of both prostaglandins and leukotrienes. It therefore seems unlikely that tartrazine intolerance is due to quantitative or qualitative alterations of arachidonic acid metabolites, and other mediators would have to be responsible for induction of symptoms.

There has been one report suggesting that the response to both ASA and tartrazine seen in patients with chronic urticaria is due to some non-specific effect on the production of metabolites leading to the development of urticarial weals (Warrin and Smith, 1982). Human leucocytes from ASA-sensitive patients have also been shown to release histamine when treated with tartrazine *in vitro*, pointing to the need for studies on the influence of ASA and tartrazine on preformed mediator release or formation (Hedman and Anderson, 1983).

The possibility that aspirin and/or tartrazine may exacerbate a pre-existing intolerance caused by natural salicylates in the diet has also been raised (Feingold, 1973). Salicylates are present in a number of foods, notably peas, prunes, rhubarb, raspberries and grapes. Many of the natural salicylates are stable and appear unchanged in food products such as pickles, tomato products, teas and wine (Poulsen, 1980).

A range of synthetic salicylates are also used to flavour sweets, ice-cream, soft drinks and cake mixes. The chemical similarity of these materials with aspirin (Fig. 4) could provide some explanation for the multiple susceptibility to other substances seen in ASA-sensitive patients, although in no way explaining the different biological mechanisms involved in intolerance to tartrazine or other food colours.

There is no evidence at present that intolerance to food colours is mediated through specific IgE antibodies normally implicated in Type I allergic reactions in man.

One recent article, however, has reported that there may be an association between clinically identified intolerance to tartrazine and an antigen-specific IgD (Weliky and Heiner, 1980). Elevated IgD antibodies have been reported in certain allergic states (Josephs and Buckley, 1980) but little is known of the functional properties of circulating IgD. However, one animal model has shown that B lymphocytes carrying IgD receptors play a major role in the ontogeny of IgE-producing cells (Bazin *et al.*, 1978). These workers also demonstrated production of specific anti-ovalbumin IgD and IgE antibodies in rats using adjuvant regimes to induce IgE synthesis (Pauwels *et al.*, 1979). Using a similar rat model, one recent study has also demonstrated the production of a tartrazine-specific reaginic antibody (Nicklin and Miller, 1985).

In this study the parenterally administered tartrazine, covalently coupled to ovalbumin, was presented in association with carrageenan. The induction of reaginic antibody to tartrazine was dependent on the par-

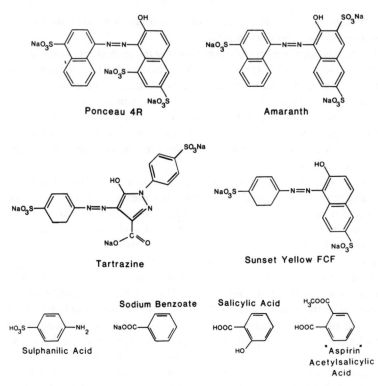

FIG. 4. Schematic structures of benzoate, acetylsalicylic acid, tartrazine and some other azo dyes.

ticular adjuvant properties of carrageenan. The response could be enhanced by a secondary challenge but declined rapidly and thereafter could not be re-elicited. As described earlier, suppressor T lymphocytes are thought to control the experimental induction of reaginic antibody, and animal models such as the one above might provide some insight as to whether tartrazine under certain conditions could bypass the normal regulatory mechanisms.

Animal experiments have also demonstrated that tartrazine conjugates can induce specific IgG antibodies after parenteral administration to rabbits (Johnson and Smith, 1972). It is of interest that these antibodies were shown to cross-react extensively with *p*-azobenzenesulphonate, particularly as the human IgD anti-tartrazine antibodies mentioned above (Weliky and Heiner, 1980) were demonstrated to react only with the sulphophenyl portion of the tartrazine molecule. Whether immunological mechanisms other than those commonly involved in food allergy play a role in intolerance to tartrazine and other food colours can only be elucidated by further investigations into basic mechanisms.

Other Food Additives

Reactions with other food additives must also be considered in the case of the aspirin- and/or tartrazine-sensitive individuals (Table 4). Such additives include preservatives such as benzoic acid and antioxidants as well as synthetic food flavourings. Sodium benzoate and benzoate esters, widely used in different foods and beverages, are the preservatives most frequently demonstrated to induce adverse reactions in patients suffering from chronic urticaria and aspirin-associated asthma (Juhlin, 1981). Similar chemical structures are shared by aspirin, the benzoate molecule and azo-dyes, and thus similarity of structure has been put forward as a reason for the multiple reactivity seen in patients (Fig. 4).

As with salicylates, benzoates occur naturally in some foods, and in berries such as cranberries and blueberries levels can reach 100 mg benzoic acid per 100 g (Poulsen, 1980). Cross-reactivity with benzoates has been reported most often in studies carried out in Scandinavia where eating of such berries may be more common than in other parts of the world. The possibility that susceptible individuals could develop benzoate intolerance through ingestion of foods with high natural amounts of the compound cannot be excluded. Benzoates also occur naturally in many other foods such as coffee beans, teas and red wine, although at about one-tenth of the levels found in blueberries.

Butylated hydroxytoluene (BHT) and butylated hydroxyanisole (BHA) are widely used antioxidants (see also Chapter 8) and have been reported to cause urticaria and asthma in some individuals. Interest in these agents stems from the observation that 14–15% of patients suffering from chronic urticaria also reacted against these additives (Juhlin, 1980), again suggesting that individuals sensitive to one substance also tend to react to a variety of other substances.

Hyperactivity

Interest in additive intolerance in children has focused on the association between food additives and hyperactivity or hyperkinesis as stated by Feingold (1975). Briefly, his principal hypothesis was that behaviour disorders in children are due to an inborn chemical reaction affecting the nervous system of certain genetically predisposed children, and that natural salicylates as well as synthetic food additives were the causative agents. Feingold accordingly developed an elimination diet (K-P diet) designed to be low in salicylates and free of food additives. Return to ordinary diet was said to result in immediate return to the hyperkinetic condition by those children who showed a marked improvement on the Feingold diet. Early studies appeared to support this hypothesis, but were severely criticized in that subjects, parents and investigators knew when the diet was administered. Several double-blind studies did not find any relationship between hyperactivity and salicylates, artificial food colours and flavours in the vast majority of hyperactive children (Stare *et al.*, 1980; Mattes and Gittelman, 1981), and in the USA the National Advisory Committee on Hyperkinesis and Food Additives (1980) stated: 'It is our opinion that studies already completed provide sufficient evidence to refute the claim that artificial food colourings, artificial flavourings and salicylates produced hyperactivity and/or learning disabilities'. It seems likely that the beneficial effects reported for the Feingold diet can be attributed to the change in the family's lifestyle caused by adherence to the diet, and the resultant changes in the hyperactive child's role in family life. Recent studies have also suggested that allergies to commonly ingested foods may cause hyperactivity in a small subgroup of children (Tryphonas and Trites, 1979), and other authors have reported a correlation between the amount of sugar ingested and levels of hyperativity in children (Prinz *et al.*, 1980). On present evidence it seems that hyperactvity, or hyperkinesis, cannot be considered a disease or a disorder, but a symptom with a variety of causes which needs to be treated by a multi-disciplinary co-operative effort involving home, school and family doctor.

Prevalence

The prevalence of intolerance to food additives is extremely difficult to assess in the general population. Defined food allergies such as cow's milk intolerance, the most common allergy in young children, have been estimated to have a prevalence between 0·2% and 7·5% (Bahna, 1978). In these studies it was possible to work with a defined population and, in the case of milk intolerance, a defined material. When it comes to assessing the frequency of intolerance to food additives, however, a number of colours and additives are often used in conjunction, and appear in a wide variety of foodstuffs. As reactivity between structurally related colours and additives apparently occurs, a given individual may not know what particular food or food component triggered the adverse reaction. Studies concerning reactivity to food additives have also generally been restricted to selected populations and, in the main, to patients attending hospital for the treatment of urticaria, asthma or 'allergy-like' diseases. These studies cannot provide true estimates of prevalence, since extrapolation from responses obtained in a given selected group to prediction of responses in the general population makes the assumption that there is no difference in susceptibility associated with the underlying disorder. It would be reasonable to assume that the susceptibility of the general population is likely to be considerably less than that of the special groups studied, and it has been estimated that in every 10 million people about 40000 will show intolerance to aspirin (0·4%), 6000 to tartrazine (0·06%) and 5000 to benzoates (0·05%) (Juhlin, 1981). A recent Danish study assessed the frequency of asthma, chronic rhinitis and chronic urticaria in the general population over 16 years of age and found them to be in the order of 3·8%, 1·9% and 0·5% respectively (Poulsen, 1980). The frequency of intolerance to food additives within each incidence group was then determined by reference to previous case histories and previous provocation tests, and 0·01–0·1% of the population were found to be sensitive to both tartrazine and benzoates. When one considers that almost everyone in the population has probably been exposed to tartrazine at some time or another, intolerance to tartrazine appears remarkably low. There is little doubt, however, that intolerance to food additives occurs in a small minority of the population. These individuals generally appear to belong to a select group that is atopic and exhibits multiple allergic or idiosyncratic responses to a variety of ingested and inhalant material.

Information about the composition of branded foods, in such a way that they can be easily identified as free from particular ingredients, would no doubt substantially assist consumers to avoid foods to which they are sensitive.

Whether food colours or other food additives are able to initiate a state of intolerance, or whether they act only on previously sensitized individuals, can only be resolved by future research into this area.

CONCLUSION

Vast quantities of antigenic material, mainly proteins and polysaccharides, are ingested daily, and therefore the main function of the gastrointestinal associated lymphoid system must be to protect the lymphoreticular system from excessive antigenic insult whilst at the same time 'sampling' the antigens so as to induce an immunologically specific unresponsiveness (oral tolerance).

Antigen exclusion functions poorly in infants and young children, in patients with IgA deficiency and in some inflammatory bowel diseases. In addition, in individuals who are already sensitized, antigens may pass between the enterocytes. Proteases, histamines and other inflammatory mediators released by degranulating mast cells destabilize the intercellular junctions between enterocytes and this general 'leakiness' induced in the gut favours the absorption of successively larger amounts of dietary constituents. In this way, hypersensitivity to a particular constituent may lead to the ingress of unrelated antigens and the establishment of allergy to a progressively expanding repertoire of antigenic epitopes from the environment. Similarly, non-specific damage to the gut by agents like alcohol or aspirin can also destabilize the intercellular junctions and permit ingress of antigenic material. The most significant point to be made about allergic reactions to food constituents is that they are comparatively rare.

Symptoms resembling allergic reactions but not elicited by immunological phenomena occur far more frequently than defined food allergies. They are due to a variety of causes. These include sensitivity to foods containing relatively high levels of histamine, such as tuna, cheese, beer and wine, or to foods such as shellfish or strawberries that cause the release of histamine from mast cells and circulating basophils without the involvement of immunological mechanisms. A number of inflammatory bowel diseases are associated with allergy-like symptoms which relate to inborn errors of enzyme metabolism as well a specific intolerance to foods such as milk, wheat and other cereals.

An increasing number of reports also associate ingestion of chemicals used to colour or preserve foods with symptoms characteristic of food intolerance. Tartrazine is the colour most frequently implicated, and there is little doubt that intolerance to food additives occurs in a small minority of the population. These individuals generally appear to belong to a select group that is also intolerant to aspirin and exhibit multiple allergic or idiosyncratic responses to a variety of ingested and inhalant material. Whether synthetic food additives are able to initiate a state of intolerance, or whether they act only on previously affected individuals, can only be resolved by future research into basic mechanisms.

REFERENCES

Aas, K. (1966). Studies of hypersensitivity to fish: a clinical study. *Int. Arch. Allergy*, **29**, 346–63.

Alun Jones, V., Dickinson, R. J., Workman, E. M., Freeman, A. H. and Hunter,

J. O. (1984). Controlled trial of diet in the management of Crohn's disease. *XII Int. Congr. Gastroenterology*, p. 943.

Asad, S. I., Youlten, L. J. F. and Lessof, M. H. (1983). Specific desensitization in 'aspirin-sensitive' urticaria: plasma prostaglandin levels and clinical manifestations. *Clin. Allergy*, 13, 459–66.

Asad, S. I., Kemeny, D. M., Youlten, L. J. F., Frankland, A. W. and Lessof, M. H. (1984). Effect of 'aspirin sensitive' patients. *Brit. Med. J.*, 288, 745–8.

Asquith, Q., Thompson, R. A. and Gooke, W. T. (1969). Serum immunoglobulins in adult coeliac disease. *Lancet*, 2, 129–31.

Bahna, S. L. (1978). Control of milk allergy: a challenge for physicians, mothers and industry. *Ann. Allergy*, 41, 1–12.

Bahna, S. L. and Gandhi, H. (1983). Milk hypersensitivity. I. Pathogenesis and symptomatology. *Ann. Allergy*, 50, 218–23.

Bazin, H., Platteau, B., Beckers, A. and Pauwels, R. (1978). Differential effect of neonatal infections of anti-mu or anti-delta antibodies on the synthesis of IgM, IgD, IgE, IgA, IgG1, IgG2a, IgG2B and IgG2c immunoglobulin classes. *J. Immunol.*, 121, 2083–7.

Brandtzaeg, P., Baklien, K., Bjerke, K., Rognum, T. O., Scott, H. and Valnes, K. (1987). Nature and properties of the human gastrointestinal immune system. In: *Immunology and the Gastrointestinal Tract*, K. Miller and S. Nicklin (Eds), CRC Press, Boca Raton (in press).

Buisseret, P. D., Youlten, L. J. F., Heinzelmann, D. I. and Lessof, M. H. (1978). Prostaglandin-synthesis inhibitors in prophylaxis of food tolerance. *Lancet*, 1, 906–8.

Challacombe, S. J. and Tomasi, T. I. (1980). Systemic tolerance and secretory immunity after oral immunization. *J. Exp. Med.*, 152, 1459–72.

Dansset, J. and Svejgaard, A. (Eds) (1977). *HLA and Disease*, Munksgaard, Copenhagen.

Durkin, H. G. and Waksman, B. H. (1979). High concentrations of IgE and IgA bearing cells in Peyer's patches of germ free rats. *Fed. Proc.*, 38, 1081.

Feingold, B. F. (1973). Food additives and child development. *Hosp. Prac.*, 8, 11–19.

Feingold, B. F. (Ed.) (1975). *Why Your Child is Hyperactive*, Random House, New York.

Ferguson, A. and Murray, D. (1971). Quantitation of intraepithelial lymphocytes in human jejunum. *Gut*, 12, 988–94.

Frazer, A. C., Fletcher, R. F., Ross, C. A., Shaw, B., Sammons, H. G. and Schneider, R. (1959). Gluten induced enteropathy. The effect of partially digested gluten. *Lancet*, 2, 252–5.

Genton, C., Frei, P. C. and Pécoud, A. (1985). Value of oral provocation tests to aspirin and food additives in the routine investigation of asthma and chronic urticaria. *J. Allergy Clin. Immunol.*, 76, 40–45.

Gerber, J. C., Payne, N. A., Velz, O., Nies, A. S. and Oates, F. A. (1979). Tartrazine and the prostaglandin system. *J. Allergy Clin. Immunol.*, 63, 289–94.

Gonzalez de la Reguera, I., Inigo, J. F. and Gehling, A. (1971). The importance of food sensitisation in atopic dermatitis. *Dermatologica*, 143, 288–91.

Gowans, J. C. and Knight, E. J. (1964). The route of re-circulation of lymphocytes in the rat. *Proc. Roy. Soc.*, B159, 257–82.

Gray, G. M. (1983). Intestinal disaccharidase deficiencies and glucose-galactose malabsorption. In: *Metabolic Basis of Inherited Disease*, J. B. Stanbury, J. B. Wyngaarden, D. S. Fredrickson, J. L. Goldstein and M. S. Brown (Eds), McGraw-Hill, New York, pp. 1729–42.

Green, M. (1974). Sublingial provocative testing for foods and FD and C dyes. *Ann. Allergy*, 33, 272–81.

Hall, J. G. and Smith, H. E. (1970). Homing of lymph-borne immunoblasts to the gut. *Nature*, 226, 226–8.

Hall, J. G., Hopkins, J. and Orlans, E. (1977). Studies on the lymphocytes of sheep. III. Destination of lymph-borne immunoblasts in relation to their tissue of origin. *Eur. J. Immunol.*, 7, 30–7.

Hedman, S. E. and Anderson, R. G. G. (1983). Release of biological mediators from human leukocytes. *Acta Pharmacol. Toxicol.*, 52, 153–4.

Hunter, J. O., Alun Jones, V., Freeman, A. H., Shorthouse, H., Workman, E. and McLaughlin, P. (1983). Food intolerance in gastrointestinal disorders. In: *Second Fison Food Allergy Workshop*, R. R. A. A. Combs (Ed.), Medicine Publishing Foundation, Oxford, pp. 69–73.

Jacobsson, I. and Lindberg, T. (1979). A prospective study of cow's protein intolerance in Swedish infants. *Acta Paediatr. Scand.*, 68, 853–9.

Johnson, H. M. and Smith, B. D. (1972). Haptenic relationships of p-azobenzene-sulphonate and some structurally related food dyes. *Immunochem.*, 9, 253–61.

Josephs, S. H. and Buckley, R. H. (1980). Serum IgD concentrations in normal infants, children and adults and in patients with elevated IgE. *J. Paediatr.*, 96, 417–20.

Juhlin, L. (1980). Incidence of intolerance to food additives. *Int. J. Dermatol.*, 19, 548–51.

Juhlin, L. (1981). Recurrent urticaria: clinical investigation of 330 patients. *Brit. J. Dermatol.*, 104, 369–81.

Juhlin, L., Michaëlsson, G. and Zetterstöm, O. (1972). Urticaria and asthma induced by food and drug additives in patients with aspirin hypersensitivity. *J. Allergy Clin. Immunol.*, 50, 92–8.

Kuitunen, P., Vasakorpi, J. K., Savilahti, E. and Pelkonen, P. (1975). Malabsorption syndrome with cow's milk intolerance. *Arch. Dis. Childhood*, 50, 351–6.

Lee, J. S. (1971). Contraction of villi and fluid transport in dog jejunal mucosa. *Amer. J. Physiol.*, 221, 488–94.

Lessof, M. H., Wraith, D. G., Merrett, T. G., Merrett, J. and Buisseret, P. D. (1980). Food allergy and intolerance in 100 patients: local and systemic effects. *Quart. J. Med.*, 49, 259–71.

Levin, B., Abraham, J. M., Burgess, E. A. and Wallis, P. G. (1970). Congenital lactose malabsorption. *Arch. Dis. Childhood*, 54, 173–7.

Lockey, S. D. (1959). Allergic reactions due to FD and C Yellow No. 5 tartrazine, an aniline dye used as a coloring and identifying agent in various steroids. *Ann. Allergy*, 17, 719–21.

Lockey, S. D., Rucknagel, D. L. and Vanselow, N. A. (1973). Familial occurrence of asthma, nasal polyps and aspirin intolerance. *Ann. Intern. Med.*, 78, 57–63.

Mattes, J. A. and Gittelman, R. (1981). Effects of artificial food colorings in children with hyperactive symptoms. A critical review and results of a controlled study. *Arch. Gen. Psychiat.*, 38, 714–8.

Mattioli, C. A. and Tomasi, T. V. B. (1973). The life span of IgA plasma cells from the mouse intestine. *J. Exp. Med.*, **138**, 452–60.

May, C. D., Fomon, R. and Remigio, D. (1982). Immunologic consequences of feeding children with cow milk and soya products. *Acta Paediatr. Scand.*, **71**, 43–51.

Mayrhofer, G., Pugh, C. W. and Barclay, A. M. (1983). The distribution, ontogeny and origin in the rat of Ia-positive cells with dendritic morphology and of Ia antigen in epithelia, with special reference to the intestine. *Eur. J. Immunol.*, **13**, 112–22.

Michaëlsson, G. and Juhlin, L. (1973). Urticaria induced by preservatives and dye additives in food and drugs. *Brit. J. Dermatol.*, **88**, 525–32.

Mike, N. and Asquith, P. (1987). Immune responses in chronic gastrointestinal diseases. In: *Immunology of the Gastrointestinal Tract*, K. Miller and S. Nicklin (Eds), CRC Press, Boca Raton (in press).

Miller, K. (1982). Sensitivity to tartrazine. *Brit. Med. J.*, **285**, 1597–8.

Moneret-Vautrin, D. A. (1983). False food allergies: non-specific reactions to foodstuffs. In: *Clinical Reactions to Food*, M. H. Lessof (Ed.), John Wiley and Sons, London, pp. 135–53.

National Advisory Committee on Hyperkinesis and Food Additives (1980). *Final Report to the Nutrition Foundation*, Nutrition Foundation, New York.

Nicklin, S. and Miller, K. (1985). Induction of a transient reagenic antibody to tartrazine in an animal model. *Int. Arch. Allergy Appl. Immunol.*, **76**, 185–8.

O'Farrelly, C., Kelly, J., Hekkens, W., Bradley, B., Thompson, A., Feighery, C. and Weir, D. G. (1983). Alpha gliadin antibody levels: a serological test for coeliac disease. *Brit. Med. J.*, **268**, 2007–10.

Owen, R. L. (1977). Sequential uptake of horse-radish peroxidase by lymphoid follicle epithelium of Peyer's patches in the normal unobstructed mouse intestine: an ultrastructural study. *Gastroenterol.*, **72**, 440–57.

Owen, R. L. and Jones, A. L. (1974). Epithelial cell specialization within human Peyer's patches: an ultrastructural study of intestinal lymphoid follicles. *Gastroentrol.*, **66**, 189–203.

Pauwels, R., Bazin, H., Platteau, B. and van der Streeter, M. (1979). The influence of different adjuvants on the production of IgD and IgE antibodies. *Ann. Immunol.*, **130C**, 49–58.

Popkiss, M. E. E., Horstman, D. A. and Harper, D. (1979). Paralytic shellfish poisoning: a report of 17 cases in Cape Town. *S. Afr. Med. J.*, **55**, 1017–23.

Porter, P., Linggood, M. A. and Chidlow, J. (1978). Elimination of *Escherichia coli* K88 adhesion determinant by antibody in porcine gut and mammary secretions following oral immunization. *Adv. Exp. Med. Biol.*, **107**, 133–42.

Poulsen, E. (1980). Danish report on allergy and intolerance to food ingredients and food additives. Toxicol. Forum, Aspen, Colorado; Danish Ministry of Environment, National Food Agency, Publ. No. 43, pp. 1–52.

Prinz, R. J., Roberts, W. A. and Hartman, E. (1980). Dietary correlates of hyperactive behaviour in children. *J. Consult. Clin. Psychol.*, **48**, 760–9.

Rice, S. L., Eitenmiller, R. R. and Koehler, P. P. (1976). Biologically active amines in food: a review. *J. Milk Food Technol.*, **39**, 353–8.

Royal College of Physicians and British Nutrition Federation, Report of Joint Committee (1984). Food intolerance and food aversion. *J. Roy. Coll. Phys.*, **18**, 83–123.

Settipane, G. A., Chafee, F. H., Postman, I. M., Levine, M. I., Saken, J. H., Barrick, R. M., Nicholas, S. S., Schwartz, H. J., Honsiger, R. W. and Klein, K. E. (1976). Significance of tartrazine sensitivity in chronic urticaria of unknown aetiology. *J. Allergy Clin. Immunol.*, **57**, 541–6.

Simpson, F. G., Bullen, A. W., Robertson, D. A. F. and Lo Sowskey, M. F. (1981). HLA-B8 and cell mediated immunity to gluten. *Gut*, **22**, 633–6.

Smith, C. K. and Durack, D. T. (1978). Isoniazid and reaction to cheese. *Ann. Interm. Med.*, **88**, 520–1.

Soothill, J. F., Stokes, C. R., Turner, M. W., Norman, A. P. and Taylor, B. (1976). Predisposing factors and the development of reagenic allergy in infancy. *Clin. Allergy*, **6**, 305–19.

Stare, F. J., Whelan, E. M. and Sheriden, M. (1980). Diet and hyperactivity: is there a relationship? *Pediatrics*, **66**, 521–5.

Stenius, R. S. M. and Lemola, M. (1976). Hypersensitivity to acetylsalicylic acid (ASA) and tartrazine in patients with asthma. *Clin. Allergy*, **6**, 119–29.

Syvanen, P. and Beckman, A. (1978). In: *Nordic Congress of Allergology*, Munksgaard, Copenhagen, p. 58.

Szczeklik, A. and Nizankowska, E. (1983). Asthma improved by aspirin-like drugs. *Brit. J. Dis. Chest*, **77**, 153–8.

Szczeklik, A., Gryglewski, R. J. and Czerniawska-Mysik, G. (1975). Relationship of inhibition of prostaglandin biosynthesis by analgesics to asthma attacks in aspirin-sensitive patients. *Brit. Med. J.*, **1**, 67–70.

Thunel, P. and Granholt, A. (1975). Provocation tests with antiphlogistica and food additives in recurrent urticaria. *Dermatologica*, **151**, 360–7.

Tomasi, T. B. (1980). Oral tolerance (an overview). *Transplantation*, **29**, 353–6.

Tryphonas, H. and Trites, R. L. (1979). Hyperactivity and food additives: facts or myths. In : *Food Toxicology: Real or Imaginary Problems*, G. G. Gibson and R. Walker (Eds), Taylor and Francis, London, pp. 246–55.

Tschaikowski, K. L. (1984). Seven years experience in allergological diagnosis and treatment of Crohn's disease. In: *XII Int. Congr. Gastroenterology*, p. 497.

Turton, C. W. G., Morris, L., Buckingham, J. A., Lawler, S. D. and Turner-Warwick, M. (1979). Histocompatibility antigens in asthma: population and family studies. *Thorax*, **34**, 670–3.

Vane, J. R. (1971). Inhibition of prostaglandin synthesis as a mechanism of action for aspirin-like drugs. *Nature (New Biol.)*, **231**, 232–5.

Vargraftig, B. B., Bessot, J. C. and Pauli, G. (1980). Is tartrazine-induced asthma related to inhibition of prostaglandin synthesis? *Respiration*, **39**, 276–82.

Verkasalu, M., Kuitunen, P., Tiilikainen, A. and Savilahti, E. (1983). HLA antigens in intestinal cow's milk allergy. *Acta Paediatr. Scand.*, **72**, 19–22.

Wakelin, D. and Giences, R. K. (1987). Immunological responses to intestinal parasite infections. In: *Immunology of the Gastrointestinal Tract*, K. Miller and S. Nicklin (Eds), CRC Press, Boca Raton (in press).

Warrin, R. P. and Smith, R. J. (1982). Role of tartrazine in chronic urticaria. *Brit. Med. J.*, **284**, 1443–4.

Weliky, N. and Heiner, D. C. (1980). Hypersensitivity to chemicals. Correlation of tartrazine hypersensitivity with characteristic serum IgD and IgE immune response patterns. *Clin. Allergy*, **10**, 375–95.

Chapter 11

METHYLXANTHINES

STANLEY M. TARKA, JR and CAROL A. SHIVELY

Hershey Foods Corporation, Hershey, Pennsylvania, USA

INTRODUCTION

Over the past decade the methylxanthines as a class of naturally occuring compounds have received a considerable amount of international, scientific, and regulatory attention because of uncertainties dealing with specific pharmacological and toxicological effects on living organisms. In 1980 FDA proposed that caffeine no longer be considered a GRAS

373

(generally recognized as safe) substance, but that it be placed in an interim food additive status pending the completion of additional studies. The areas which raised the most concern were the potential reproductive, teratogenic, mutagenic, carcinogenic, and behavioral effects of the methylxanthines. In addition, better estimates of intake patterns and amounts, as well as pharmacokinetic and metabolic data, were needed to assess the safety of these compounds in the food supply. The tremendous upsurge in recent scientific investigations with the methylxanthines has provided much vital information in these questionable areas.

In this chapter, we will not attempt to provide an exhaustive review of the literature since there are numerous other sources for this information. Instead, our eforts will focus on identifying the various sources of dietary methylxanthines, their disposition in mammalian species including man, and a current review of what is known about the toxicological aspects of this unique group of related purine alkaloids.

OCCURRENCE

The most common methylxanthines found in our food supply are caffeine (1,3,7-trimethylxanthine) and theobromine (3,7-dimethylxanthine). Theophylline (1,3-dimethylxanthine) is only a minor dietary constituent, although it is ingested commonly as a therapeutic agent. These compounds are all methylated derivatives of xanthine, a dioxypurine, and differ only in the number and placement of their methyl groups.

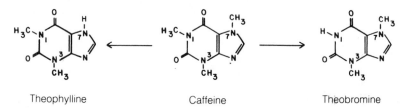

Theophylline   Caffeine   Theobromine

By far, caffeine is the most prevalent methylxanthine in our diet. It is thought to exist in as many as 60 plant species throughout the world. Historically, caffeine from natural sources has been consumed and enjoyed from very early times, with tea being the oldest recorded caffeine-containing beverage.

Dietary caffeine is consumed almost entirely in beverages, with coffee accounting for about 75% of the per capita US caffeine usage and tea 15%

(Graham, 1978). It was also estimated that caffeine was ingested on a daily basis by 82% of the population over 18 years of age. Although coffee and tea are the major sources of dietary caffeine, cocoa and cola beverages also contribute to the total amount of methylxanthines in our diet. A recent review on the history and use of caffeine (Roberts and Barone, 1983) is recommended as a detailed reference for information on caffeine content of food/beverage products and intake patterns.

Coffee

The consumption of coffee as a hot beverage was not known until the 11th century. Prior to that time caffeine-containing berries from native plants were crushed and eaten as a food, or fermented into a type of juice or wine. After the introduction of coffee into Europe its use grew rapidly, and today it is estimated that one-third to one-half of the US population drinks coffee.

Caffeine levels in freshly ground roasted coffee beans have been reported to vary from 0·8 to 1·8% (Kaplan et al., 1974). Caffeine concentrations in brewed coffee also vary with factors such as method of brewing, type and form of the coffee, brewing time, and amount of coffee used. Preparation of coffee by the dripolator method yields the highest caffeine levels (124–137 mg/cup), whereas the percolator method gives somewhat lower values (108–117 mg/cup) (Blauch and Tarka, 1983).

Data assembled by Burg (1975) on over 2000 caffeine analyses of coffee reported average values of 83, 59 and 3 mg caffeine per 5 oz cup of percolated, instant and decaffeinated coffee, respectively. Gilbert et al. (1976) reported similar values of 74, 66 and 1 mg caffeine per 5 oz cup, respectively.

Tea

Caffeine consumption estimates by Morgan et al. (1982) indicated that tea is the major caffeine source for children (34% of total ingested caffeine). According to Blauch and Tarka (1983) the caffeine content of American Black tea ranged from 41 to 65 mg/cup and the theobromine level ranged from 1·8 to 3·6 mg/cup. The caffeine content of brewed tea was cited at 30–48 mg/cup by Burg (1975) and 8–91 mg/cup by Gilbert et al. (1976).

Cocoa and Chocolate

The total methylxanthine content of eight commercial brands of cocoa powder was reported to range from 1·66 to 2·91% (Zoumas et al., 1980). Of this total, theobromine accounted for 1·46–2·66% (mean 1·89%) and caffeine content ranged from 0·08 to 0·35% (mean 0·21%). Theobromine and caffeine levels in hot cocoa prepared from five brands of mix were 54–77 and 2–7 mg/cup, respectively, while hot cocoa from a home mix contained 94 mg theobromine and 10 mg caffeine (Zoumas *et al.*, 1980).

Later estimates by Blauch and Tarka (1983) in nine instant hot cocoa mixes indicated similar values. Burg (1975) reported theobromine levels of 232–272 mg/cup of cocoa. However, since HPLC methodology was not employed to separate theobromine and caffeine accurately, these values are most likely too high.

Other dietary sources of theobromine and caffeine include commercial milk chocolate and sweet dark chocolate. Theobromine and caffeine levels in sweet dark chocolate (0·463 and 0·069%) are significantly higher than those present in milk chocolate (0·153 and 0·022%). For additional information on the methylxanthine composition of cocoa and chocolate products, as well as on consumption patterns, the reader is referred to a recent book chapter on this subject by Shively and Tarka (1984).

Cola-type Beverages

Caffeine was included in the original GRAS (generally recognized as safe) list by FDA under the conditions of its intended use in cola-type beverages. In these drinks the maximum allowable caffeine level is 0·02%. In general, only cola-type soft drinks contain caffeine, although some non-cola types also do. Caffeine levels in regular cola beverages range from about 15 to 23 mg per 6 oz serving. Morgan *et al.* (1982) estimate that caffeine-containing soft drinks comprise 26% of the total caffeine intake in children 5 to 18 years old.

METHYLXANTHINE DISPOSITION

Metabolism

Because of the frequent exposure of humans to methylxanthines through dietary sources, the metabolism of these compounds is of significant interest. In addition, a familiarity with the basic metabolic processes of the methylxanthines is necessary for meaningful extrapolation and interpretation of toxicological effects. The following summary is intended to provide an overview of the current knowledge on methylxanthine metabolism in man, as well as in various animal species employed in safety assessment studies.

A useful index of the rate of metabolism for any given compound is its plasma half-life, the time required for plasma concentrations to be reduced by 50% as a result of biotransformation and excretion. The plasma half-life of caffeine and theobromine varies considerably among animal species and man as shown in Table 1. In addition, the major metabolite excreted by each species is quite diverse indicating that all species may not be truly representative of human patterns. These factors must be carefully considered when selecting an appropriate animal model for toxicological research and evaluating this data in risk assessment to the human population.

Caffeine

Animal studies. Khanna *et al.* (1972) published the first caffeine metabolism study in rats using radiolabelled (^{3}H) compound. Following intraperitoneal administration, 64–67% of the radioactivity was excreted in the urine during the first 24 h. Using preparative thin-layer chromatography, the following metabolites were detected in the chloroform–methanol extract: theophylline (1·2%), theobromine (5·1%), paraxanthine (8·8%), and trace amounts of 1,3,7-trimethyluric acid and 3-methyluric acid. Two unknown metabolites and unchanged caffeine were also observed. Later studies by this group (Rao *et al.*, 1973) tentatively identified these unknown caffeine metabolites as 1,3,7-trimethyldihydrouric acid and 3,6,8-trimethylallantoin. The 1,3,7-trimethyldihydrouric acid was difficult to isolate in pure form and readily dehydrated to caffeine with heat. In solution this metabolite was in equilibrium with its open-chain N-formyl analog, subsequently named 6-amino-5-(N-methylformylamino)-1-methyluracil by other investigators. Rao *et al.* (1973) proposed that 1,3,7-trimethyldihydrouric acid was an intermediate in the formation of 1,3,7-dimethyluric acid and 3,6,8-trimethylallantoin.

Arnaud (1976) investigated the metabolism of caffeine in rats using [2-^{14}C]- and [1-Me-^{14}C]-caffeine. Fecal elimination accounted for 2–7% of the dose, while labelled CO_2 produced by 1-demethylation processes accounted for 15% of the dose. Urine metabolites identified and quantitated for the first time were 1-methylxanthine, 3-methylxanthine, 7-methylxanthine, 1,3-dimethyluric acid, 1,7-dimethyluric acid, 3,7-dimethyluric acid, methylurea and dimethylurea. A larger amount of water-soluble derivatives (3,7-dimethyluric acid, trimethylallantoin, 6-amino-5-(N-methylformylamino)-1,3-dimethyluracil) were reported than in previous studies (Khanna *et al.*, 1972; Rao *et al.*, 1973), since quantitation was done using whole urine instead of extracted samples. In

TABLE 1

Interspecies Comparison of Caffeine and Theobromine Metabolism and Kinetics

| Species | Plasma half-life (h) | | Major metabolite | |
	Theobromine	Caffeine	Theobromine	Caffeine
Mouse	$-^a$	1·5	6-Amino-5-(N-methyl-formylamino)-1-methyluracil	1,7-Dimethylxanthine
Rat	4	2	6-Amino-5-(N-methyl-formylamino)-1-methyluracil	6-Amino-5-(N-methylamino)-1,3-dimethyluracil
Rabbit	2	1	7-Methylxanthine	1,7-Dimethylxanthine
Monkey	$-^a$	6^b	$-^a$	1,3-Dimethylxanthine^b
Dog	17	4	3-Methylxanthine	3-Methylxanthine
Man	10	5	7-Methylxanthine	1-Methyluric acid

^{a}Not investigated.
^{b} *Macaca fascicularis.*

contrast to the report of Rao *et al.* (1973), the uracil metabolite was shown to be stable and easy to isolate.

Burg and Stein (1972) quantitated caffeine metabolism in the urine, feces and expired air of male CD-1 mice after oral administration of 5 or 25 mg/kg. The major metabolites identified were 1,7-dimethylxanthine, 3-methylxanthine, 7-methylxanthine, 1,3-dimethyluric acid and 1-methyluric acid, with 3–6% of the dose excreted as unchanged caffeine. No consistent differences in urinary radioactivity were reported between mice exposed to caffeine since weaning and those not exposed to caffeine, although fecal excretion of caffeine was greater in the exposed mice.

Although the presence of the diaminouracil derivatives of caffeine was not reported by Burg and Stein (1972), recent *in vitro* (Ferrero and Neims, 1983) and *in vivo* studies (Arnaud, 1985) have confirmed their formation in the mouse. Arnaud (1985) found the major metabolite of caffeine in the mouse to be an unknown polar metabolite X_3 (22% of urine radioactivity) while 1,7-dimethylxanthine or paraxanthine was the primary identifiable compound (17%).

Welch *et al.* (1977) and Aldridge *et al.* (1977) published two similar studies on the effect of phenobarbital, 3-methylcholanthrene, benzo[a]-pyrene and polychlorinated biphenyls on the plasma clearance of caffeine given either orally or intravenously to rats. Their results indicated a marked increase in caffeine elimination by inducers known to increase a form of cytochrome P-450 known as P-448.

Caffeine metabolic studies in beagle dogs (Aldridge and Neims, 1979; Tse and Valia, 1981) and mongrel dogs (Warszawski *et al.*, 1977) have reported caffeine half-lives of 4–7 h, respectively, in adult dogs and 47·5 h in 1-day old mongrel puppies. The major metabolite in beagle dogs was 3-methylxanthine (21% of the administered dose); no attempt was made at quantitation of the diaminouracil derivatives. Phenobarbital and β-naphthoflavone were found to be equipotent as inducing agents of caffeine elimination in beagle dogs with half-lives decreasing from 4 to 1·5 h.

Data for the metabolism of caffeine in the rabbit are limited. Garattini *et al.* (1982) showed that caffeine is eliminated from the plasma of adult rabbits by first-order kinetics up to doses of at least 10 mg/kg. Paraxanthine was the major urinary metabolite. While the rabbit, like man, initiates biotransformation by an N^3-demethylation process, the rabbit metabolizes the resultant paraxanthine slowly. Thus, the major metabolites in the human such as 7-methylxanthine, 1-methyluric acid, and 1,7-dimethyluric acid are less prominent in the rabbit. The potential production of the diaminouracil derivatives is virtually unexplored.

Burg *et al.* (1974) studied caffeine metabolism in the squirrel and rhesus monkey. The chronic toxicity of caffeine in the squirrel monkey appears to be related to its long half-life of 11 h, compared to a half-life of 2·4 h in the rhesus monkey. Although the exact reason for the inability of the squirrel monkey effectively to metabolize caffeine has not been identified, the rhesus monkey provides a better animal model for extrapolation of toxicological findings to man.

Caldwell *et al.* (1981) administered [8-¹⁴C]caffeine to adult chimpanzees, rhesus monkeys and galagos and collected urine and feces for 24 h. Although only 38–56% of the dose was recovered in the urine and <1% in the feces, this study indicated that caffeine is extensively metabolized with <1% excreted unchanged. Considerable species differences in metabolic profile were reported.

Christensen *et al.* (1981) examined caffeine metabolism in the baboon using [1-Me-¹⁴C]caffeine and found that the major metabolite was theophylline (25% of the administered dose). Excretion of 6-amino-5-(N-methylformylamino)-1,3-dimethyluracil, the major metabolite in the rat, amounted to only 2·8% of the dose. The excretion of this metabolite was studied quantitatively in the rat, monkey (*Macaca cynomologus*) and man by Latini *et al.* (1981). They confirmed that the rat excretes a much larger fraction of this uracilic derivative than does the monkey or man.

Caffeine metabolism in monkeys (*Macaca fascicularis*) chronically consuming caffeine at doses comparable to humans was recently reported by Gilbert *et al.* (1985). No overt toxicity was noted after exposure to caffeine in the drinking water at levels of 0·30 mg/ml. The high plasma levels of theophylline which were present indicate that caffeine metabolism in the monkey differs from that in humans. Theophylline was the major metabolite in the urine. After withdrawal of caffeine, plasma caffeine levels declined with a half-life of 5·5 h and theophylline with a half-life of 12·7 h.

Human studies. Early studies by Cornish and Christman (1957) reported that the principal urinary metabolite of caffeine in man was 1-methyluric acid resulting from the N^7-demethylation of paraxanthine followed by C^8-oxidation. Recent investigations (Callahan *et al.*, 1982, 1983; Tang-Liu *et al.*, 1983) confirmed that the paraxanthine pathway predominates in man for the first demethylation of caffeine and that greater than one-half of the urinary metabolites are 1-methylxanthine and its derivatives. A new polar caffeine metabolite in adult male volunteers was identified by Callahan *et al.* (1982) as 5-acetylamino-6-amino-3-methyluracil. Amounts excreted in the urine ranged from 7 to 35% of the administered dose. The half-life of caffeine in both saliva and serum was about 3 h, with the concentration of caffeine in saliva ranging from 65 to 85% of that found in serum samples.

Identification and chemical characterization studies of 5-acetylamino-6-formylamino-3-methyluracil were published by two groups (Tang *et al.*, 1983; Branfman *et al.*, 1983). Structure determinations were made using UV, NMR and mass spectral data with an authentic standard for comparison. This metabolite was shown to be unstable in the presence of dilute base and/or methanol, giving rise to a deformylated compound, 5-acetylamino-6-amino-3-methyluracil, which was recently reported as a major metabolite of caffeine in man (Tang *et al.*, 1983). Branfman *et al.* (1983) demonstrated that the acetyl group of 5-acetylamino-6-amino-3-methyluracil did not originate from caffeine.

Additional investigations into the variability of caffeine metabolism in man demonstrated that formation of this newly discovered uracil was bimodally distributed and interethnically variable between Caucasian and Oriental populations (Grant *et al.*, 1983*a*). Correlation of 5-acetylamino-6-formylamino-3-methyluracil production and acetylation of sulfamethazine in a group of 20 subjects strongly suggested a connection with the well-known acetylation polymorphism (Grant *et al.*, 1983*b*).

Theobromine

Animal studies. Arnaud and Welsch (1979) were the first to investigate theobromine metabolism in rats using a radiolabeled compound. After an oral dose of [7-Me-^{14}C]-theobromine, compounds identified in rat urine were theobromine (49% of the radioactivity), 7-methylxanthine (6%) and 7-methyluric acid (4%). Two metabolites—3,7-dimethyluric acid (2·7%) and 6-amino-5-(N-methylformylamino)-1-methyluracil (36%)—were identified for the first time. Minor amounts (<1%) of dimethylallantoin and N-methylurea were also detected.

Biotransformation of theobromine in five mammalian species (rats, mice, hamsters, rabbits, dogs) was recently investigated by assaying urinary metabolites after oral [8-^{14}C]theobromine administration (Miller *et al.*, 1984). Excretion patterns of theobromine and its metabolites were qualitatively similar among species, indicating that theobromine is probably metabolized along similar pathways. However, quantitative measurements showed that the major theobromine metabolite excreted by the rat and mouse was 6-amino-5-(N-methylformylamino)-1-methyluracil, while the rabbit and dog formed primarily N-demethylated products. The plasma elimination of theobromine in the dog ($t_{1/2}$ 17–19 h) was reported to be substantially longer than in other species (Gans *et al.*, 1980).

Bonati *et al.* (1984) performed extensive kinetic and metabolic studies in male rats using [8-¹⁴C]theobromine as a radiotracer. Doses ranging from 1 to 100 mg/kg were given either acutely or after chronic theobromine administration for a 2-week period. No significant differences in elimination kinetics or metabolic profiles were found between the treatments. Unchanged theobromine (50%) was the major compound excreted in the urine; 6-amino-5-(*N*-methylformylamino)-1-methyluracil (25%) was the predominant metabolite.

Latini *et al.* (1984) performed similar kinetic and metabolic studies in male and female rabbits following theobromine doses of 1 to 100 mg/kg. The major compound eliminated in the urine was 7-methylxanthine (40%) with 25% of the administered dose excreted as unchanged theobromine. This pattern of elimination is quantitatively similar to that in man. No qualitative differences in metabolic profile were present between males and females. A trend toward accumulation was detected at 100 mg/kg in male rabbits and at 50 mg/kg in female rabbits.

Theobromine metabolism and kinetics were investigated in female pregnant and non-pregnant rats after [8-¹⁴C]theobromine doses of 5–100 mg/kg (Shively and Tarka, 1983*a*). No qualitative differences were observed in urinary metabolites between pregnant and non-pregnant animals; 6-amino-5-(*N*-methylformylamino)-1-methyluracil was the major metabolite. A higher percentage of the dose was excreted as unchanged theobromine in all animals at 100 mg/kg, indicating a saturation of bio-transformation mechanisms at that dose level.

Human studies. The landmark study on human methylxanthine metabolism by Cornish and Christmas (1957) identified and quantitated monomethylxanthines and methyluric acids after ingestion of caffeine, theobromine and theophylline. The major urinary metabolites of theobromine in man were 7-methylxanthine (28–30% of the dose), 3-methylxanthine (14–21%) and 7-methyluric acid (3–4%), with 11–12% of the dose being excreted unchanged. Since more 7-methylxanthine was excreted than 3-methylxanthine, the authors suggested that demethylation of theobromine occurs more readily at the 3-position.

Arnaud and Welsch (1979) more recently identified 3,7-dimethyluric acid and 6-amino-5-(*N*-methylformylamino)-1-methyluracil as two additional metabolites of theobromine in human urine. Tarka *et al.* (1983) defined theobromine plasma elimination kinetics and quantitated urinary excretion rate constants of theobromine and its metabolites in normal male subjects. The major theobromine metabolite was 7-methylxanthine (42%), although approximately 10% of the dose was converted to 6-

amino-5-(N-methylformylamino)-1-methyluracil. Theobromine half-lives ranged from 7·2 to 11·5 h.

Miners *et al.* (1982) investigated the role of xanthine oxidase in human theobromine metabolism by quantitating urine metabolites under multiple-dosing conditions with and without allopurinol administration. When theobromine was administered alone, 44% of the recovered dose was excreted as 7-methylxanthine and 11% as 7-methyluric acid. When allopurinol was given for 7 days, no 7-methyluric acid was found in the urine, but excretion of 7-methylxanthine was significantly higher (59%).

Pharmacokinetics
Recent studies have shown that, unlike caffeine (Latini *et al.*, 1978) and theophylline (Teunissen *et al.*, 1985), dose-dependent theobromine kinetics do not exist in rats (Shively and Tarka, 1983*a*; Bonati *et al.*, 1984) or in rabbits (Latini *et al.*, 1984; Traina and Bonati, 1985) when oral doses as high as 100 mg/kg are given. Kinetic parameters in rats and rabbits were also found to be similar whether theobromine was given by oral or intravenous routes (Bonati *et al.*, 1984; Latini *et al.*, 1984; Traina and Bonati, 1985). Unlike the rat, caffeine disposition in man was reported to be unaltered after doses of 1, 5 and 10 mg/kg (Bonati *et al.*, 1982). A comparative pharmacokinetic study of caffeine in young and elderly men indicated very similar elimination parameters (Blanchard and Sawers, 1983).

Caffeine kinetics were studied in 40-day and 1-year old rats by Latini *et al.* (1980). Elimination was slower in old rats ($t_{1/2}$ 332 min) than in young ones ($t_{1/2}$ 120 min). This was an important contribution to the literature and may explain the findings of Peters and Boyd (1967) who found that older rats were more sensitive to the toxic effects of caffeine.

Several studies have investigated the influence of dietary methylxanthines on theobromine (Drouillard *et al.*, 1978; Miners *et al.*, 1982; Shively *et al.*, 1985) and theophylline (Caldwell *et al.*, 1977; Monks *et al.*, 1979, 1981) kinetics and metabolism in man. Drouillard *et al.* (1978) found that the mean metabolic clearance of a single, oral dose of theobromine (6 mg/kg) given to male volunteers on a methylxanthine-free diet was reduced after theobromine was administered for 4 days prior to dosing. This reduction in clearance was reversible when theobromine was withdrawn. In a second phase of this study, theobromine plasma half-lives were also shown to be shortened when methylxanthines were removed from the diet. A recent study by Shively *et al.* (1985) found that [8-^{14}C]theobromine clearance and metabolic disposition in 8 normal male volunteers was unaltered when theobromine (6 mg/kg) was given for 7 days in dietary form as chocolate. These kinetic differences between chemical and dietary form of theobromine were explained by the reduced bioavailability of theobromine from chocolate.

Other studies in human volunteers with theophylline have shown that clearance was increased when all methylxanthines were removed from the diet (Caldwell *et al.*, 1977; Monks *et al.*, 1979). However, inclusion of additional methylxanthines in the diet of subjects consuming their usual amount of methylxanthines had no effect on theophylline disposition (Monks *et al.*, 1981).

Metabolism during Pregnancy

Pregnancy was shown to have only minor effects on theobromine disposition in rats and rabbits (Shively and Tarka, 1983*a*; Latini *et al.*, 1984), while theophylline metabolism was impaired during late pregnancy in rats (Arnaud *et al.*, 1982). Studies in pregnant women have documented that caffeine elimination was significantly reduced during pregnancy (Aldridge *et al.*, 1981; Knutti *et al.*, 1981; Parsons and Pelletier, 1982), thus increasing the possible risk of toxicity to both mother and fetus.

Neonatal Metabolism

Caffeine and theophylline are currently the drugs of choice in the treatment of premature infant apnea, a disorder in which spontaneous breathing ceases for short periods of time. These drugs are also now used for the management of young infants with near-miss sudden infant death syndrome. Until recently very little was known about the metabolism and disposition of these compounds in the fetus and growing child.

A number of studies have shown a marked reduction in the elimination of caffeine (Parsons *et al.*, 1976; Aranda *et al.*, 1977, 1979; Aldridge *et al.*, 1979; Parsons and Neims, 1981) and theophylline (Aranda *et al.*, 1976; Giacoia *et al.*, 1976; Grygiel and Birkett, 1980; Hilligoss *et al.*, 1980) in premature and full-term newborn humans. During the first month of life caffeine represented 85% of the identifiable metabolites in urine (Aldridge *et al.*, 1979). By the age of 7–9 months, the percentage decreased gradually to the adult value of 2%. The 4-day plasma half-life of caffeine in the newborn (compared to adult values of 2–4 h) was dependent on the slow urinary excretion of unchanged caffeine, since little or no metabolism was present. The decrease in half-life to about 4 h by the age of 8 months correlated closely with increased metabolite production. Extensive pharmacokinetic studies in 32 premature infants with apnea reported a similar reduction in caffeine clearance and found the mean caffeine plasma elimination half-life to be 103 ± 18 h (Aranda et al., 1979). Recent studies by Aranda et al. (1984) indicated that a rapid maturational process occurs for caffeine during the first 3 months of postnatal life with C^8-oxidation and N^3-demethylation being the major biotransformation pathways in early life.

In premature neonates only theophylline and caffeine could be detected in urine even after 6 weeks of theophylline therapy, confirming a lack of activity in the enzymes responsible for theophylline N-demethylation and C^8-oxidation (Grygiel and Birkett, 1980). Aranda et al. (1984) also reported unchanged theophylline as the major excretory compound in the urine. However, in addition to caffeine, they detected 1,3-demethyluric acid in the urine. Thus, theophylline is poorly metabolized and its elimination in neonates is dependent almost exclusively on renal excretion of unchanged drug. The presence of caffeine in the plasma and urine of infants undergoing theophylline treatment has raised the possibility that newborns possess a novel biotransformation mechanism (Bada et al., 1979; Bory et al., 1979; Boutroy et al., 1979; Grygiel and Birkett, 1980). Scalais et al. (1983) conclusively established the production of caffeine from theophylline in the neonate by using the stable isotope ^{15}N. The excreted metabolites of theophylline (expressed as the molar fraction of 15·6% of the dose recovered after 72 h) were unchanged theophylline (60%), caffeine (13%) and 1,3-demethyluric acid (18%). This methylation process has not yet been demonstrated in adults and may represent a unique developmental pathway.

TOXICOLOGICAL ASPECTS

Acute Toxicity
In order to understand the toxicity of foodstuffs containing the methylxanthines, it is important first to understand their acute toxicological properties. Salant and Rieger (1912) reported that the minimum fatal dose of caffeine administered intraperitoneally to rabbits, guinea pigs and cats varied from 150 to 250 mg/kg. Kisskalt (1915) reported the LD_{50} of caffeine to be approximately 260 mg/kg for white rats. Later studies by Poe and Johnson (1953) demonstrated that lethal doses of caffeine or theophylline were approximately 200 mg/kg when given intraperitoneally to young rats and that caffeine was slightly more toxic in older rats (LD_{50} 167 mg/kg).

The contributions of Boyd (1960) and Boyd et al. (1965) represent the most comprehensive evaluation of the toxicity of caffeine. The LD_{50} of caffeine administered orally to guinea pigs and albino rats was 230 and 192 mg/kg, respectively. The common cause of death was attributed to respiratory failure following convulsions. The toxicity of caffeine was determined after daily administration via intragastric cannula to female albino rats over a 100-day period (equivalent to 1/10 of the animals' life span). Rats given daily doses slightly above the maximum LD_{50} (110 mg/ kg) exhibited a stressor reaction in the form of hypertrophy of the salivary glands, liver, heart, kidneys and lungs, inhibition of oogenesis, minor changes in organ water levels, and an occasional death apparently from bronchiopneumonia. Although major changes in growth rates, eating and drinking habits were not apparent, some polydipsia, diuresis, nephritis, thyroiditis, occasional dermatitis, and loss of red pulp in the spleen were seen. Peters and Boyd (1967) reported that the sensitivity of rats to the lethal effects of caffeine increased with age, confirming earlier observations. Older rats exhibited more frequent hypokinetic-convulsive deaths than the psychotoxic deaths seen in young rats. Caffeine was also more toxic in male than in female rats.

A thorough review of the literature on factors affecting caffeine toxicity was published by Peters (1967). The minimal non-lethal toxic dose for rats and mice was between 25 and 50 mg/kg. After subcutaneous injection of caffeine in rats death followed severe convulsions, whereas after oral administration rather mild tetanic convulsions were seen with death being attributed to respiratory failure or in some cases to cardiovascular collapse. High daily doses (185 mg/kg) of caffeine killed susceptible rats in 2–3 days, leaving only those that were resistant. No explanation was provided for these differences. The stress sequence can be followed by recording changes in the weight of the adrenals and thymus gland. A net increase in relative adrenal weight and a decrease in relative thymus weight were observed within 7 days of administration. This effect became more pronounced as the time sequence increased. Diet and metabolic conditions also markedly influenced the magnitude of toxicity. Acute starvation was reported to augment the susceptibility of albino rats to the lethal effect of caffeine. Rats fed two synthetic diets consisting of either raw egg white or sucrose were more susceptible to the lethal effects of caffeine than when they were fed a commercial laboratory chow. This seems to be a common observation with synthetic diets, and therefore toxicological researchers recommend using defined commercial chow in short- and long-term evaluations. For humans, the minimal non-lethal toxic dose was reported to be between 2 and 5 mg/kg, a figure which appears quite dubious since these concentrations would be well within the range achieved from the consumption of 8–10 cups of coffee.

Behavioral effects have also been reported in the previously discussed toxicity studies (Peters, 1967; Peters and Boyd, 1967). Oral doses of 185 mg/kg caffeine to rats resulted in depressed activity for 2 days, after which time stereotyped movements such as running backwards in circles and fumbling developed. In isolated rats, tail chasing and finally severe mutilation of the tail or hind feet were noted. Death followed hemorrhagic shock. An interesting observation was that aggregation of rats protected against the self-aggression of isolated rats, but this was replaced sometimes by lethal fighting. With doses of 0·5–1·5 g in humans, early hypermotility due to rapid peak caffeine plasma concentrations, anxiety, hallucinations, delirium, convulsions and drowsiness were described.

The literature contains only a handful of reports on the acute toxicological effects of cocoa and chocolate waste products. Of particular concern is how toxic effects were correlated with the respective theobromine contents of each of these materials. Clough (1942) reported the death of three dogs following the ingestion of 2 g/kg theobromine in a commercial ration within a 48-hour period, and Decker and Myers (1972) diagnosed theobromine poisoning in a single dog due to the consumption of excessive baking chocolate (19 g/kg). They diagnosed this as theobromine toxicity by the presence of whole melted chocolate found in the stomach. The methodology employed, as well as the presence of other complicating dietary factors, unfortunately allowed no firm conclusion from this study. Hoskam and Haagsma (1974) reported chocolate poisoning in two dachshunds presumably due to a theobromine content equivalent of 15 g/kg. While the sample size was limited, it could be concluded that theobromine toxicity was the cause of death, since this experimental dose of theobromine was 750 times larger than the therapeutic dose used for dogs (20 mg/kg) at that time by veterinarians. The field trials of Black and Barron (1943) reported toxicity of cacao waste products in poultry when fed at dietary levels of 15% or above. Unfortunately, no data were given on the theobromine and caffeine content of the material, and thus it was not possible to correlate the toxicity with methylxanthine consumption.

Braude and Foot (1942) found that cocoa meal containing 2·5% theobromine caused digestive disturbances and death in weanling pigs when fed at 8% of the ration. The toxic effect was less apparent as age and weight increased. Braude (1943) further evaluated the toxic effects of feeding cocoa meal to pigs as a partial substitute for grain as part of the war effort in

1943. When the dietary ration contained 7·5% cocoa meal there was a high degree of toxicity and consequent mortality which was preceded by poor growth, unthrifty appearance, lethargy, scours and loss of equilibrium. At the 5% level the material was not noticeably toxic, but the author felt there was no advantage to include it in the diet of fattening pigs since its nutritive value was small. While it was not possible analytically to support the conclusion that theobromine was the cause of death, Braude reported that the extraction of theobromine from the meal rendered it harmless to younger pigs and it could be fed with satisfactory results at 8% of the diet.

In humans, methylxanthine toxicity has rarely occurred. There are several cases reported in the literature, and in nearly every case the xanthine toxicity was iatrogenic (White and Daeschner, 1956; Jokela and Vartiainen, 1959; Smith, 1972; Dimaio and Garriott, 1974; Banner and Czajka, 1980: McGee, 1980; Winek et al., 1980). The syndrome described for caffeine and theophylline typically manifests itself as a disturbed state of consciousness—restlessness later followed by drowsiness leading to coma, profuse vomiting, convulsions and, least often, proteinuria and haematuria.

Studies by Tarka (1980) indicated that the oral LD_{50} for theobromine was approximately 950 mg/kg in the rat. The basis for the remarkable difference between caffeine (200 mg/kg), theophylline (206 mg/kg) and theobromine (950 mg/kg) is unclear, although it may be due to differences in absorption kinetics or to the presence of the methyl group at the C-1 position in the purine ring. McColl et al. (1955) reported the intraperitoneal LD_{50} of theobromine sodium acetate in mice to be 789 mg/kg while the oral LD_{50} was 1356 mg/kg. A summary of the acute toxicity and route of administration of the methylxanthines in all animal species and man is presented in Table 2. Table 3 compares the acute toxicity of methylxanthine derivatives. Note that 1-allyltheobromine is the most toxic compound, with the unsaturated double bond playing a critical role.

Neuroendocrine Actions

Neuroendocrine effects from the methylxanthines have been shown to occur in dogs (Amiragova, 1962), rats (Wolff and Varrone, 1969; Peytremann et al., 1973; Spindel et al., 1980, 1983; Scammell and Fregly, 1982; Clozel et al., 1983; Shively and Tarka, 1983b) and man (Spindel et al., 1984). In dogs, caffeine (20–30 mg/kg) stimulated the secretory function of the thyroid gland and depressed hormone production following administration of I^{131} (Amiragova, 1962). Experiments in rats also indicated an effect of the methylxanthines on thyroid hormones. Wolff and Varrone

TABLE 2
Acute Toxicity of Methylxanthines (from Tarka, 1982)

Compound	Species	LD$_{50}$ (mg/kg)			Clinical signs
		p.o.	i.p.	i.v.	
Caffeine	Man	150–200[a]	—	57[a]	Convulsions, emesis, coma
	Rat	200	200	105	Convulsions, respiratory failure
	Mouse	127	220[b]	100	Convulsions
	Hamster	230	—	—	Convulsions
	Guinea pig	230	235	—	Convulsions, stupor
	Rabbit	246	—	—	Convulsions
	Cat	125[b]	190[b]	—	Convulsions
	Dog	145[b]	—	175	Convulsions
Theobromine[c]	Rat	950	—	—	—
	Mouse	1 350[b]	789	—	—
Theophylline	Rat	—	206	—	Delayed convulsions, tetanic spasm
	Mouse	332	217	—	—

[a] Fatal dose
[b] Median lethal dose.
[c] Theobromine sodium acetate was used due to poor solubility of theobromine.

TABLE 3

Comparative Acute Toxicity of Methylxanthine Derivatives in the Mouse (from Tarka, 1982)

Compound	LD_{50} (mg/kg)		Clinical signs
	p.o.	i.p.	
Caffeine	127	220[a]	Convulsions
Caffeine and sodium benzoate	878	525	
Theobromine	950	—	
Theobromine and sodium acetate	1 356	789	Emesis
1-Allyl theobromine [$H_2C = CHCH_2-$]	191	102	
1-Butyl theobromine [$CH_3CH_2CH_2CH_2-$]	667	230	Convulsions
1-Isoamyl theobromine [$(CH_3)_2CHCH_2CH_2-$]	772	222	Emesis
Theophylline	332	217	Convulsions
Theophylline ethylenediamine (aminophylline)	391	257	Profuse salivation, emesis, convulsions
7-Allyl theophylline	315	299	Convulsions
7-Butyl theophylline	617	272	Convulsions
7-Isoamyl theophylline	723	211	Convulsions, emesis

[a]Median lethal dose.

(1969) found that rats developed goiters when fed methylxanthines in low iodine diets. The order of potency of the tested compounds was theophylline = aminophylline > caffeine > theobromine.

A recent study by Spindel et al. (1980) reported a dose-dependent depression of serum thyrotropin (TSH) and growth hormone (GH) after intraperitoneal administration of caffeine in rats. ED_{50} values for TSH and GH were 30 and 50 mg/kg, respectively. TSH concentrations were significantly depressed for 1–6 h after treatment, with the extent of the reduction related to caffeine blood levels. Decreases in serum $3,5,3'$-triiodothyronine (T_3) and thyroxine (T_4) followed the TSH response, occurring 4 h after the caffeine dose. Similar effects were ascribed to theophylline and theobromine although these compounds were administered in doses two-fold higher than caffeine. A subsequent study by Spindel et al. (1983) confirmed the reduction in TSH and found that caffeine also increased serum corticosterone concentrations (ED_{50} 40–50 mg/kg), although a tolerance developed over a 1-week period such that further caffeine doses elicited no effect on TSH or corticosterone. Theophylline was shown to be equipotent to caffeine, while theobromine and paraxanthine were less potent. The lower activity of the latter compounds was attributed to the lower serum concentrations achieved.

Both acute and chronic endocrinological effects following caffeine, theobromine and cocoa powder administration were assessed by Shively and Tarka (1983b) and Shively et al. (1984a). In confirmation of the findings of Spindel et al. (1980, 1983), high intraperitoneal doses of caffeine (100 mg/kg) significantly depressed TSH secretion up to 6 h after administration, while markedly elevating plasma corticosterone. This reduction in TSH did not statistically alter the plasma levels of T_3 and T_4, although a 34% reduction in T_3 occurred between 2 and 6 hours following caffeine dosing. However, in contrast to previous findings of Spindel et al. (1980), similar theobromine doses (100 mg/kg) exerted no effect. Ingestion of caffeine, theobromine or cocoa powder for 28 days at levels equivalent to a methylxanthine intake of 500 mg/kg/day produced no endocrinological effects in rats (Shively and Tarka, 1983b). These results are consistent with Spindel et al. (1983) who demonstrated a tolerance effect for the methylxanthines when administered chronically.

Scammell and Fregly (1982) reported decreased serum T_4 concentrations and T_4 5'-deiodinase activities in rats after feeding theophylline ad libitum at 0.25% dietary levels for 14 days. These results were in contrast to the studies of Shively and Tarka (1983b) who found no change in T_4 plasma concentrations in rats after feeding caffeine and theobromine for 4 weeks at dietary levels producing plasma methylxanthine levels similar to Scammell and Fregly (1982).

Studies similar to those of Spindel *et al.* (1980, 1983) were performed in newborn rats by Clozel *et al.* (1983). Significant elevations in GH were observed following a single caffeine dose (5 or 50 mg/kg), while multiple caffeine doses for 14 days elicited no effect. A biphasic T_4 response was present, with high caffeine doses increasing T_4 at 4 h and decreasing T_4 at 24 h after dosing. In contrast to previous findings in adult rats, caffeine significantly increased both basal and TRH-stimulated TSH release in newborn rats. The relevance of these findings to human neonates remains to be explored.

Endocrine responses to caffeine in human subjects have recently been examined after administration of 250 and 500 mg doses (Spindel *et al.*, 1984). No effects on prolactin, T_3, TSH, GH or cortisol were observed at either dose level, while 500 mg caffeine doses elevated plasma levels of β-endorphin-like immunoreactivity in both men and women. Since these caffeine dose levels translate to only 3–8 mg/kg, and effects in rats were produced at 30 mg/kg, it is unlikely that consumption of caffeine from food and beverage sources will elicit any endocrinological response in man.

Immunotoxicity

Although the methylxanthines have been reported to have adverse effects on many organ systems when ingested in high doses by experimental animals, there is a paucity of data regarding their action on lymphoid organs and immune function.

Decreased thymic weights have been reported in rats following dietary exposure to large amounts of caffeine and theobromine (Tarka *et al.*, 1979; Gans, 1982, 1984). Tarka *et al.* (1979) found that thymic atrophy became prominent in male Sprague-Dawley rats consuming 0·6% theobromine in the diet for 28 days. Progressive decreases in thymic cortical lymphocytes were observed with increasing intake of theobromine. At dietary levels of 1% the shrunken thymus gland was composed only of stromal cells with scattered medullary lymphocytes. It should be noted that this dietary level corresponded to a methylxanthine intake of more than 200 mg/kg/day which is 50–100 times higher than the maximum human consumption from cocoa-containing products.

Gans (1982) reported the occurrence of thymic atrophy in rats maintained on either semi-purified or chow diets. A subsequent study (Gans, 1984) demonstrated caffeine to be equipotent to theobromine in inducing these effects.

Geber *et al.* (1975) found that administration of high caffeine doses (200 mg/kg, i.p.) to mice increased their circulating interferon levels in response to viral infection. However, lower doses of salicylate (100 mg/kg, i.p.) were significantly more effective than caffeine. These results suggested that both compounds may serve as prophylactic agents against virus-related diseases.

Recent studies by Saxena *et al.* (1984) and Singh *et al.* (1984) assessed the effects of acute caffeine administration on the lymphoid organs in rats and on specific immune functions in mice. Caffeine increased adrenal gland and peripheral lymph node weights, while causing a non-significant decrease in thymic weight at doses equivalent to 1/5 of the LD_{50}. In mice, the highest dose of caffeine (1/5 of LD_{50}) produced significant impairment of humoral immune response as shown by decreased IgM antibody plaque-forming cells in the spleen. Furthermore, the cell-mediated immune response was suppressed in a dose-dependent manner. Caffeine-treated mice were also more susceptible to *E. coli* endotoxin as demonstrated by increased mortality following infection. In bone marrow cells of mice, caffeine caused a dose-dependent reduction in cell viability. A decrease in lymphocyte count and an increase in granulocyte count was also observed in peripheral blood.

Several recent studies have shown immunological effects of theophylline on human white blood cells (Shapira *et al.*, 1982; Pardi *et al.*, 1984). The possible use of aminophylline as an *in vivo* immunomodulating agent to reduce allograft rejection in humans has raised much interest. The ability of theophylline to activate suppressor systems *in vivo* may contribute to these observed properties, but it is still not certain whether this previously unknown pharmacological action is obtainable with the usual therapeutic drug blood levels. The results of Pardi *et al.* (1984) demonstrated that a single dose of aminophylline (5 mg/kg i.v. for 20 min) altered the response of peripheral blood leukocytes to polyclonal mitogens, as well as re-distributing circulating helper and suppressor lymphocyte subpopulations. These marked influences on circulating lymphocyte populations by theo-phylline suggest that additional studies should be performed with other methylxanthines commonly ingested in comparable doses (5 mg/kg).

Because of the widespread use of theophylline in the treatment of premature infant apnea and its reported effects on lymphocytes, the potential effect on lymphocyte proliferation and immunoglobin production was determined in newborn infants (Baley *et al.*, 1982). Although no significant *in vivo* immunological effects could be demonstrated, these authors suggested that additional studies be performed in theophylline-treated infants to assess fully whether any such effects occur due to its frequent use in the clinical environment.

Renal Effects and Urinary Mineral Excretion

The diuretic properties of the methylxanthines have been known by pharmacologists for over 50 years. The reader is referred to the extensive early studies of Bliss and Morrison (1933), Blumgart *et al.* (1934), Dorfman and Jarvik (1970) and McColl *et al.* (1956) for details. Xanthine diuretics induce a relatively smaller response than a comparable dose of mercurial diuretics and as a result have been completely replaced by more efficacious drugs. Huang *et al.* (1958) reported that xanthine diuresis was due to reduced reabsorption of sodium and chloride in the proximal tubules rather than to any change in renal hemodynamics, and proposed that methylxanthines may increase the membrane permeability of renal tubular cells, causing ions to leak out.

The idea that methylxanthines may affect renal dynamics because of their diuretic properties has led researchers to evaluate the role of these compounds on mineral excretion. It was reported previously by Lemann *et al.* (1979) and Yu *et al.* (1981) that other diuretics have a profound effect on increasing urinary output of calcium and magnesium as well as sodium and potassium. Heaney and Recker (1982) reported that such an effect was correlated with caffeine consumption by pre-menopausal females and manifested itself in the form of a decreased calcium balance which was attributed to both urinary and intestinal calcium losses. Recently, Massey and Wise (1984) performed a pilot study in 12 female college students who consumed decaffeinated coffee or tea with 150 or 300 mg added caffeine and reported that the total urinary 3-hour excretion of calcium, magnesium and sodium, but not potassium, was significantly increased. This effect on mineral excretion was attributed to the changes in mineral concentration and increased urinary volume. Colin *et al.* (1984) examined the effects of acute theophylline administration at therapeutic doses of 5 mg/kg i.v. on urinary excretion of cyclic adenosine monophosphate (cAMP), calcium and phosphorus in normal subjects. Theophylline exerted a pronounced biological effect on renal tubular activity, with an increase in nephro-genous cAMP accompanied by a rise in phosphate and calcium urinary excretion. The data suggested that the phosphaturic and calcituric effects of theophylline on the renal tubules may be mediated by cAMP rather than parathyroid hormone.

Recent clinical studies by Hollingbery *et al.* (1985) and Massey and Berg (1985) on the effects of caffeine in healthy males and in pre- and post-menopausal women support earlier observations of increased urinary mineral excretion. In addition, these studies suggested an involvement of the prostaglandins in increased urinary calcium concentration following caffeine consumption.

It is apparent from the foregoing studies that the methylxanthines appear to play a role in urinary mineral excretion in heavy methylxanthine consumers and in individuals on therapeutic treatment regimens containing methylxanthines. The clinical relevance of this finding has not been assessed to date and is deserving of additional research to elucidate the significance of these observations.

Reproduction/Teratogenicity

Extensive reviews of the literature on the reproductive and teratogenic effects of caffeine and the methylxanthines have been previously prepared by Collins (1979) and Tarka (1982). In September 1980, the Food and Drug Administration as a follow-up to its concerns about caffeine initiated several regulatory activities, including the cautioning of pregnant women to limit their consumption of foods and drugs containing caffeine. They also proposed to remove caffeine from the list of substances that are generally recognized as safe (GRAS) for addition to food and to place it on an interim list pending the outcome of additional research currently underway at that time.

Recent animal safety studies conducted on the methylxanthines during the late 1970s indicated that the testes and thymus were selective target organs for the toxicity of these compounds. Friedman et al. (1979) reported testicular atrophy and aspermatogenesis in 85–100% of Osborne-Medel rats fed caffeine, theophylline or theobromine at dietary levels of 0·5% for 64 weeks. In the same study these findings were confirmed in a second rat strain (Holtzman). The order of relative potency as determined from these studies was caffeine > theobromine > theophylline. Tarka et al. (1979) reported that atrophy of the testes, as well as the thymus, became prominent in both mature and immature Sprague-Dawley rats after a 28-day dietary exposure to 0·6% theobromine. Lower concentrations of 0·2% and 0·4% theobromine had no effect on the testes, but thymic weights were reduced by at least 10% in males and 50% in females. Testicular changes included seminiferous tubular cell degeneration and necrosis with formation of multinucleate (giant) cells. A low protein diet enhanced the severity of this effect. The daily dose of theobromine which produced retrogressive growth and histopathological changes was approximately 200–300 mg/kg in mature rats and 500 mg/kg in immature rats. Hamsters and mice were found to be more resistant than rats.

Additional rodent studies undertaken by Tarka et al. (1981), to examine whether these changes in rat testes were reversible after a 7-week recovery period, indicated that 70–90% of the seminiferous tubules from the 0·6% and 0·8% theobromine groups still lacked well-formed spermatozoa. However, a recent study by Tarka *et al.* (1984), which examined testicular atrophy and impaired reproductive function after a longer recovery period of 12 weeks, revealed that testicular atrophy and subsequent infertility were reversible in rats fed 0·6% but not 0·8% theobromine.

Gans (1982) compared theobromine-induced thymic and testicular atrophy in rats at 8, 16, 21 and 28 days after feeding 0·6% and 0·8% theobromine in semi-synthetic or pulverized commercial rodent chow diets. Atrophy of the thymus gland occurred earlier than testicular damage irrespective of the basal composition of the diet containing theobromine. In contrast, testicular atrophy was less severe and developed later in animals fed theobromine in commercial chow diet. This attenuation in toxicity could have been due either to the lower plasma theobromine concentrations present in rats fed commercial chow diet or to a reduction in a specific metabolite which may be responsible for the toxicity.

A subsequent study by Gans (1984) examined the comparative toxicity of dietary caffeine and theobromine in the rat and reported that, although caffeine was more potent than theobromine as an anorexic agent, it was equivalent to theobromine in its potential ability to induce thymic and testicular atrophy with spermatogenic cell destruction.

Toxicological studies performed in dogs by Gans *et al.* (1980) showed that theobromine doses of 100–150 mg/kg did not induce thymic or testicular atrophy when given for up to 1 year. However, degenerative fibrotic lesions of the right atrial appendage of the heart were detected. A direct comparison of the effects of theobromine in rats and dogs was limited by the inability to attain plasma theobromine concentrations in the dog as high as those in the rat. This was due to the greater toxicity of theobromine in the dog whose half-life is longer (17–19·5 h) than that of the rat (4–6 h).

Recently, Dahlback *et al.* (1984) studied testicular toxicity of several xanthine derivatives in the rat and reported that the 1-methylated xanthine derivatives were the most toxic. No definitive mechanism was provided to explain the testicular atrophy, but the authors speculated that it may be in part related to a stress syndrome and not to an accumulation of the parent compound. The relevance of the effects on the rodent testes needs to be put into proper clinical perspective, since the atrophy appears to be species-specific. In spite of the widespread consumption of methyl-xanthine-containing products, the reproductive capability of man has not been adversely affected. The dietary level of methylxanthines required to induce testicular atrophy in the rat is extremely high (250–300 mg/kg/day) and far exceeds maximum human consumption levels. Additionally, the dominant-lethal study of Shively *et al.* (1984*b*), in which theobromine was administered at doses 25–225 times the maximum human consumption level, provided support for the reproducttive safety of theobromine. No significant dose-dependent induction of dominant lethal mutations or adverse effects on pregnancy rate were observed.

Elmazar *et al.* (1981, 1982) conducted acute studies investigating the mechanism of action of caffeine as a teratogen in mice, and what effects different oral preparations of caffeine had on induction of terata. They reported that oral doses of caffeine at 200 and 300 mg/kg (but not 100 mg/kg) on day 14 caused cleft palate while all dose levels elevated plasma corticosterone. Since corticosteroids are a known cleft palate inducer in mice but not in humans, even when women were treated throughout pregnancy with large doses (Schardein, 1976), the authors concluded that the findings in mice did not predict a hazard from normal caffeine consumption in man. The form in which caffeine was administered determined whether a teratogenic response was observed. Retarded ossification of the supraoccipital bones was observed in fetuses when caffeine (150 mg/kg) was administered in the drinking water, but not when the same dose was given as a sustained-release tablet. The most important effect observed at high doses, irrespective of the form of treatment, was a reduction in fetal weight. Dunlop and Court (1981) evaluated the effect of dietary caffeine fed to rats throughout pregnancy and lactation at a level of 10 mg/kg/day and reported that offspring of successive pregnancies showed growth reduction. This finding was not accompanied by teratogenicity, but after four pregnancies offspring growth and neonatal mortality was severely reduced.

Nolen (1981) evaluated the effect of brewed and instant coffees on reproduction and teratogenesis in the rat either at full strength (100%) or as 50 or 25% dilutions beginning at weaning and continuing for about 30 weeks through two pregnancies. These levels provided caffeine intakes of 80, 40 and 20 mg/kg/day respectively, with the high dose being equivalent to 50-60 cups of coffee/day in man. No deleterious effects on reproduction or embryogenesis were observed, but fetuses in the groups given 100 or 50% solutions of brewed coffee and 100% instant coffee had a significantly higher incidence of unossified sternebrae, suggesting a retardation of the fetal calcification process.

Nolen (1982) also performed a similar reproduction/teratology study of brewed and instant decaffeinated coffees in rats given full strength or 50 or 25% dilutions for about 6 months post-weaning. These levels are equivalent to human consumption of 50, 25 or 12 cups of coffee per day. Again no effects on reproduction or embryogenesis were seen except for the significant increase in unossified sternebrae which was not considered to be a teratogenic response.

The work and subsequent publication of the rat 'gavage' study of caffeine by Collins et al. (1981) was responsible for the initial concern expressed by the US Food and Drug Administration regarding over-consumption of caffeinated products by pregnant women and the possibility of birth defects. A subsequent rat study by Collins et al. (1983) evaluated caffeine dissolved in drinking water which provided daily caffeine intakes of 10, 27, 51, 87, 116 and 205 mg/kg. This 'sipping' study demonstrated that the effects on maternal mortality, fetal weight, fetal ossification and development were less severe after ad libitum sipping than after oral intubation. There were no dose-related gross anomalies and ectrodactyly was only seen at the highest doses. However, the delay in ossification reported in the gavage study was also observed here but at much higher doses. These data contributed significantly to understanding the threshold required for induction of teratogenic effects. The question of whether the teratogenic effects observed in mice treated with caffeine were due to caffeine per se or to one of its metabolites was recently addressed by York et al. (1985). While administration of caffeine alone caused similar types and rates of malformations as observed in previous studies, induction of maternal drug-metabolizing enzymes with β-naphthoflavone protected the embryos from the congenital anomalies induced by large doses of caffeine. The rapid elimination of caffeine resulting from increased metabolism and the reduction in toxicity/teratogenicity indicated that caffeine, and not a metabolite, was the toxicant.

Recently, Tarka et al. (1986a,b) conducted definitive evaluations on the peri/postnatal and teratogenic effects of cocoa powder and theobromine in rats and of the teratogenic potential of these compounds in rabbits. Feeding 2·5 or 5% cocoa powder or 0·0675 or 0·135% theobromine to rats had no effect on peri/postnatal parameters or teratogenicity, but fetuses of the 0·135% theobromine group had a significantly higher incidence of incompletely ossified or absent sternebrae and pubic bones suggesting a delay in osteogenesis. Skeletal variants observed in these studies were attributed to a potentially salient maternal or fetal toxicity that was unrelated to a specific compound/treatment. The consumption at the high dose level (100 mg/kg/day theobromine) was 50 times greater than the maximum human consumption level. The data from the rabbit studies are even more meaningful, since in the rabbit the metabolism of theobromine is quantitatively similar to man. Feeding cocoa powder at 2·5, 5 and 7·5% and theobromine at 0·0625, 0·125 and 0·1875% of the diets, respectively, resulted in neither fetotoxicity nor teratogenicity. However, fetuses exposed to 0·125% theobromine had a significantly higher incidence of incompletely ossified or absent sternebrae while exposure to either 0·1875% theobromine or 7·5% cocoa powder resulted in corresponding effects on metacarpal bones, again indicating a delay in osteogenesis.

Thus, a tremendous amount of animal research has been conducted to allay any reproductive/teratogenic concerns voiced by regulatory authorities. These studies also addressed concerns raised in earlier reported animal experiments.

Since 1980 the issue of caffeine consumption by pregnant women also gained considerable attention from both the media and scientific investigators. Linn et al. (1982) retrospectively analyzed interview and medical record data of 12 205 non-diabetic, non-asthmatic women in order to evaluate the relation between coffee consumption and adverse outcomes of pregnancy. After controlling for smoking and other potential confounding factors, no association was found between coffee consumption and low birth weights, and there was no relationship with the occurrence of malformations. Kurppa et al. (1982) in an ongoing perspective study at the University of Helsinki also found no relationship between coffee/tea consumption and congenital defects. Van't Hoff (1982) in a small prospective study at Guy's Hospital found no correlation of umbilical cord plasma caffeine levels as high as 62 μmol/liter with adverse outcomes of pregnancy. Rosenberg et al. (1982) performed a definitive case-control study on selected birth defects in relation to caffeine-containing beverages. They examined 2030 malformed infants for six selected birth defects in relation to maternal caffeine ingestion during pregnancy from tea, coffee and cola beverages, beginning in 1976 in a case-control surveillance. Results indicated that caffeine intake was not associated with large increases in the rates of inguinal hernia, cardiac defects, pyloric stenosis, oral clefts and neural tube defects. The authors pointed out, however, that large samples would need to be evaluated to rule out smaller increases, as well as to permit adequate evaluation of less common malformations. Martin (1982) reviewed the literature on maternal nicotine and caffeine consumption and offspring outcome and concluded that smoking was undoubtedly the major detriment to fetal health and that evidence for caffeine damage is neither compelling nor consistent. He concluded that, unless a pregnant woman ingests extremely large quantities daily, the fetus is probably not at risk.

It is obvious from the foregoing review that we are now in a much better position to provide pregnant women with recommendations/advice on caffeine consumption. The scientific data available provide a relief to pregnant women in that moderate consumption of naturally occurring or added caffeine in our food supply will not harm either them or their unborn child. They do need to be cautioned, however, to modify their intake during the last trimester of pregnancy since metabolism and clearance of caffeine from the body becomes influenced by endocrine parameters resulting in a decreased rate of metabolism and elimination.

Fibrocystic Breast Disease
Worldwide, a significant percentage of women are affected by non-cancerous lumpy breast tissue which has been termed fibrocystic breast disease. With this condition they are thought to be at a greater risk of developing breast cancer.

The hypothesis that consumption of methylxanthines in coffee, tea, cola and chocolate is associated with benign breast disease in women has gained considerable interest since it was first proposed by Minton et al. (1979) who reported that abstention from all forms of methylxanthines resulted in resolution of the signs and symptoms of fibrocystic disease of the breast. This study has been severely criticized for the small number of participants (13 of 20 women reported disappearances of lesions upon abstention from all forms of dietary methylxanthines) and for their theory that chronic methylxanthine consumption permanently elevated cyclic AMP levels in breast epithelial cells, either as a direct result of inhibition of cyclic nucleotide phosphodiesterase activity or indirectly via catecholamine release. Additional clinical and biochemical studies in a larger patient population also implicated methylxanthines as a causative factor of fibrocystic breast disease by indicating that abstention from methylxanthines resulted in complete resolution of the disease in 82·5% of the subjects (Minton et al., 1981a). A biochemical subgrouping of benign breast disease was also proposed by Minton et al. (1981b) to define the potential for premalignant disease. Benign breast lesions with increased cAMP levels were correlated with eventual malignant change. None of these effects was demonstrated by Butcher (1984) who performed similar studies.

Ernster et al. (1982) subsequently conducted a controlled trial using 159 women with various degrees of fibrocystic breast disease and were unable to validate statistically the clinical relevance of discontinuing all forms of ingestion of dietary methylxanthines in order to observe regression of benign breast disease. They did, however, observe a limited decrease in symptoms in those participants abstaining from methylxanthine but after comparison of before/after mammograms concluded that there was little support for the methylxanthine hypothesis.

Heyden and Muhlbaier (1984) conducted a prospective study of fibro-cystic breast disease in 72 women with palpable breast nodules over a 6-month period with monthly examinations and questionnaires on intake of coffee, tea, soft drinks, chocolate, candies and caffeine-containing drugs. They concluded that in the condition of fibrocystic breast disease, which has such a high degree of waxing and waning and so much variety of subjective sensitivity and objective clinical palpation, it is difficult to draw any association with the amount of methylxanthines consumed and the condition of fibrocystic breast disease.

There have been six case-control studies published on the relationship between various forms of dietary methylxanthines and fibrocystic disease of the breast. Lawson *et al.* (1981) studied coffee and tea consumption and fibrocystic breast disease as part of the Boston Collaborative Drug Surveillance Program in 451 women hospitalized for fibrocystic or malignant disease of the breast. They reported a modest positive associa-tion between hot beverage consumption but no apparent dose-response effect. All the data for this study were collected prior to publication of the Minton article, so any bias in reporting was eliminated. Marshall *et al.* (1982) could not find any difference in incidence of fibrocystic breast disease and coffee and tea consumption when they evaluated data collected from 1957 to 1965 at the Roswell Park Memorial Institute. Odenheimer *et al.* (1984) found a significant positive association between benign breast disease and coffee consumption in a case-control study of discordant twins. The data of a recent study by Boyle *et al.* (1984) based on a hospital case-control study including 634 women with fibrocystic breast disease and 1066 comparison controls in Connecticut demonstrated a positive association between average daily caffeine consumption and fibrocystic breast disease. There was a 1·5-fold increased risk of fibrocystic breast disease in moderate coffee drinkers and a 2·3-fold increase in heavy drinkers. On the other hand, Lubin *et al.* (1985) found no association between methylxanthine or coffee consumption and fibrocystic breast disease in a dietary case-control study of 854 histologically diagnosed cases of fibrocystic breast disease, 372 matched surgical controls and 723 matched neighborhood controls in Israel between 1977 and 1980. Finally, La Vecchia *et al.* (1985) conducted a case-control study of 288 women with histologically confirmed benign breast lumps (203 dysplastic lesions and 85 benign tumors) and two groups of control women (285 in-patients and 291 out-patients) at the Milan Tumor Institute between November 1981 and March 1983. A positive association was demonstrated between methylxanthine consumption in the form of coffee and tea intake and dysplastic disease of the breast, with heavy consumers having the greatest risk. Methylxanthine consumption, however, was not associated with an increased risk of developing benign tumors (fibroadenomas) of the breast.

While caffeine has been the predominant methylxanthine on which fibrocystic breast disease studies have been based, the recent pilot study of Hindi-Alexander et al. (1985) focused on the possible contribution of theophylline to this effect over a 9-month period. The study group consisted of 62 women with asthma, 43 of whom were taking theophylline for asthma therapy, and two comparison groups, one of which had 66 women who were allergic but not asthmatic and a second group of 72 non-allergic, non-asthmatic women. Their results suggest that total methylxanthines were a contributing factor in fibrocystic breast disease severity with or without adjustment for relevant variables. Theophylline was significant only with adjustments for age, pregnancy and menopause, in contrast to caffeine which was only significant with no adjustments.

The controversy over the characterization and description of fibrocystic disease of the breast has led Love et al. (1982) to question whether fibrocystic breast disease is really a 'non-disease'. After reviewing the existing literature relative to clinical and histologic definitions of fibrocystic breast disease and cancer, they concluded that the term fibrocystic breast disease has lost its specificity and should be abandoned for more descriptive terms. This would provide a clear definition of terminology so that large, well-controlled prospective studies could clinically and histologically evaluate hormonal variations in the breast as potential indicators of future malignant disease.

The specific role of dietary methylxanthines in the onset and/or aggravation of fibrocystic breast disease continues to be a controversial area requiring much needed future research. Several of the studies reviewed suggested some degree of association between methylxanthine consumption and fibrocystic breast disease, but on a biochemical basis both the cyclic AMP theory, as well as that relating to catecholamine release, cannot be substantiated. Other avenues must be explored in a definitive long-term clinical study evaluating the role of methylxanthines in fibrocystic breast disease and the involvement of specific clinical, biochemical and endocrinological parameters in this condition.

Behavioral and Central Nervous System Effects

The pharmacological mode of action of methylxanthines appears to be due to the antagonism of adenosine receptors as shown by Bruns *et al.* (1980), Fredholm (1980), Daly *et al.* (1981), Fredholm and Persson (1982) and Boulenger *et al.* (1982), but this is not to suggest that other possible actions including phosphodiesterase inhibition are not involved. Curatolo and Robertson (1983) have extensively reviewed this subject for caffeine, and data from earlier methylxanthine-related research has been covered elsewhere (Tarka, 1982).

Recent work in experimental animals focused on the effects of methylxanthines on specific behavioral parameters after administration of these purines. Lloyd and Stone (1981) compared the effects of chronic administration of caffeine, theophylline or aminophylline to Wistar and Fischer 344 male rats and noted that food restriction resulted in self-injurious behavior particularly in the Fischer rat. They postulated that this was due to activation of dopamine and 5-hydroxytryptamine neuron systems. Caffeine sensitivity in the neonatal rat was demonstrated as young as 1-day old and the basic response was similar to that observed in adults (Holloway and Thor, 1982). An increase in schedule-controlled responding to food presentation has also been reported following intraperitoneal administration of 6 or 12 mg/kg caffeine to immature rats (Meliska and Brown, 1982).

While caffeine has been the focus of most behavioral research on methylxanthines, the effects of theophylline have also received attention. Denenberg *et al.* (1982) studied the sleep/awake behavioral states of newborn rabbits given 10 mg/kg theophylline by intubation and found that this drug sharply reduced active sleep patterns as well as the development of quiet sleep. This effect was most probably due to the delay in ability effectively to metabolize theophylline in the neonatal rabbit.

In order to bring the effect of caffeine on behavior and development into perspective, Butcher *et al.* (1984) evaluated the behavioral and physical development of rats chronically exposed to caffeinated fluids prior to breeding and in the subsequent F_1 generation by providing 25 and 100% brewed coffee solutions and 0·014 and 0·056% caffeine solutions as the sole fluid source. No effects were seen on reproductive performance, and most of the behavioral effects observed were consistent with the expected effects of caffeine administration. Post-weaning exposure effects, including delayed incisor eruption, increased open field activity and reduced running wheel activity, suggested a longer-term change in activity. There were no effects on learning, memory or motor functioning.

The development of tolerance to specific drugs has also been evaluated experimentally for caffeine. Holtzman (1983) found that chronic caffeine administration to rats resulted in the development of tolerance to caffeine-induced stimulation of locomotor activity that was virtually complete, specific and fully reversible when caffeine treatment was stopped.

The obvious question is: How does this relate to man? Sawyer *et al.* (1982) reviewed the effects of caffeine on human behavior and identified several areas for future evaluation dealing with arousal, stress, anxiety and performance. There has been more research conducted on caffeine relative to these questions than on any other single component of our diet, and we are all aware of cases of 'caffeinism' from overindulgence. This condition is recognized by clinicians in the form of anxiety, insomnia and headaches, as well as other non-specific symptoms, and is readily treated. Researchers should continue to evaluate the role of caffeine since it is such a ubiquitous component of our diet.

Mutagenesis/Carcinogenesis

While methylxanthines have been reported to exhibit mutagenic activity at high concentrations, the available experimental data from mutagenicity studies do not indicate that this is a potential health problem. The literature on mutagenicity has been reviewed by Tarka (1982). Recently, Aeschbacher *et al.* (1984) discussed the risk evaluation of coffee based on *in vitro* and *in vivo* mutagenicity testing. While constituents of coffee are known to have mutagenic activity *in vitro*, it has also been demonstrated that these components can be metabolically deactivated in the presence of the liver microsomal enzyme system both *in vitro* and *in vivo*. This explains the negative results for coffee in a recent carcinogenicity bioassay in mice (Stalder *et al.*, 1984).

The potential genotoxicity of theobromine and cocoa powder has recently been reported by Brusick *et al.* (1986a,b) who found that the genotoxic potential of theobromine in some assays was qualitatively and quantitatively similar to caffeine but the levels of this methylxanthine found naturally in cocoa powder were devoid of mutagenic potential.

The carcinogenic potential of caffeine has prompted a great deal of research both in laboratory animals and in epidemiological studies. Curatolo and Robertson (1983) have carefully reviewed pertinent studies to evaluate the proposed association between coffee intake and malignancy. They concluded that there is no clear evidence that coffee consumption is even casually related to cancer of the bladder, urinary tract, ovary, kidney or pancreas.

Recent long-term animal studies have also evaluated the potential carcinogenicity of caffeine. Takayama and Kuwabara (1982) administered caffeine in drinking water for 78 weeks to Wistar rats and evaluated its tumorigenicity. No evidence of carcinogenicity was noted. Mohr et al. (1984) reported that long-term administration of caffeine in the drinking water of Sprague-Dawley rats did not enhance, promote or cause neoplasia. Similar observations had been reported by Brune et al. (1981). To date, only one long-term study has been reported on theobromine (S. Takayama, personal communication); the usefulness of this study is limited by the fact that it only encompassed a 78-week period of administration in drinking water, and it was further hampered because of the relative insolubility of theobromine in water.

There are also reports on the suppressive effects of tumor induction by caffeine. Denda et al. (1983) reported that high doses of caffeine following administration of 4-hydroxyaminoquinoline 1-oxide decreased pancreatic tumorigenesis in rats. Hosaka et al. (1984) demonstrated that the induction of hepatic tumors by 2-acetylaminofluorene in rats was suppressed by administration of caffeine. Finally, Allen et al. (1985) reported that caffeine enhanced the anti-tumor effects of the phleomycins PLM-CHP and PLM-PEP and Blenoxane in rats carrying Walker 256 carcinosarcoma and/or in mice carrying Ehrlich ascites tumor. While caffeine alone has no marked anti-tumor properties, the clinical significance of its enhancement of other anti-tumor agents on cytotoxicity of selected tumor cells needs to be pursued through additional research.

Respirogenic Action
The ability of methylxanthines to increase alveolar ventilation in experimental animals has been known for many years and it is not the intent of this review to cover the history of this pharmacological property. The clinical efficacy of methylxanthine preparations in the treatment of bronchial distress in asthmatics was first reported in 1922 by Dr. Samson Hirsch who rectally administered a mixture of theophylline and theobromine to a severe asthmatic and observed a bronchospasmolytic action (Schultze-Werninghaus and Meier-Sydow, 1982). This action was also confirmed in isolated bovine bronchial muscle and led to the conclusion by Hirsch that dimethylxanthines could be used prophylactically in a long-term treatment regimen of bronchial asthma.

Because of their efficacy in the treatment of neonatal apnea, theophylline and caffeine are the pharmacological agents of choice in the management and prevention of this condition. Aranda et al. (1981)

recently prepared an excellent review on the pharmacological considerations required in the therapy of neonatal apnea with theophylline and caffeine. The methylxanthines are well known for their varying degrees of ability to inhibit phosphodiesterase, and this property is most frequently cited for their efficacy in some physiological actions. Langercrantz *et al.* (1984), however, have postulated that the therapeutic effect of theophylline on neonatal apnea may be due to adenosine antagonism rather than via inhibition of phosphodiesterase. Their rationale for this hypothesis is that apnea is often triggered by hypoxemia and that adenosine released during hypoxia mediates this effect.

Recently, Simons *et al.* (1984) demonstrated that caffeine, theobromine and theophylline are all effective bronchodilators in children with asthma, and they recommended that ingestion of all methylxanthine-containing foods and medication be avoided in studies of anti-asthma drugs. They also speculated that caffeine and theobromine in any commonly available form might have temporary value as a bronchodilator in situations where prescribed anti-asthma medications are not readily available. This would entail a 50 kg patient ingesting three cups of brewed coffee, or two cups of strong cocoa, or ingesting two 4-ounce chocolate bars to get the appropriate methylxanthine dose. Thus, dietary methylxanthines can exert a positive potentiating bronchodilator effect in combination with therapeutic methylxanthines, and these sources could be considered in the treatment of asthmatics.

Gastrointestinal Effects

Early investigations on the effects of methylxanthines on gastric secretion concentrated on the role of acid production and the pathogenesis of ulcers after methylxanthine ingestion. Roth and Ivy (1944*a*,*b*) demonstrated that caffeine administered orally or parenterally was a potent stimulant of both the acid and pepsin content of gastric juice in the cat and in man. Roth *et al.* (1944) further related these observations to peptic ulcers in the cat and made recommendations including avoidance of caffeine and caffeine-containing beverages in the management of peptic ulcers. A moderate but statistically significant increase in the volume and acidity of gastric juice was reported following intravenously or orally administered aminophylline, glucophylline and theobromine by Steigmann *et al.* (1952), but no such changes were observed when these xanthines were given orally in solid form. Brady and Bayless (1975) demonstrated in the rat that the methylxanthines were potent intestinal secretagogues when administered intraluminally, and suggested they play a similar role in man. This hypothesis has never been fully investigated in man and thus the relationship is uncertain.

A frequent gastrointestinal symptom after the consumption of coffee is heartburn. Cohen (1980) suggested that coffee-induced gastrointestinal symptoms may result from reflux esophagitis, secondary to acid hypersecretion or to a less-than-normal increase in lower esophageal sphincter pressure. Price et al. (1978) in their studies of reflux esophagitis found that patients who experienced heartburn after infusion of 0·01N HCl into the esophagus also experienced heartburn after infusion of coffee. They suggested that coffee may be a direct non-specific esophageal irritant. An earlier study by Babka and Castell (1973) evaluated the effects of several foods and beverages on the lower esophageal sphincter muscle and the induction of heartburn. They found that whole milk (but not non-fat milk), orange and tomato juices and chocolate syrup produced decreases in sphincter pressure associated with symptomatic reflux in some subjects and that chocolate syrup (1·2% fat) produced the most dramatic effect. Since this is such a common problem, the definitive effects of suspect foods and beverages need to be thoroughly researched in order to ascertain what specific dietary component is responsible.

Cardiovascular and Circulatory Effects
The actions of the methylxanthines on the circulatory system are complex, with the effects dependent upon the conditions prevailing at the time of their administration and the dosage employed (Rall, 1985). These effects are also covered in reasonable detail elsewhere (Tarka, 1982).

Heart disease manifested as acute myocardial infarction is a risk often associated with coffee consumption. Curatolo and Robertson (1983) reviewed numerous retrospective and prospective studies on the consumption of coffee and the alleged increased risk of ischemic heart disease. Careful evaluation of the literature consistently failed to show a direct association between coffee intake and myocardial infarction and did not provide supportive evidence that coffee intake is a risk factor in this disease. Coffee and tea are known to increase the incidence of premature ventricular contraction and cardiac arrhythmias in susceptible individuals (Prineas et al., 1980). Dobmeyer et al. (1983) verified the arrhythmogenic effects of caffeine in normal volunteers and in patients with heart disease by determining cardiac electrophysiologic effects.

The relationship between methylxanthine consumption and lipid homeostasis is one that has great significance in light of the suggested correlation between serum cholesterol and coronary heart disease. The methylxanthines are thought to effect lipolysis by increasing cyclic AMP levels. This could occur by effectively blocking adenosine receptor sites resulting in metabolic changes in cyclic AMP levels, catecholamine levels and sympathetic nerve activity (Dews, 1984). Several rabbit and rodent studies with coffee, tea, cocoa, theophylline, caffeine and theobromine (Heyden *et al.*, 1969; Myasnikov, 1958; Cholerva, 1973; Woosley and Will, 1973; Akinyanju and Yudken, 1967; Fears, 1978; Tobin *et al.*, 1976; Johansson, 1981; Palm *et al.*, 1984; Salamatullah *et al.*, 1984; Yokogoshi *et al.*, 1983; Norihisma and Akira, 1981) have reported elevations in serum cholesterol and phospholipid levels. Generally, dietary methylxanthines and their food sources either reduced or had no effect on serum triglyceride levels.

There have been several prospective and retrospective studies where the effects of coffee and caffeine on lipid parameters were studied (Naismith *et al.*, 1969, 1970; Stullar and Pickler, 1976; Thelle *et al.*, 1983; Sherlow and Mathers, 1984; Little *et al.*, 1966; Phillips *et al.*, 1981; Klatsky *et al.*, 1985; Williams *et al.*, 1985; Thoragood and Mann, 1975; Lang *et al.*, 1983). The host of factors which must be taken into account in assessing effects of methylxanthines includes age, sex, adiposity, alcohol consumption, dietary habits, exercise, smoking habits, ethnicity, occupational stress, additives to caffeine-containing beverages and method of preparation. These factors all tend to confound the relationship of methylxanthines to coronary heart disease and may be the reason for the discrepancies between various studies.

The effect of prolonged caffeine administration on blood pressure in hypertensive subjects was evaluated in a double-blind placebo-controlled study by Robertson *et al.* (1984). The results of this study suggest that long-term caffeine use probably does not cause hypertension in the general population. Subjects with borderline hypertension have neither a greater susceptibility to the pressor effect of caffeine nor resistance to developing a tolerance to the drug that characteristically occurs with long-term use.

The effects of caffeine on the blood pressure and heart rate were also examined in 12 patients with autonomic failure (Onrot *et al.*, 1985). They concluded that caffeine was a pressor agent and attenuated postprandial hypotension in autonomic failure. In this respect caffeine may serve as a useful agent in the treatment of orthostatic hypotension due to autonomic failure.

Based on examination of the existing data, one can conclude that under normal conditions methylxanthines do not pose a threat in the development of coronary heart disease and need only be avoided by those diagnosed as being already at risk to coronary heart disease because of hypertension or elevated serum cholesterol or triglycerides.

SUMMARY

Caffeine is by far the most prevalent methylxanthine in our diet, with lesser amounts of theobromine consumed primarily through cocoa and chocolate sources. Although only a minor amount of theophylline is consumed via the diet, this compound is frequently ingested for therapeutic purposes. Because of the frequent exposure of humans to methylxanthines in food and beverages, as well as in drug formulations, the metabolism of these compounds is of significant interest. Recent studies have extensively defined the metabolism and kinetics of caffeine and theobromine in man and in various animal species employed in toxicological evaluations. The reduced ability of pregnant women and human neonates to eliminate caffeine and theophylline has also been well documented.

The acute toxicity of caffeine and theobromine has been thoroughly characterized in several animal species, including the rat. The most common cause of death was attributed to respiratory failure following convulsion. Dogs are more sensitive to the toxic effects of theobromine than other animal species, presumably due to their slower elimination rate. In humans, methylxanthine toxicity manifests itself as a disturbed state of consciousness, followed by convulsions, vomiting and coma. Death has been reported following ingestion of massive doses.

Neuroendocrine effects have been reported in rats primarily with caffeine at doses of 30 mg/kg or greater. Comparable effects have not been seen in humans, although the doses employed were much lower (5 mg/kg). Immunotoxicological effects have also occurred in rats and mice following high doses of caffeine, and some effects on white blood cells in humans have been observed after theophylline administration. Further neuro-endocrine and immunotoxicological studies are needed since these areas are relatively unexplored at the present time.

Although the diuretic properties of the methylxanthines have been known for decades, recent studies in man have shown increased urinary mineral excretion following caffeine administration. The clinical relevance of this finding has not been assessed to date.

Extensive reproductive studies in rats with caffeine and theobromine have reported toxic effects on the testes at high dietary levels (0·6%). In the case of theobromine, these effects were shown to be reversible. No specific effects on the female reproductive system have been demonstrated, although an overall maternal toxicity stress-like syndrome does occur after high doses.

Teratogenicity evaluations of the methylxanthines in rats and rabbits indicated a higher incidence of unossified sternebrae suggesting a retardation of the fetal calcification process. In pregnant women, while this effect has not been demonstrated, it is known that caffeine disposition is significantly impaired during the later stages of pregnancy. Because the consequences of this altered caffeine elimination could have deleterious effects on the fetus, it is advisable to caution pregnant women to maintain a moderate caffeine intake during their pregnancy.

Numerous studies have evaluated the role of methylxanthine in the occurrence of fibrocystic breast disease. While some reports suggested a regression of the disease following methylxanthine abstinence, others have found no effect. It is presently difficult to draw any firm conclusion between dietary methylxanthine intake and fibrocystic breast disease because of the high degree of waxing and waning of the disease, and the lack of well defined and consistent clinical and pathological criteria. The specific role of dietary methylxanthines in the onset and/or aggravation of fibrocystic breast disease continues to be a controversial area requiring future research.

Evidence continues to accumulate that behavioral differences exist between caffeine consumers and abstainers. These differences may be attributed to effects of methylxanthines at the adenosine receptor site, since ingestion of caffeine from dietary sources could potentially produce blood caffeine levels high enough to compete with endogenous adenosine at its receptor site.

While methylxanthines have been reported to exhibit mutagenic activity at high doses, the available data from these studies indicate that a potential health problem does not occur from the levels of methylxanthine ingested through dietary sources. The carcinogenic potential of caffeine has prompted a great deal of research both in laboratory animals and in epidemiological studies. At present, there is no clear evidence that caffeine or theobromine produces cancer either in experimental animals or in man.

Recent studies have demonstrated that caffeine, theobromine and theophylline are all effective bronchodilators in children with asthma. The dose levels of caffeine and theobromine which were investigated could be readily consumed in three cups of brewed coffee, two cups of strong cocoa or two 4-ounce chocolate bars. These results led the authors to recommend that dietary methylxanthines (caffeine and theobromine) should not be consumed in combination with therapeutic methylxanthines (theophylline) due to a possible potentiating bronchodilator action.

Ingestion of coffee has been frequently associated with heartburn, a gastrointestinal effect which may be due to reflux esophagitis following a reduction in lower esophageal sphincter pressure. Other foods/beverages such as whole milk, orange and tomato juices and chocolate syrup were also associated with decreased sphincter pressure and symptomatic reflux in experimental subjects. Since this is a common problem, the definitive effects of suspect foods/beverages should be thoroughly researched in order to ascertain what specific dietary component is responsible.

Finally, the relationship between methylxanthine consumption and lipid homeostasis is one of great significance in light of the suggested correlation between coronary heart disease and serum cholesterol and triglyceride concentrations. Based on existing data, one can conclude that, under normal conditions of consumption, methylxanthines from dietary sources do not pose a threat in the development of coronary heart disease and need only be avoided by those individuals diagnosed as having preexisting hypertension or elevated serum cholesterol or triglycerides.

REFERENCES

Aeschbacher, H. U., Meier, H., Ruch, E., Wolleb, U. and Wurzner, H. P. (1984). Risk evaluations of coffee based on *in vitro* and *in vivo* mutagenicity testing. In: *Coffee and Health*, Banbury Report 17, B. McMahon and T. Sugimura (Eds), Cold Spring Harbor Laboratory, Cold Spring Harbor, New York, pp. 89–98.

Akinyanju, P. and Yudken, J. (1967). Effect of coffee and tea on serum lipids in the rat. *Nature*, **214**, 426–7.

Aldridge, A. and Neims, A. H. (1979). The effects of phenobarbital and β-naphthoflavone on the elimination kinetics and metabolite pattern of caffeine in the beagle dog. *Drug Metab. Dispos.*, **7**, 378–82.

Aldridge, A., Parsons, W. D. and Neims, A. H. (1977). Stimulation of caffeine metabolism in the rat by 3-methylcholanthrene. *Life Sci.*, **21**, 967–74.

Aldridge, A., Aranda, J. V. and Neims, A. H. (1979). Caffeine metabolism in the newborn. *Clin. Pharmacol. Ther.*, **25**, 447–53.

Aldridge, A., Bailey, J. and Neims, A. H. (1981). The disposition of caffeine during and after pregnancy. *Semin. Perinatol.*, **5**, 310–4.

Allen, T. E., Aliano, N. A., Cowan, R. J., Grigg, G. W., Hart, N. K., Lamberton, J. A. and Lane, A. (1985). Amplification of the antitumor activity of phleomycins and bleomycins in rats and mice by caffeine. *Cancer Res.*, **45**, 2516–21.

Amiragova, M. G. (1962). Effect of caffeine and barbamyl on the secretory cycle of the thyroid gland. *Bull. Exp. Biol. Med.*, **54**, 763–6.

Aranda, J. V., Sitar, D. S., Parsons, W. D., Loughnan, P. M. and Neims, A. H.

(1976). Pharmacokinetic aspects of theophylline in premature newborns. *New Engl. J. Med.*, **295**, 413–6.

Aranda, J. V., Gorman, W., Outerbridge, E. W. and Neims, A. H. (1977). Pharmacokinetic disposition of caffeine in premature neonates with apnea. *Pediatr. Res.*, **11**, 414.

Aranda, J. V., Cook, C. E., Gorman, W., Collinge, J. M., Loughnan, P. M., Outerbridge, E. W., Aldridge, A. and Neims, A. H. (1979). Pharmacokinetic profile of caffeine in the premature newborn infant with apnea. *J. Pediatr.*, **94**, 663–8.

Aranda, J. V., Grondin, D. and Sasynuik, B. I. (1981). Pharmacologic considerations in the therapy of neonatal apnea. *Pediatr. Clin. North Am.*, **28**, 113–33.

Aranda, J. V., Scalais, E., Papageorgiou, A. and Beharry, K. (1984). Ontogeny of human caffeine and theophylline metabolism. *Dev. Pharmacol. Ther.*, 7, 18–25.

Arnaud, M. J. (1976). Identification, kinetic and quantitative study of [2-^{14}C]- and [1-Me-^{14}C]-caffeine metabolites in rat's urine by chromatographic separations. *Biochem. Med.*, **16**, 67–76.

Arnaud, M. J. (1985). Comparative metabolic disposition of [1-Me-^{14}C]caffeine in rats, mice, and Chinese hamsters. *Drug Metab. Dispos.*, **13**, 471–8.

Arnaud, M. J. and Welsch, C. (1979). Metabolic pathway of theobromine in the rat and identification of two new metabolites in human urine. *J. Agric. Food Chem.*, **27**, 524–7.

Arnaud, M. J., Bracco, I. and Welsch, C. (1982). Metabolism and distribution of labeled theophylline in the pregnant rat. Impairment of theophylline metabolism by pregnancy and absence of a blood-brain barrier in the fetus. *Pediatr. Res.*, **16**, 167–71.

Babka, J. C. and Castell, D. O. (1973). On the genesis of heartburn. The effects of specific foods on the lower esophageal sphincter. *Dig. Dis.*, **18**, 391–7.

Bada, H. S., Khanna, N. N., Somani, S. M. and Tin, A. A. (1979). Interconversion of theophylline and caffeine in newborn infants. *J. Pediatr.*, **94**, 993–5.

Baley, J. E., Ruuskanen, O., Miller, K. and Pittard, W. B. (1982). Effects of theophylline on the neonatal immune response. *Pediatr. Res.*, **16**, 649–52.

Banner, W., Jr. and Czajka, P. A. (1980). Acute caffeine overdose in the neonate. *Am. J. Dis. Child*, **134**, 495–8.

Black, D. J. G. and Barron, N. S. (1943). Observations on the feeding of a cacao waste product to poultry. *Vet. Rec.*, **55**, 166–7.

Blanchard, J. and Sawers, S. J. A. (1983). Comparative pharmacokinetics of caffeine in young and elderly men. *J. Pharmacokin. Biopharm.*, **11**, 109–26.

Blauch, J. L. and Tarka, S. M., Jr. (1983). HPLC determination of caffeine and theobromine in coffee, tea, and instant hot cocoa mixes. *J. Food Sci.*, **48**, 745–50.

Bliss, A. R. and Morrison, R. W. (1933). A comparative study of certain xanthine diuretics. *J. Lab. Clin. Med.*, **19**, 248–65.

Blumgart, H. L., Gilligan, D. R., Levy, R. C., Brown, M. G. and Volk, M. C. (1934). Action of diuretic drugs. 1. Action of diuretics in normal persons. *Arch. Int. Med.*, **54**, 40–81.

Bonati, M., Latini, R., Galletti, F., Young, J. F., Tognoni, G. and Garattini, S. (1982). Caffeine disposition after oral doses. *Clin. Pharmacol. Ther.*, **32**, 98–106.

Bonati, M., Latini, R., Sadurska, B., Riva, E., Galletti, F., Borzelleca, J. F.,

Tarka, S. M., Jr., Arnaud, M. J. and Garattini, S. (1984). Kinetics and metabolism of theobromine in male rats. *Toxicology*, **30**, 327–41.

Bory, C., Baltassat, P., Porthault, M., Bethenod, M., Frederich, A. and Aranda, J. V. (1979). Metabolism of theophylline to caffeine in premature newborn infants. *J. Pediatr.*, **94**, 988–93.

Boulenger, J. P., Patel, J. and Marangos, P. J. (1982). Effects of caffeine and theophylline on adenosine and benzodiazepine receptors in human brain. *Neurosci. Lett.*, **30**, 161–6.

Boutroy, M. J., Vert, P., Royer, R. J., Monin, P. and Royer-Morrot, M. J. (1979). Caffeine, a metabolite of theophylline during the treatment of apnea in the premature infant. *J. Pediatr.*, **94**, 996–8.

Boyd, E. M. (1960). The acute oral toxicity in guinea pigs of acetylsalicylic acid, phenacetin, and caffeine alone and combined. *Toxicol. Appl. Pharmacol.*, **2**, 23–32.

Boyd, E. M., Dolman, M., Knight, L. M. and Sheppard, E. P. (1965). The chronic oral toxicity of caffeine. *Can. J. Physiol. Pharmacol.*, **43**, 995–1007.

Boyle, C. A., Berkowitz, G. S., Li Volsi, V. A., Ort, S., Merino, M. J., White, C. and Kelsey, J. L. (1984). Caffeine consumption and fibrocystic breast disease: a case-control epidemiologic study. *J. Nat. Cancer Inst.*, **72**, 1015–9.

Brady, P. G. and Bayless, T. M. (1975). Methylxanthines induced small intestine secretion. *Johns Hopkins Med. J.*, **136**, 251–3.

Branfman, A. R., McComish, M. F., Bruni, R. J., Callahan, M. M., Robertson, R. and Yesair, D. W. (1983). Characterization of diaminouracil metabolites of caffeine in human urine. *Drug Metab. Dispos.*, **11**, 206–10.

Braude, R. (1943). Toxic effects in the feeding of cocoa meal to pigs. *Brit. Vet. J.*, **99**, 302–7.

Braude, R. and Foot, A. S. (1942). Cacao by-products in pig feeding. *Emp. J. Exp. Agric.*, **10**, 182–8.

Brune, H., Deutsch-Wenzel, R. P., Habr, M., Ivankovic, S. and Schmähl, D. (1981). Investigations of the tumorigenic response to benzo(a)pyrene in aqueous caffeine solutions applied orally to Sprague-Dawley rats. *J. Cancer Res. Clin. Oncol.*, **102**, 153–7.

Bruns, R. D., Daly, J. W. and Snyder, S. H. (1980). Adenosine receptors in brain membranes: binding of N^6-cyclohexyl-(^{3}H)-adenosine and 1,3-diethyl-8-(^{3}H)-phenylxanthine. *Proc. Nat. Acad. Sci.*, **77**, 5547–51.

Brusick, D., Myhr, B., Galloway, S., Rundell, J., Jagannath, D. R. and Tarka, S. M., Jr. (1986a). Genotoxicity of theobromine in a series of short-term assays. *Mutat. Res.*, **169**, 105–14.

Brusick, D., Myhr, B., Galloway, S., Rundell, J., Jagannath, D. R. and Tarka, S. M., Jr. (1986b). Genotoxicity of cocoa in a series of short-term assays. *Mutat. Res.*, **169**, 115–21.

Burg, A. W. (1975). How much caffeine in the cup? *Tea Coffee Trade J.*, **147**, 40–2, 88. ✳

Burg, A. W. and Stein, M. E. (1972). Urinary excretion of caffeine and its metabolites in the mouse. *Biochem. Pharmacol.*, **21**, 909–22.

Burg, A. W., Burrows, R. and Kensler, C. J. (1974). Unusual metabolism of caffeine in the squirrel monkey. *Toxicol. Appl. Pharmacol.*, **28**, 162–6.

Butcher, R. (1984). Theories and mechanisms of breast disease. *Proc. Fifth Int.*

ILSI Caffeine Workshop, Cancun, Mexico, 17–21 June.

Butcher, R. E., Vorhees, C. V. and Wootten, V. (1984). Behavioral and physical development of rats chronically exposed to caffeinated fluids. *Fund. Appl. Toxicol.*, **4**, 1–13.

Caldwell, J., Lancaster, R., Monks, T. J. and Smith, R. L. (1977). The influence of dietary methylxanthines on the metabolism and pharmacokinetics of intra-venously administered theophylline. *Brit. J. Clin. Pharmacol.*, **4**, 637–8.

Caldwell, J., O'Gorman, J. and Adamson, R. H. (1981). Urinary metabolites of caffeine in the chimpanzee, rhesus monkey, and galago. *Pharmacologist*, **23**, 212.

Callahan, M. M., Robertson, R. S., Arnaud, M. J., Branfman, A. R., McComish, M. F. and Yesair, D. W. (1982). Human metabolism of [1-methyl-^{14}C]- and [2-^{14}C]-caffeine after oral administration. *Drug Metab. Dispos.*, **10**, 417–23.

Callahan, M. M., Robertson, R. S., Branfman, A. R., McComish, M. F. and Yesair, D. W. (1983). Comparison of caffeine metabolism in three nonsmoking populations after oral administration of radiolabeled caffeine. *Drug Metab. Dispos.*, **11**, 211–7.

Cholerva, J. (1973). Morphological studies on the influence of caffeine on experi-mental coronary cholesterol atherosclerosis in rabbits. *Mater. Med. Pol.*, **5**, 235–8.

Christensen, H. D., Manion, C. V. and Kling, O. R. (1981). Caffeine kinetics during late pregnancy. In: *Drug Metabolism in the Immature Human*, L. F. Soyka and F. P. Redmond (Eds), Raven Press, New York, pp. 163–81.

Clough, G. W. (1942). Theobromine poisoning in the dog. *Vet. J.*, **74**, 196–7.

Clozel, M., Branchaud, C. L., Tannenbaum, G. S., Dussault, J. H. and Aranda, J. V. (1983). Effect of caffeine on thyroid and pituitary function in newborn rats. *Pediatr. Res.*, **17**, 592–5.

Cohen, S. (1980). Pathogenesis of coffee-induced GI symptoms. *New Engl. J. Med.*, **303**, 122–4.

Colin, A. A., Kraiem, Z., Kahana, L. and Hochberg, Z. (1984). Effect of theo-phylline on urinary excretions of cyclic AMP, calcium, and phosphorus in normal subjects. *Min. Electrol. Metab.*, **10**, 359–61.

Collins, T. F. X. (1979). Review of reproduction and teratology studies of caffeine. *FDA By-Lines*, **9**, 352–73.

Collins, T. F. X., Welsh, J. J., Black, T. N. and Collins, E. V. (1981). A study of the teratogenic potential of caffeine given by oral intubation to rats. *Regul. Toxicol. Pharmacol.*, **1**, 355–78.

Collins, T. F. X., Welsh, J. J., Black, T. N. and Ruggles, D. I. (1983). A study of the teratogenic potential of caffeine ingested in drinking water. *Food Chem. Toxicol.*, **21**, 763–7.

Cornish, H. H. and Christman, A. A. (1957). A study of the metabolism of theobromine, theophylline, and caffeine in man. *J. Biol. Chem.*, **228**, 315–23.

Curatolo, P. W. and Robertson, D. (1983). The health consequences of caffeine. *Am. Int. Med.*, **98**, 641–53.

Dahlback, M., Heintz, L., Ryrfeldt, A., Stenberg, K. (1984). Toxic effects of some xanthine derivatives with special emphasis on adverse effects on the rat testis. *Toxicology*, **32**, 23–35.

Daly, J. W., Bruns, R. F. and Snyder, S. H. (1981). Adenosine receptors in the central nervous system: relationship to the central action of methylxanthines.

Life Sci., **28**, 2083–97.

Decker, R. A. and Myers, G. H. (1972). Theobromine poisoning in a dog. *J. Am. Vet. Assoc.*, **161**, 198–9.

Denda, A., Yokose, Y., Emi, Y., Murata, Y., Ohara, T., Sunagawa, M., Mikami, S., Takahashi, S. and Konishi, Y. (1983). Effects of caffeine on pancreatic tumorigenesis by 4-hydroxyaminoquinoline 1-oxide in partially pancreatectomized rats. *Carcinogenesis*, **4**, 17–22.

Denenberg, V. H., Zeidner, L. P., Thoman, E. B., Kramer, P., Rowe, J. C., Philipps, A. F. and Raye, J. R. (1982). Effects of theophylline on behavioral state development in the newborn rabbit. *J. Pharmacol. Exp. Ther.*, **221**, 604–8.

Dews, P. B. (1984). *Caffeine*, Springer-Verlag, New York.

Dimaio, V. J. M. and Garriott, J. C. (1974). Lethal caffeine poisoning in a child. *Forensic Sci.*, **3**, 275–8.

Dobmeyer, D. J., Stine, R. A., Leier, C. V., Greenburg, R. and Schaal, S. F. (1983). The arrhythmogenic effects of caffeine in human beings. *New Engl. J. Med.*, **308**, 814–6.

Dorfman, L. J. and Jarvik, M. E. (1970) Comparative stimulant and diuretic actions of caffeine and theobromine in man. *Clin. Pharmacol. Ther.*, **11**, 869–72.

Drouillard, D. D., Vesell, E. S. and Dvorchik, B. H. (1978). Studies on theobromine disposition in normal subjects. *Clin. Pharmacol. Ther.*, **23**, 296–302.

Dunlop, M. and Court, J. M. (1981). Effect of maternal caffeine ingestion on neonatal growth in rats. *Biol. Neonat.*, **39**, 178–84.

Elmazar, M. M. A., McElhatton, P. R. and Sullivan, F. M. (1981). Acute studies to investigate the mechanism of action of caffeine as a teratogen in mice. *Human Toxicol.*, **1**, 53–63.

Elmazar, M. M. A., McElhatton, P. R. and Sullivan, F. M. (1982). Studies on the effects of different oral preparations of caffeine in mice. *Toxicology*, **23**, 57–71.

Ernster, V. L., Mason, L., Goodson, W. H., III, Sickles, E. A., Sacks, S. T., Selvin, S., Dupey, M. E., Hawkinson, J. and Hunt, T. K. (1982). Effect of caffeine-free diet on benign breast disease: a randomized trial. *Surgery*, **91**, 263–7.

Fears, R. (1978). The hypercholesterolemic effect of caffeine in rats fed on diets with and without supplementary cholesterol. *Brit. J. Nutr.*, **39**, 363–4.

Ferrero, J. L. and Neims, A. H. (1983). Metabolism of caffeine by mouse liver microsomes: GSH or cytosol causes a shift in products from 1,3,7-trimethylurate to a substituted diaminouracil. *Life Sci.*, **33**, 1173–8.

Fredholm, B. B. (1980). Are methylxanthine effects due to antagonism of endogenous adenosine? *Trends Pharmacol. Sci.*, **1**, 129–32.

Fredholm, B. B. and Persson, G. A. (1982). Xanthine derivatives as adenosine receptor antagonists. *Eur. J. Pharmacol.*, **81**, 673–6.

Friedman, L., Weinberger, M. A., Farber, T. M., Moreland, F. M., Peters, E. L., Gilmore, C. E. and Khan, M. A. (1979). Testicular atrophy and impaired spermatogenesis in rats fed high levels of the methylxanthines caffeine, theobromine, or theophylline. *J. Envir. Pathol. Toxicol.*, **2**, 687–706.

Gans, J. H. (1982). Dietary influences on theobromine-induced toxicity in rats. *Toxicol. Appl. Pharmacol.*, **63**, 312–20.

Gans, J. H. (1984). Comparative toxicities of dietary caffeine and theobromine in the rat. *Biochem. Toxicol.*, **22**, 365–9.

Gans, J. H., Korson, R., Cater, M. R. and Ackerly, C. C. (1980). Effects of short-term and long-term theobromine administration to male dogs. *Toxicol. Appl. Pharmacol.*, **53**, 481–96.

Garattini, S., Bonati, M. and Latini, R. (1982). Caffeine kinetics and metabolism in several animal species. *Proc. Fourth Int. Caffeine Workshop*, Athens, Greece, 17–21 October.

Geber, W. F., Lefkowitz, S. S. and Hung, C. Y. (1975). Effect of ascorbic acid, sodium salicylate, and caffeine on the serum interferon level in response to viral infection. *Pharmacology*, **13**, 228–33.

Giacoia, G., Jusko, W. J., Menke, J. and Koup, J. R. (1976). Theophylline pharmacokinetics in premature infants with apnea. *J. Pediatr.*, **89**, 829–32.

Gilbert, R. M., Marshman, J. A., Schwieder, M. and Berg, R. (1976). Caffeine content of beverages as consumed. *Can. Med. Assoc. J.*, **114**, 205–8.

Gilbert, S. G., Stavric, B., Klassen, R. D. and Rice, D. C. (1985). The fate of chronically consumed caffeine in the monkey (Macaca fascicularis). *Fund. Appl. Toxicol.*, **5**, 578–87.

Graham, D. M. (1978). Caffeine—its identity, dietary sources, intake, and biological effects. *Nutr. Rev.*, **36**, 97–102.

Grant, D. M., Tang, B. K. and Kalow, W. (1983a). Variability in caffeine metabolism. *Clin. Pharmacol. Ther.*, **33**, 591–602.

Grant, D. M., Tang, B. K. and Kalow, W. (1983b). Polymorphic N-acetylation of a caffeine metabolite. *Clin. Pharmacol. Ther.*, **33**, 355–9.

Grygiel, J. J. and Birkett, D. J. (1980). Effect of age on patterns of theophylline metabolism. *Clin. Pharmacol. Ther.*, **28**, 456–62.

Heaney, R. P. and Recker, R. R. (1982). Effects of nitrogen, phosphorus and caffeine on calcium balance in women. *J. Lab. Clin. Med.*, **99**, 46–55.

Heyden, S. and Muhlbaier, L. H. (1984). Prospective study of 'fibrocystic breast disease' and caffeine consumption. *Surgery*, **96**, 479–83.

Heyden, M. D., DeMaria, W., Johnston, W. W. and O'Fallon, W. M. (1969). Caffeine effects on cholesterol and development of aortic and coronary atherosclerosis in rabbits. *J. Chron. Dis.*, **21**, 677–85.

Hilligoss, D. M., Jusko, W. J., Koup, J. R. and Giacoia, G. (1980). Factors affecting theophylline pharmacokinetics in premature infants with apnea. *Dev. Pharmacol. Ther.*, **1**, 6–15.

Hindi-Alexander, M. C., Zielezny, M. A., Montes, N., Bullough, B., Middleton, E., Rosner, D. H. and London, W. M. (1985). Theophylline and fibrocystic breast disease. *J. Allergy Clin. Immunol.*, **75**, 709–15.

Hollingbery, P. W., Bergman, E. A. and Massey, L. K. (1985). Effect of dietary caffeine and aspirin on urinary calcium and hydroxyproline excretion in pre- and post-menopausal women. *Fed. Proc.*, **44**, 1149.

Holloway, W. R., Jr. and Thor, D. H. (1982). Caffeine sensitivity in the neonatal rat. *Neurobehav. Toxicol. Teratol.*, **4**, 331–3.

Holtzman, S. G. (1983). Complete, reversible, drug-specific tolerance to stimulation of locomotor activity by caffeine. *Life Sci.*, **33**, 779–87.

Hosaka, S., Nagayama, H. and Hirono, I. (1984). Suppressive effect of caffeine in the development of hepatic tumors induced by 2-acetylaminofluorene in ACI rats. *Gann*, **75**, 1058–61.

Hoskam, E. G. and Haagsma, J. (1974). Chocolate poisoning in two dachshunds terminating fatally. *Tijdschr. Diergeneeskd.*, **99**, 523–5.

Huang, K. C., King, N. B. and Genazzani, E. (1958). Effect of xanthine diuretics on renal tubular transport of PABA. *Am. J. Physiol.*, **192**, 373–8.

Johansson, S. (1981). Cardiovascular lesions in Sprague-Dawley rats induced by long-term treatment with caffeine. *Acta Pathol. Microbiol. Scand.*, **89**, 185–91.

Jokela, S. and Vartiainen, J. (1959). Caffeine poisoning. *Acta. Pharmacol. Toxicol.*, **15**, 331–4.

Kaplan, E., Holmes, J. H. and Sapeika, N. (1974). Caffeine content of tea and coffee. *S. African J. Nutr.*, **10**, 32–3.

Khanna, K. L., Rao, G. S. and Cornish, H. H. (1972). Metabolism of caffeine-^{3}H in the rat. *Toxicol. Appl. Pharmacol.*, **23**, 720–30.

Kisskalt, K. (1915). Über die Beziehungen der tödlichen Dosis zur Oberfläche. *Biochem. Z.*, **71**, 468–80.

Klatsky, A. L., Petitti, D. B., Armstrong, M. and Friedman, G. D. (1985). Coffee, tea and cholesterol. *Am. J. Cardiol.*, **55**, 577–8.

Knutti, R., Rothweiler, H. and Schlatter, C. (1981). Effect of pregnancy on the pharmacokinetics of caffeine. *Eur. J. Clin. Pharmacol.*, **21**, 121–6.

Kurppa, K., Holmberg, P. C., Kuosma, E. and Saxén, L. (1982). Coffee consumption during pregnancy. *New Engl. J. Med.*, **306**, 1548.

Lang, T., Degoulet, P., Aime, F., Fouriaud, C., Jacquinet-Salord, M., Laprugne, J., Main, J., Oeconomos, J., Phalente, J. and Prades, A. (1983). Relationship between coffee drinking and blood pressure: analysis of 6321 subjects in the Paris region. *Am. J. Cardiol.*, **52**, 1238–42.

Langercrantz, H., Yamamoto, Y., Fredholm, B. B., Prabhakar, N. R. and von Euler, C. (1984). Adenosine analogues depress ventilation in rabbit neonates. Theophylline stimulation of respiration via adenosine receptors. *Pediatr. Res.*, **18**, 387–90.

Latini, R., Bonati, M., Castelli, D. and Garattini, S. (1978). Dose-dependent kinetics of caffeine in rats. *Toxicol. Lett.*, **2**, 267–70.

Latini, R., Bonati, M., Marzi, E. and Garattini, S. (1980). Caffeine disposition and effects in young and one year old rats. *J. Pharm. Pharmacol.*, **32**, 596–9.

Latini, R., Bonati, M., Marzi, E. and Garattini, S. (1981). Urinary excretion of a uracilic metabolite from caffeine by rat, monkey, and man. *Toxicol. Lett.*, **7**, 267–72.

Latini, R., Bonati, M., Gaspari, F., Traina, G. L., Jiritano, L., Bortolotti, A., Borzelleca, J. F., Tarka, S. M., Jr., Arnaud, M. J. and Garattini, S. (1984). Kinetics and metabolism of theobromine in male and female pregnant and nonpregnant rabbits. *Toxicology*, **30**, 343–54.

La Vecchia, C., Franceschi, S., Parazzini, F., Regallo, M., Decarli, A., Gallus, G., Di Pietro, S. and Tognoni, G. (1985). Benign breast disease and consumption of beverages containing methylxanthines. *J. Nat. Cancer Inst.*, **74**, 995–1000.

Lawson, D. H., Jick, H. and Rothman, K. J. (1981). Coffee and tea consumption and breast disease. *Surgery*, **90**, 801–3.

Lemann, J., Adams, N. D. and Gray, R. W. (1979). Urinary calcium excretion in human beings. *New Eng. J. Med.*, **301**, 535–41.

Linn, S., Schoenbaum, S. C., Monson, R. R., Rosner, B., Stubblefield, P. G. and Ryan, K. J. (1982). No association between coffee consumption and adverse outcomes of pregnancy. *New Engl. J. Med.*, **306**, 141–5.

Little, J. A., Shanoff, H. M., Csima, A. and Yano, R. (1966). Coffee and serum lipids in coronary heart disease. *Lancet*, **1**, 732–4.

Lloyd, H. G. E. and Stone, T. W. (1981). Chronic methylxanthine treatment in rats: a comparison of Wistar and Fischer 344 strains. *Pharmacol. Biochem. Behav.*, **14**, 827–30.

Love, S. M., Gelman, R. S. and Silen, W. (1982). Fibrocystic 'disease' of the breast—a nondisease? *New Engl. J. Med.*, **307**, 1010–4.

Lubin, F., Ron, E., Wax, Y., Black, M., Funaro, M. and Shitrit, A. (1985). A case-control study of caffeine and methylxanthines in benign breast disease. *J. Amer. Med. Assoc.*, **253**, 2388–92.

McColl, J. D., Parker, J. M. and Ferguson, J. K. W. (1955). A comparison of the relative toxic, emetic, and convulsive actions of a series of methylated xanthine derivatives. *J. Pharmacol. Exp. Ther.*, **116**, 343–50.

McColl, J. D., Parker, J. M. and Ferguson, J. K. (1956). Evaluation of some 1- and 7-substituted methylated xanthines as diuretics in the rat. *J. Pharmacol. Exp. Ther.*, **118**, 162–7.

McGee, M. B. (1980). Caffeine poisoning in a 19-year-old female. *J. Forensic Sci.*, **25**, 29–32.

Marshall, J., Graham, S. and Swanson, M. (1982). Caffeine consumption and benign breast disease: a case-control comparison. *Am. J. Public Health*, **72**, 1015–9.

Martin, J. C. (1982). An overview: maternal nicotine and caffeine consumption and offspring outcome. *Neurobehavioral Toxicol. Teratol.*, **4**, 421–7.

Massey, L. K. and Berg, T. (1985). Effect of dietary caffeine on urinary mineral excretion in healthy males. *Fed. Proc.*, **44**, 1149.

Massey, L. K. and Wise, K. J. (1984). The effect of dietary caffeine on urinary excretion of calcium, magnesium, sodium, and potassium in healthy young females. *Nutr. Res.*, **4**, 43–50.

Meliska, C. J. and Brown, R. E. (1982). Effects of caffeine on schedule-controlled responding in the rat. *Pharmacol. Biochem. Behav.*, **16**, 745–50.

Miller, G. E., Radulovic, L. L., Dewit, R. H., Brabec, M. J., Tarka, S. M., Jr. and Cornish, H. H. (1984). Comparative theobromine metabolism in five mammalian species. *Drug. Metab. Dispos.*, **12**, 154–60.

Miners, J. O., Attwood, J. and Birkett, D. J. (1982). Theobromine metabolism in man. *Drug Metab. Dispos.*, **10**, 672–5.

Minton, J. P., Foecking, M. K., Webster, D. J. and Matthews, R. H. (1979). Caffeine, cyclic nucleotides, and breast disease. *Surgery*, **86**, 105–9.

Minton, J. P., Abou-Issa, H., Reicher, N. and Roseman, J. M. (1981a). Clinical and biochemical studies on methylxanthine-related fibrocystic breast disease. *Surgery*, **90**, 299–304.

Minton, J. P., Abou-Issa, H., Elliot, J. B., Foecking, M. K., Roseman, J. M. and Matthews, R. H. (1981b). Biochemical subgrouping of benign breast disease to define premalignant potential. *Surgery*, **90**, 652–6.

Mohr, V., Althoff, J., Ketkar, M. B. and Conradt, P. (1984). The influence of caffeine on tumor incidence in Sprague-Dawley rats. *Food Chem. Toxicol.*, **22**, 377–82.

Monks, T. J., Caldwell, J. and Smith, R. L. (1979). Influence of methylxanthine-containing foods on theophylline metabolism and kinetics. *Clin. Pharmacol. Ther.*, **26**, 513–24.

Monks, T. J., Lawrie, C. A. and Caldwell, J. (1981). The effect of increased caffeine intake on the metabolism and pharmacokinetics of theophylline in man. *Biopharm. Drug Dispos.*, **2**, 31–7.

Morgan, K. J., Stults, V. J. and Zabik, M. E. (1982). Amount and dietary sources of caffeine and saccharin intake by individuals aged 5 to 18 years. *Regul. Toxicol. Pharmacol.*, **2**, 295–307.

Myasnikov, A. L. (1958). Influence of some factors on development of experimental cholesterol atherosclerosis. *Circulation*, **17**, 99–113.

Naismith, D. J., Akinyanju, P. A. and Yudken, J. (1969). The influence of coffee drinking on plasma lipids and fasting blood glucose in healthy human volunteers. *Proc. Nutr. Soc.*, **28**, 12A.

Naismith, D. J., Akinyanju, P. A., Szanto, S. and Yudken, J. (1970). The effect in volunteers of coffee and decaffeinated coffee on blood glucose, insulin, plasma lipids, and some factors involved in blood clotting. *Nutr. Metab.*, **12**, 144–51.

Nolen, G. A. (1981). The effect of brewed and instant coffee on reproduction and teratogenesis in the rat. *Toxicol. Appl. Pharmacol.*, **58**, 171–83.

Nolen, G. A. (1982). A reproduction/teratology study of brewed and instant decaffeinated coffees. *J. Toxicol. Environ. Health*, **10**, 769–83.

Norihisma, K. and Akira, Y. (1981). Effects of various dietary xenobiotics on serum total cholesterol and high density lipoprotein cholesterol in rats. *Nutr. Rep. Int.*, **23**, 825–31.

Odenheimer, D. J., Zunzunegui, M. V., King, M. C., Shipler, C. P. and Friedman, G. D. (1984). Risk factors for benign breast disease: a case-control study of discordant twins. *Am. J. Epidemiol.*, **120**, 565–71.

Onrot, J., Goldberg, M. R., Biaggioni, I., Hollister, A. S., Kincaid, D. and Robertson, D. (1985). Hemodynamic and humoral effects of caffeine in autonomic failure: therapeutic implications for postprandial hypotension. *New Engl. J. Med.*, **313**, 549–54.

Palm, P. E., Arnold, E. P., Nick, M. S., Valentine, J. R. and Doerfler, T. E. (1984). Two-year toxicity/carcinogenicity study of fresh-brewed coffee in rats initially exposed in utero. *Toxicol. Appl. Pharmacol.*, **74**, 364–82.

Pardi, R., Zocchi, M. R., Ferrero, E., Ciboddo, G. F., Inverardi, L. and Rugarli, C. (1984). *In vivo* effects of a single infusion of theophylline on human peripheral blood lymphocytes. *Clin. Exp. Immunol.*, **57**, 722–8.

Parsons, W. D. and Neims, A. H. (1981). Prolonged half-life of caffeine in healthy term newborn infants. *J. Pediatr.*, **98**, 640–1.

Parsons, W. D. and Pelletier, J. G. (1982). Delayed elimination of caffeine by women in the last two weeks of pregnancy. *Can. Med. Assoc. J.*, **127**, 377–80.

Parsons, W. D., Aranda, J. V. and Neims, A. H. (1976). Elimination of transplacentally acquired caffeine in full-term neonates. *Pediatr. Res.*, **10**, 333.

Peters, J. M. (1967). Factors affecting caffeine toxicity: a review of the literature. *J. Clin. Pharmacol.*, **7**, 131–41.

Peters, J. M. and Boyd, E. M. (1967). The influence of sex and age in albino rats given a daily oral dose of caffeine at a high dose level. *Can. J. Physiol. Pharmacol.*, **45**, 305–11.

Peytremann, A., Nicholson, W. E., Liddle, G. W., Hardman, J. G. and Sutherland, E. W. (1973). Effects of methylxanthines on adenosine $3',5'$-monophosphate and corticosterone in the rat adrenal. *Endocrinology*, **92**, 525–30.

Phillips, N. R., Havel, R. J. and Kane, J. P. (1981). Levels and interrelationships of serum and lipoprotein cholesterol and triglycerides; association with adiposity and the consumption of ethanol, tobacco, and beverages containing caffeine. *Arteriosclerosis*, **1**, 13–24.

Poe, C. F. and Johnson, C. C. (1953). Toxicity of caffeine, theobromine and theophylline. *Acta Pharmacol. Toxicol.*, **9**, 267–74.

Price, S. F., Smithson, K. W. and Castell, D. O. (1978). Food sensitivity in reflux esophagitis. *Gastroenterology*, **75**, 240–3.

Prineas, R. J., Jacobs, D. R., Jr., Crow, R. S. and Blackburn, H. (1980). Coffee, tea, and VPB. *J. Chronic Dis.*, **33**, 67–72.

Rall, T. W. (1985). Central nervous system stimulants: the xanthines. In: *The Pharmacological Basis of Therapeutics*, A. G. Gilman, L. S. Goodman, T. W. Rall and F. Murad (Eds), 7th edn, Macmillan Publishing Co., New York, pp. 589–603.

Rao, G. S., Khanna, K. L. and Cornish, H. H. (1973). Identification of two new metabolites of caffeine in rat urine. *Experientia*, **19**, 953–5.

Roberts, H. R. and Barone, J. J. (1983). Biological effects of caffeine. *Food Technol.*, **37**, 32–9.

Robertson, D., Hollister, A. S., Kincaid, D., Workman, R., Goldberg, M. R., Tung, C. S. and Smith, B. (1984). Caffeine and hypertension. *Am. J. Med.*, **77**, 54–60.

Rosenberg, L., Mitchell, A. A., Shapiro, S. and Slone, D. (1982). Selected birth defects in relation to caffeine-containing beverages. *J. Amer. Med. Assoc.*, **247**, 1429–32.

Roth, J. A. and Ivy, A. C. (1944*a*). The effect of caffeine upon gastric secretion in the dog, cat, and man. *Am. J. Physiol.*, **141**, 455–61.

Roth, J. A. and Ivy, A. C. (1944*b*). The experimental production of acute and subacute gastric ulcers in cats by intramuscular injection of caffeine in beeswax. *Gastroenterology*, **2**, 274–85.

Roth, J. A., Ivy, A. C. and Atkinson, A. J. (1944). Caffeine and peptic ulcer: relation of caffeine and caffeine-containing beverages to the pathogenesis, diagnosis, and management of peptic ulcer. *J. Amer. Med. Assoc.*, **126**, 814–20.

Salamatullah, Q., Masahiro, T., Hidahiko, Y. and Akira, Y. (1984). Effects of dietary PCB and caffeine on serum and liver lipids and urin..ry ascorbic acid in rats after different times. *Agric. Biol. Chem.*, **40**, 1581–6.

Salant, W. and Rieger, J. B. (1912). *The Toxicity of Caffeine* (an experimental study of different species of animals). Bulletin No. 148, US Department of Agriculture, Bureau of Chemistry, pp. 5–98.

Sawyer, D. A., Julia, H. L. and Turin, A. C. (1982). Caffeine and human behavior: arousal, anxiety, and performance effects. *J. Behav. Med.*, **5**, 415–39.

Saxena, A. K., Singh, K. P., Srivastava, S. N., Khanna, S., Shukla, L. J. and Shanker, R. (1984). Immunomodulating effects of caffeine (1,3,7-trimethyl-xanthine) in rodents. *Indian J. Exp. Biol.*, **22**, 298–301.

Scalais, E., Papageorgiou, A. and Aranda, J. V. (1983). Biotransformation of theophylline during the first six weeks of life. *Pediatr. Res.*, **17**, 155A.

Scammell, J. G. and Fregly, M. J. (1982). Effect of theophylline on thyroid status in the rat. *Pharmacology*, **25**, 160–9.

Schardein, J. L. (1976). *Drugs as Teratogens*, CRC Press, Cleveland, Ohio, pp. 217–9.

Chapter 12

USE AND SAFETY OF NOVEL FOODS

A. E. BENDER

Fetcham, Surrey, UK

INTRODUCTION

The definition of a novel food cannot be precise since the degree of novelty can range from so small a change as a new cultivar or the temperature of processing to an entirely new food or process. The most recent official definition (DHSS, 1980) is: 'produced from raw material which has not hitherto been used for human consumption or which has been consumed in only small amounts, or produced by new or extensively modified processes not previously used in the production of food'. The Institute of Food Science and Technology (1975) provided a definition, repeated in 1983, namely: 'foods which have not previously formed a part of human diets or are made by novel processes for which there is no previous experience to draw on'.

It seems to be generally accepted that established foods are safe, which may not be true, and that if a food is already consumed in quantity in one part of the world it may be safely introduced elsewhere. The disease of favism shows that this is also not true. Favism is acute haemolytic anaemia caused by eating broad beans in people who are genetically deficient in the red cell enzyme glucose-6-phosphate dehydrogenase. The genetic defect is common in Mediterranean and Middle East countries and rare or virtually absent in north European countries. So the definition of novel foods should include the phrase 'not hitherto eaten in the region in question'.

The amount consumed is also of importance since food ingredients such as yeasts and moulds have long been ingested in small amounts but would not be readily recommended in large amounts.

An early proposed novel food was 'food yeast', *Torulopsis utilis*, grown on molasses and intended in the 1940s as a protein-rich food supplement (MRC, 1945). It would appear that the investigators proceeded directly to human feeding trials, and the literature contains several conflicting conclusions. These range from safe consumption of 85–110 g per day to reports of digestive disturbances following the consumption of as little as 3 g per day. The cause of these diverse findings has not been explained but it was suggested some years later that the ill-effects may have been caused by residues of the anti-foaming agent used at that time in the growth of the yeast culture rather than by the yeast itself.

From the time of the establishment of the Food and Agriculture Organisation far more attention was paid to food in many regions of the world and to the so-called 'protein gap'. It was thought that, while carbohydrate could be fairly readily produced, protein sources were not so easy, and it did not seem to be realised that by far the greater part of man's protein supplies comes from plant foods. Another reason for emphasis on proteins was the problem of infant feeding, particularly weaning from breast milk to suitable foods. In many parts of the world it was said that such suitable foods were not available whereas later experience showed that foods were available but little used. One difficult problem was caused by maize which absorbs so much water that the energy density of maize gruel is too low for infant feeding. Apart from this problem there was little evidence, limited to certain regions, that infants were short of protein as such, i.e. obtaining enough energy but not enough protein.

Emphasis on 'world shortage of protein' led to the development of a large number of novel foods intended as sources of protein. These varied from making waste materials such as oilseed residues suitable for human food to growing or collecting algae and plankton. For the purposes of discussion, they can be classed into five groups: synthetic foods, substitute foods, use of primary sources, use of non-food resources, and growth of

TABLE 1
Classification of Novel Foods

Type	Examples
Synthetic	Fats (but more easily produced by traditional methods)
	Vitamins
	Amino acids
Substitute foods	Textured vegetable proteins
	Fabricated enriched rice and wheat grains
	Milk substitute
Primary foods	Mycoprotein
	Leaf protein
	Plankton
	Krill
Non-food sources	Sugars from sawdust and waste paper pulp
	Protein from wool
Microbiological group	Yeasts
	Moulds
	Algae
	Bacteria
Upgrading	Oilseed residues
	Fish meal
	Plant waste and residues
	Seaweed
'New' plants	Marama bean
	Leucaena
	Yam bean
	Grain amaranth
	Ye-eb

microorganisms, together with the upgrading of materials hitherto regarded as animal feedstuffs (Table 1).

Most of these were based on sound scientific principles and most have been a failure. There are two basic problems. First, people want food not powders, and food of the type that they have been used to eating, not something new. Secondly, especially where infant foods are involved, those who need them cannot afford them, and those who can afford them usually do not need them.

Fish meal epitomises some of the major problems. In the late 1940s fish-house waste and small, bony fish unsuitable for human consumption were used as animal feed and were plentiful and cheap. The problem was to prepare them hygienically and to remove the unwanted parts and the unpleasant smell and taste. Enormous efforts were devoted to these ends, including numerous expensive biological assays of protein quality, since the preparations were thought of in terms of protein. It took some 20 years to achieve a product suitable in all respects—except price. Fish protein concentrate, as it came to be called, was prepared as a white odourless and tasteless powder but, apart from the fact that powders have no appeal until they are made into desirable foods, the price increased in proportion to the effort devoted to the problem until, when it did become available, it approached that of good-quality meat. Expectations of shortages and high prices for meat were not fulfilled and the major objection, that people want the type of food they are used to eating, remained. So hardly any of these brave hopes have been fulfilled.

Numerous problems were encountered and overcome in laboratory trials, such as the presence of toxic substances in the starting material (e.g. gossypol in cotton seed residues), reaction between solvent and foodstuff (as in defatting of oily fish), and nucleic acid in 'single cell protein'.

It is interesting to note that few of these novel ideas were new. The blue-green alga Spirulina has been known locally for some thousands of years, fish meal was used, at least as a flavouring, in ancient Rome, and biscuits enriched with fish meal were made in Norway in 1880. Leaf protein was first suggested in 1773, the growth of bacteria on methane was carried out in 1906, and the conversion of wheat gluten into a substitute lamb chop was effected by John Kellogg in 1907. This is part of the difficulty in defining novel food.

Historical Problems

Major problems have arisen in the past which, although unlikely to arise in such a form in the future, indicate potential hazards. Pellagra was the result of introducing a novel food, and beri-beri the result of a novel process. In both examples the food involved constituted so large a part of the food eaten that its shortcomings were reflected in the diet. Such circumstances would not arise among the general population of industrialised communities with their varied diets, but little is known about the bizarre eating habits of individuals. It is always necessary for public health authorities to take into account specially vulnerable sections of the community. For example, while the average consumption of canned baked beans in Great Britain is about 100 g per week, two individuals were found to be consuming 10 kg per week and to have continued this practice for 5 years at the time of observation (D. Bender, personal communication).

Maize was the novel food that caused pellagra. When it was introduced into Europe in the 17th century, it formed a relatively small proportion of the diet and there were no observed effects. Later, owing to increased poverty, more people began to rely on maize as a major food, and this appears to be the reason why a 'new disease' traced to the diet was observed by Casal in Spain in 1730. The same economic depression led to outbreaks of the disease in parts of Italy in the 18th century, and spread through southern Europe. Pellagra in Europe and the southern states of the United States did not give way to modern nutritional knowledge until the 1930s and is still a problem in areas of the world where maize or certain types of sorghum constitutes a large part of the diet.

Beri-beri had been recognised by early Chinese medical writers but occurred sporadically until a sudden large increase during the last quarter of the 19th century. The reason was the advent of steam-powered mills which processed the rice more 'efficiently' and removed the greater part of the thiamin.

These examples of disasters caused by a novel food and a novel process were due to the heavy reliance on those foods. The replacement of stone grinding of wheat by steel roller mills in Great Britain in the second half of the 19th century led to the widespread consumption of white bread in place of wholemeal bread but did not result in malnutrition (apart, possibly, from the reduced intake of dietary fibre). This was presumably because sufficient B vitamins were supplied by other foods so that the relative deficiencies of white bread were not important.

A more recent and relevant example is that of vitamin B_6. It had been known since 1936 to be essential to various animal species but was not found to be essential to human beings until 1954. This came about through the introduction (even if in error) of a 'novelty' in the process of manufacturing an infant formula milk in which the temperature was high enough to destroy most of the vitamin B_6. Since the consumers, infants, were relying on this product as their sole food they became deficient in vitamin B_6 and some 70 cases of convulsions were reported. Such a small change can hardly be termed novel but it does exemplify the difficulties that can arise.

SAFETY AND NUTRITIONAL VALUE

The criteria of quality which induce people to consume a food must be obvious to the consumer, such as appearance, smell, and qualities based on tradition, culture and experience. Nutritional value cannot be seen, and only the general knowledge of the consumer, knowing that certain foods are 'good' for him, can influence his nutritional choice. So it is often necessary to legislate for the protection of the consumer by controlling the compositional standards or by enrichment of the food. Similarly the presence of toxic substances and microbiological contamination may not be apparent, and here again legislation is necessary to protect the consumer.

Many foods and processes that were introduced before there was very much knowledge of nutrition and toxicity would not be permitted with our present state of knowledge. The presence of cyanide in butter beans, oxalates in rhubarb and solanine in potatoes would give rise to as much alarm if they were introduced today as would the proposal to smoke or even to salt foods. Yet they have long been consumed without ill-effects.

Much effort has been devoted in recent years to ascertain nutritional changes that take place during processes such as canning, drying and even cooking food, yet there is no evidence that the introduction of any of our established methods of processing has had any detrimental effect on the nutritional status of the population. Indeed, since processing and allied food production have made available a much greater variety of foods at all times of the year, it is likely that nutritional status is higher than previously. However, knowing what we now do, novel foods such as moulds and novel processes such as irradiation must be investigated before marketing.

Some of the Problems
The proposed introduction of a novel food or process raises the questions: (1) who is likely to consume the food; (2) how much is any section of the population likely to consume; (3) what traditional foods—accepted as providing wholesome sources of nutrients—might be replaced? (Table 2.)

In protecting the consumer, authority must take into account individuals who may be relying heavily on certain foods as their source of nutrients, and who might therefore be at risk if that food is replaced by a nutritionally inferior food (Table 3). Reference has already been made to bizarre diets but there are also people who subsist on very restricted diets. We have observed (unpublished) elderly individuals who relied entirely for their vitamin C on such unlikely sources as jam and milk. These do supply sufficient to prevent the appearance of clinical signs but it is possible that a minor change in processing could destroy the nutrient. When jam was made in copper vessels all the vitamin C was destroyed; the introduction of stainless steel vessels preserved the small amount present. It is not difficult to visualise the opposite: if copper had replaced some inert construction

TABLE 2
Major Sources of Nutrients in Great Britain (% of total)

	Protein	Calcium	Iron	Vitamin C
Cheese				
Milk	22	59		
Potatoes	4	7		22
Cereals	24	24	38	
Meat products	32		24	

TABLE 3
Proportion of Total Nutrient and Energy Intake Supplied by Meat and Milk in UK
Diet (% total) (National Food Survey, 1982)

	Meat products	Liquid milk
Energy	16	10
Protein	32	15
Iron	24	
Calcium		42
Zinc	36[a]	
Thiamin	15	12
Riboflavin	20	32
Niacin equivalents	36	10
Retinol equivalents	34	13
Vitamin B$_6$	23[a]	
Vitamin B$_{12}$	59[a]	

[a]Figures from MAFF (1974).

material the small but, in this instance, vital amount of vitamin C would have been lost.

In attempting to assess how much of a traditional food might be replaced by the novel food, average intakes provide little useful information. The average intake of meat products is 1 kg per week but many people eat none at all. The average intake of vitamin C is 57 mg per day but this covers a range from a few milligrams to several hundred milligrams. Potatoes supply just over 20% of the vitamin C intake of the average British diet, so it is clear that some people rely very largely on potatoes as their source of this vitamin. Changes such as new varieties or new sources of supply in times of local shortage will obviously affect such people to a far greater extent than the average.

Progress and Development

The general principle is: 'any manufactured food which simulates a natural food should, in all important respects, have the same nutritional value as the natural food it simulates' (DHSS, 1974). It was accepted that with advancing knowledge there might be changes in what are to be regarded as 'all important aspects' and, as discussed below, this term is open to different interpretations.

The report on novel foods (DHSS, 1974) was written when it was expected that the field bean would be used as the raw material for the meat substitute. Since this is relatively poor in the sulphur amino acids it was suggested that methionine should be added to bring the levels up to those of meat. This was not included in the nutrients listed in the other report (DHSS, 1980) but it did specify that the quality of the TVP (texturised vegetable protein) should be not less than 65% of that of casein [PER (protein efficiency ratio) 1·6 and NPU (net protein utilisation) 0·6], while stating that quality is only of importance when intake is marginal and that this might become a problem only in particular individuals such as some elderly people or those who suffer some chronic illness.

Protein content and quality have been unnecessarily emphasised because the earlier preparations were designed as protein-rich supplements to infant weaning foods. The later expected use of novel foods as ingredients of an adult diet tended to continue this emphasis. The quality of the protein of individual foods is unimportant in the diet as a whole. In many developing countries by far the greater part of the protein is obtained from cereals and the average quality of the dietary protein is 0·7, rarely as low as 0·6. In Western countries three foods, cereals, milk and meat, supply about three-quarters of the protein (Table 3), yet the protein quality is increased only from 0·7 to 0·8. This indicates that the quality of the protein of a novel food is of little if any importance. Indeed, there could be a protein which completely lacks an essential amino acid (and so has NPU zero) but which could make a significant contribution to the diet if the remaining essential amino acids fulfil any inadequacy in the rest of the diet.

In earlier discussions of the substitution of TVP for meat (DHSS, 1974), the type of meat was not specified and 'good quality' meat was taken as the standard. However, different cuts of meat have different amounts of the sulphur amino acids; generally the lower the quality the more connective tissue and the less sulphur amino acids. Fourteen different types of meat products are listed in the National Food Survey, ranging from beef, pork, liver and sausage to cooked chicken, rabbit and 'other canned and cooked meat', with a fifteenth category for 'other meat products'. This point was subsequently rectified (DHSS, 1980) and it was stated: 'ideally, each new food requires individual nutritional assessment'.

The most important aspect is that of substitution. One canned TVP product on the market had NPU much lower than that of good-quality meat, namely 0·45 compared with 0·75, and even lower than that of good soya at 0·7, yet this value was identical with the product 'canned meat with onions and gravy' that it was intended to compete with.

Table 2 shows how heavily the average consumer relies on few foods as the principal source of nutrients. About 40% of the average calcium intake comes from milk; potatoes alone contribute 22% of the vitamin C together with 15% of the niacin equivalent and 10% of the thiamin; carrots supply 16% of the retinol equivalent. On the other hand, fish supplies only 5% of the protein intake but 13% of the dietary vitamin D.

MAJOR NUTRIENTS

The interpretation of the term 'major nutrients' or 'the nutritional equivalent in all but unimportant respects of the natural food which it would simulate' is largely a matter of opinion. The European Economic Community (CEC, 1978) recommended 10 mg iron, 2 mg thiamin, 0·8 mg riboflavin and 5 μg vitamin B_{12} per 100 g dry matter, as in the UK. Canadian recommendations are based on the following amounts per gram of protein: 4·4 μg copper, 0·45 μg folic acid, 0·25 mg iron, 1·1 mg magnesium, 0·34 mg niacin, 0·04 mg pantothenic acid, 20 mg potassium, 0·02 mg pyridoxine, 0·01 mg riboflavin, 0·02 mg thiamin, 0·08 μg vitamin B_{12} and 0·2 mg zinc (quoted by CEC, 1978). The same report includes a list from the US Department of Agriculture interim regulations based on the following amounts per gram of protein: vitamin A 13–20 i.u., thiamin 0·02–0·03 mg, riboflavin 0·01–0·02 mg, pantothenic acid 0·04–0·06 mg, vitamin B_6 0·10–0·15 mg, iron 0·15–0·25 mg, magnesium 1·15–1·75 mg, zinc 0·5–0·75 mg, copper 17–25 μg, and potassium 17–25 mg.

These last two sets of figures indicate the tendency in some advisory bodies to attempt to make any given novel food a more complete source of nutrients than natural foods. It is never clear how far political considerations influence scientific recommendations.

Dietary Fat

Fat offers an example of changing attitudes towards quality of food. Until recent years milk was partly valued on its fat content and producers were penalised for milk below the standard level. Now that fats are regarded as contributory to coronary heart disease they are no longer particularly valued. The DHSS (1974) report on novel foods recommended that TVP should contain no more fat than is present in raw lean beef stewing steak but this recommendation was withdrawn in the 1980 report as being unnecessary. It is, of course, possible to produce a meat substitute that is lower in fat and so presumably of better nutritional value than the meat it simulates. The same is true of dietary fibre; white bread is available with bran added to a level higher than that found in wholemeal breads.

Bioavailability of Nutrients

It is difficult and sometimes even impossible to determine how much of a nutrient chemically present in a food is biologically available to the consumer (Bender, 1983). Furthermore, it is noteworthy that only recently (Brubacher et al., 1985) were approved methods published for the determination of vitamin A, β-carotene, vitamin B_1, vitamin C and vitamin E, with the statement that 'unfortunately only tentative methods could be chosen for vitamins B_2, B_6 and D'. For niacin and folate only references were given because none of the methods satisfied the requirement that they have been used successfully in experienced hands. It was not considered possible even to give references for vitamins B_{12} and K, pantothenate and biotin. This refers to the total amount present.

The availability of vitamins and minerals is influenced by a variety of factors, including the chemical form of the nutrient, the presence of other substances in the food and in other foods eaten at the same time, and even the physical state of the food (Bender, 1983).

It was shown in the Sheffield experiment (Hume and Krebs, 1949) that only one-third of the carotene was available from coarsely minced carrot, and that this was increased to 75% as the particle size was reduced. It was also shown that carotene was better absorbed from vegetables if cooked in fat. Iron provides an even more difficult example since its absorption is influenced by the physiological state of the individual, as well as the presence of other substances in the digestive tract, and the chemical form of the iron in the food.

When comparing nutrient losses in foods processed in different ways, often little attention is paid to the final cooking process. Indeed, comparisons have been reported in the literature between raw foods and the processed version completely forgetting that the raw food may require cooking while the processed food is already partly or even completely cooked.

Current considerations of novel foods should, but do not always, take this into account by comparing the substitute food with the traditional food 'on the plate', i.e. at the time of eating. Some processes have been shown to make it more difficult to recover a particular added nutrient while, on the contrary, the breakdown of vegetable cell walls in canning and heating of the food increased the recovery of some nutrients. The problem of iron availability is even more complicated since it has been shown that cooking of some meat products reduces the availability of iron while the reverse might have been expected.

All that can be done in considering novel foods is to ensure that the product contains the same total amount (or more) of nutrient as the one it is expected to replace. Only if a novel food is expected to replace a major traditional source of a nutrient on a significant scale would it become necessary to determine the availability of the nutrient in human beings, but such a possibility could arise.

Dietary Fibre

The possible substitute of soya preparations for meat has given rise to concern that the phytate and fibre present in the soya might interfere with the absorption of minerals, including iron, calcium, magnesium, zinc and phosphate. Moreover, the iron in meat (haem iron) is not only better absorbed than iron from plant foods but assists the absorption of iron from other foods.

The problems of reduced mineral absorption are not restricted to novel preparations but encountered in such 'natural' foods as wholemeal and unleavened bread. This concern is repeatedly expressed in all discussions involving dietary fibre.

The earliest indications of a nutritional problem arose from the observations of zinc deficiency in Middle East countries including Iran. Measurements were made on volunteers where unleavened wholemeal bread replaced their white, leavened bread, and two-thirds of their meat was replaced by cheese and beans. This caused losses from the body of iron, zinc, calcium and phosphate, and certain blood changes (Reinhold *et al.*, 1973, 1976). Since there are population groups consuming some five times as much dietary fibre as western Europeans there would seem to be some adaptation to this type of diet, but the picture is not clear.

While some workers have reported that the negative calcium balances caused by a high intake of wholemeal bread or brown rice reverted to positive after 3 weeks, the Iranian group, admittedly feeding higher levels of phytate, showed no diminution of losses of zinc and calcium after 60 days on the experimental diet (Reinhold et al., 1973, 1976).

This group suggested that the consumption of large amounts of unleavened bread was the cause of the high incidence of mineral deficiencies in certain regions of Iran. An earlier conclusion that phytate was the main factor was subsequently amended to the fibre, but animal experimentation laid the blame on phytate (Davies and Nightingale, 1975; Davies and Reid, 1979). It was on this basis, namely consideration of the phytate/zinc ratio, that figures for zinc enrichment of TVP were suggested (DHSS, 1980). More recent work makes it clear that both fibre and phytate inhibit mineral absorption.

The amount of zinc absorbed from bran-enriched wholemeal bread steadily increased as the phytate was reduced by prolonged periods of leavening the dough. However, the final levels of absorption were still indicating that the dietary fibre was also inhibitory (Nävert et al., 1985).

Further problems have arisen from the introduction of mould mycelium since the effect of the chitin present on mineral absorption has been little investigated.

Mineral absorption is perhaps the most serious aspect in any consideration of nutritional value of novel foods since there is no certainty that everyone is adequately supplied with available minerals at the present time. As the wealth of literature on dietary fibre indicates, this is not an easy problem to resolve.

Available Energy

It might be thought that compared with nutrients the energy content of foods can be measured with precision but this is not so. Small errors are incurred in the incomplete and variable digestibility of fats and proteins but carbohydrates involve much greater errors.

The carbohydrate content of foods is measured in three ways: 'by difference', 'by difference allowing for dietary fibre', and by estimation of the glucose liberated from available carbohydrate. In the US Food Composition Tables energy values are calculated using digestibility factors for various groups of foods (Watt and Merrill, 1975). These range from 98% for foods rich in fats and proteins to as little as 56% for wheat bran. This accounts for the considerable differences between figures quoted, especially for foods rich in dietary fibre (Tables 4 and 5). The formation of resistant starch in the extrusion process increases the error.

TABLE 4

Energy Value of Foods Calculated by Two Methods (kcal/100 g) (Paul and Southgate, 1978)

	(1)	(2)
White flour	352	353
Wholemeal flour	339	327
Butter	793	748
Apples	45	55
Dried apricots	183	297
Bananas	77	103
Blackcurrants	29	79
Grapefruit	22	32

(1) Using factors 4·1 for proteins; 9·3 for fat; 3·75 for available carbohydrate as glucose (UK Food Composition Tables).
(2) Using specific factors for different foods (US Food Composition Tables).

TABLE 5

Calculation of the Metabolisable Energy Value of Foods by Use of Different Equations to Allow for Incomplete Digestion and Urinary Losses (Miller and Judd, 1984)

	Atwater factors (a)	Miller & Payne (b)	Southgate (c)	Miller & Judd (d)
Bran	240	334	306	303
Beans	235	247	239	238
Wholemeal bread	212	242	217	220
Potatoes	69	78	69	76
Carrots	23	35	28	34
All-bran	309	373	325	291

(a) $25 \times N + 3.75 \times C + 9 \times F + 7 \times$ alcohol
(b) $0.95 \times$ gross combustible energy $- 7.5 \times N$
(c) $0.98 \times$ gross energy $- 6.6 \times N - 4 \times F$
(d) $(0.95 -$ dietary fibre per g dry wt$) \times$ gross energy $- 7.4 \times N$

The errors are compounded by the observation that individuals differ in their ability to make partial use of 'unavailable' carbohydrates. Since some novel foods are relatively rich in unavailable carbohydrates and substances such as chitin, the comparison of energy sources is not as simple as might be expected.

SAFETY

Food hazards are often ranked in the following order of risk: microbiological contamination, nutritional hazards, natural toxicants, environmental contaminants, pesticide residues and, at the bottom of the list, food additives. The first two are regarded as a far greater risk than the next two, while the risks from pesticide residues and additives are considered to be very much lower than those from natural toxicants and contaminants. Hall (1985) ranked the hazards as popularly conceived; this places food additives and pesticide residues first, followed by environmental contaminants, nutritional and microbiological risks, with natural toxicants at the bottom of the list.

The testing for safety of substances in the diet presents enormous problems. There are two virtually unresolvable difficulties, namely the attempt to prove a negative and the extrapolation from very large doses fed to animals to small amounts ingested by man.

The attempt to prove that a given substance is not harmful has led over the years to more and more trials on greater numbers of animals for longer and longer periods of time. The amounts both of natural non-nutritive substances in foods and of additives are too small to have any observable effects on test animals, so greatly exaggerated doses have to be administered. Indeed, the basis of the acceptable daily intake of an additive is usually one-hundredth of the maximum no-effect dose. It is obviously not possible to feed such levels of food. However, attempts have been made to do so by feeding test foods at very high dose levels for prolonged periods.

In animal experiments the same routine as employed in examining single chemicals has been followed, namely to examine every possible function and tissue of the animal, including offspring, for every possible parameter together with detailed post-mortem examination.

When a similar approach is used to examine the effects of the highest tolerable dose in human subjects the major problem is to decide what the investigator is searching for. Chemical tests have already shown the absence of toxic substances, animal tests have provided evidence of safety in their case, so what can serve as an index of risk in the human subject? Generally blood, urine and any tissues available are examined for every enzyme and parameter known to biochemists, but there are no standards for comparison. We have average values for a limited number of parameters measured on a limited number of apparently healthy people but these cannot be regarded as 'normal' values, certainly not for any specific individual, so what differences from accepted average values can be regarded as deviations from normality? If they are deviations, are they caused by the test diet? Are they necessarily harmful?

The paucity of information about what is 'normal' is exceeded by the paucity of information about fluctuations in measurable physiological and biochemical 'constants' that may take place over periods of weeks, days or hours in normal, healthy subjects. One report serves to indicate the potentially false conclusions that can arise from such physiological fluctuations. This was a series of fortnightly measurements made over a period of 32 weeks on 6 healthy young volunteers who continued to eat their normal diets. In all 6 subjects serum albumin fluctuated by 10%, urea by ±20% while cholesterol, so often measured in relation to coronary heart disease, ranged between ±5% in the most consistent individual and −17% to +15% in the least consistent individual (Bender, 1976).

Had a peak or trough in these measurements coincided with any treatment, such as feeding a novel food, this would presumably have been interpreted as a harmful effect—or even, in the instance of reduced cholesterol, a beneficial effect!

The difficulties in testing novel foods and the differences between them and food additives were pointed out by Hall (1985). In the WHO report on 'wholesomeness of irradiated foods' half of the 53 animal tests that included a control group showed adverse effects *from the unirradiated food* when compared with stock diet. The same problem would obviously arise if traditional foods were subjected to the same type of testing. The method of feeding single substances at one-hundred times the expected dose cannot be considered for foods. Apart from the impossibility of literally doing so, abnormal amounts of any acceptable food fed for prolonged periods will give rise to adverse effects. This was not appreciated over the 20–30 years spent in feeding trials of irradiated foods.

Guide-lines

These problems are taken into account in the most recent British publication on the subject (MAFF, 1984). Here it is suggested that feeding trials can be planned only when detailed chemical investigation throws up problems of toxicity and nutritional value that can be identified. For example, if the novel process of irradiation leads to the formation of unique radiation products, these substances would need to be identified and examined for toxicity. If feeding trials of the food itself become necessary, the intended use of the food and the upper limit of its likely intake would be taken into consideration. For example, the protein quality of a food is of no interest if the food is not intended or expected to replace a traditional source of protein.

One of the earliest of the guide-lines for testing novel foods was that of the Protein Advisory Group of the United Nations (PAG, 1970). At that time some 25 years of research had resulted in the development of about 80 protein-rich weaning foods in various countries. While many of these were made from foods entirely suitable for human consumption, some were prepared from oilseed residues used as animal feed; guidance was felt necessary to establish hygiene standards and nutritional objectives, and to ensure the complete removal of any toxins that might be present.

Many of these preparations were already in use by the time the guide-lines were published, and the foods used as components were not con-sidered to be particularly novel. Indeed, the recommendations were entitled 'Guide lines for human testing of supplementary food mixtures' which was changed to 'Human testing of novel foods' only when revised (PAG, 1983). The approach is illustrated by the recommendation that the foods should be tested on infants and young children in order to determine growth rates and nitrogen balance more effectively than on older children or adults. This is in sharp contrast to the most recent guide-lines (DHSS, 1984) where a preliminary trial consisting of a single meal fed to one volunteer is suggested. Although this cautious approach is mentioned specifically with reference to 'extremely novel products' it is only for such products that human tests are considered necessary.

Conclusions

Traditional foods and established processes are accepted as the standard, despite problems of natural toxins, the production of toxins in roasting, smoking and frying of foods, and problems of availability of nutrients.

With our present knowledge, no novel food could be marketed without careful examination. This inevitably leads to the conclusion that novel materials and novel processes will provide safer and more nutritious foods than the ones they may replace.

REFERENCES

Bender, A. E. (1983). The important difference between chemical analysis and biological availability. In: *Chemistry and World Food Supplies; The New Frontier*, L. W. Shemilt (Ed.), Chemrawn II, Pergamon Press, pp. 537–46.

Bender, D. A. (1976). Variations in serum chemistry in normal subjects without change of diet. *Proc. Nutr. Soc.*, **35**, A146–7.

Brubacher, G., Müller-Mulot, W. and Southgate, D. A. T. (1985). *Methods for Determination of Vitamins in Food*. Recommended by COST 91. Elsevier Applied Science Publishers, London/New York.

Commission of European Communities (1978). *Report of the Study Group on Vegetable Proteins in Foodstuffs for Human Consumption* (in particular, in meat products), Brussels.

Davies, N. T. and Nightingale, R. (1975). The effect of phytate on intestinal absorption and secretion of zinc, and whole-body retention of zinc, copper, iron and manganese in rats. *Brit. J. Nutr.*, **34**, 243–58.

Davies, N. T. and Reid, H. (1979). An evaluation of the phytate, zinc, copper, iron and manganese contents of, and zinc availability from, soya-based textured vegetable protein meat-substitutes or meat-extenders. *Brit. J. Nutr.*, **41**, 579–89.

Department of Health and Social Security (1980). *Foods Which Simulate Meat.* Report on Health and Social Subjects No. 17, HMSO, London.

Department of Health and Social Security (1974). *Testing of Novel Foods.* Memorandum, HMSO, London.

Hall, R. (1985). *Proceedings of the XIII International Congress of Nutrition*, T. G. Taylor and N. K. Jenkins (Eds), pp. 816–19.

Hume, E. M. and Krebs, H. A. (1949). *Vitamin A Requirements*. Spec. Rep. Ser. Med. Res. Council (London), No. 264, HMSO, London.

Institute of Food Science and Technology (1975). Technical Advisory Committee Report No. 139.

Medical Research Council (1945). Accessory Food Factors Committee. MRC (War) Memorandum No. 16, HMSO, London.

Miller, D. S. and Judd, P. A. (1984). The metabolisable energy of food. *J. Sci. Food Agric.*, **35**, 111–6.

Ministry of Agriculture, Fisheries and Food (1984). Report of the Working Party on Novel Foods; Committee on Medical Aspects of Food Policy. In: *Report on Novel Protein Foods*, HMSO, London.

Nävert, B., Sandstrom, B. and Cederblad, A. (1985). Reduction of the phytate content of bran by leavening in bread and its effects on zinc absorption in man. *Brit. J. Nutr.*, **53**, 47–53.

PAG (1970). Protein Advisory Group of the United Nations System. *Human Testing of Supplementary Food Mixtures*, PAG Guideline No. 7, United Nations, New York.

PAG (1983). Human testing of novel foods. Protein Advisory Group Guideline No. 7. *Food and Nutrition Bulletin*, Vol. 15, No. 2, United Nations University.

Paul, A. A. and Southgate, D. A. T. (1978). McCance and Widdowson's *The Composition of Foods*, 4th edn, HMSO, London.

Reinhold, J. G., Lahimgarzadeh, A., Nasr, K. and Hedayati, H. (1973). Effects of purified phytate and phytate-enriched bread upon metabolism of zinc, calcium, phosphorus and nitrogen in man. *Lancet*, **i**, 283–8.

Reinhold, J. G., Faradji, B., Abadi, P. and Ismail-Beigi, F. (1976). Decreased absorption of calcium, magnesium, zinc and phosphorus by humans due to increased fibre and phosphorus consumption as wheat bread. *J. Nutr.*, **106**, 493–503.

Watt, B. K. and Merrill, A. L. (1975). *Composition of Foods*. Agriculture Handbook No. 8, US Dept. of Agriculture, Washington, DC, p. 160.

Chapter 13

THE FUTURE OF FOOD TOXICOLOGY

D. M. CONNING

The British Nutrition Foundation, London, UK

Food toxicology, as currently perceived, has arisen from the legislation found necessary during the second half of the nineteenth century, to curb the practice of food adulteration. With the coming of the industrial revolution and the migration, on a substantial scale, of people to the towns and cities (the beginning of urbanisation) the problems of food distribution began. No system of distribution of food on a sufficient scale existed, and it became common for unscrupulous vendors to eke out their supplies and substantially improve their profits by the addition of filler materials. Several of these were poisonous and deaths occurred.

Legislation was first enacted in the UK in 1860 but its enforcement was largely ineffectual because of the backward state of analytical chemistry in respect of food contaminants. As the technical expertise improved, so it became feasible to estimate the concentration of a particular material that might be associated with adverse effects—the beginnings of food toxicology. Originally the analyses were conducted to detect fraud but some of the adulteration proved of value. For example, the dilution of coffee with chicory resulted in an acceptable material if sold at its true, cheaper price. It then became a question of the permissible amounts of adulteration, and this in part was related to issues of public health.

The development of toxicology as a science has always trailed behind the continued progress in analytical chemistry. It was therefore inevitable that the biologist had great difficulty in asserting that a given compound at a given concentration could induce adverse effects, except in the circumstance of high dosage. For this reason the early toxicological studies were confined to acute poisoning and lethality determined by studies in laboratory animals. These animals were very variable in quality, quantity and species, so the biological results exhibited wide ranges.

It was thus impossible for the biologist (toxicologist) to be precise or

443

specific about his findings, a position unacceptable to regulatory lawyers who would have no way of defining or enforcing limits of adulteration. As a consequence, the concept of a 'no effect' level of dosage was devised. This recognised that a given compound added to the diet at various concentrations would exhibit a concentration at which none of the biological effects observed at higher dose would be detectable. This 'no effect' level could be taken as the dose that would be without definable effect in man. At a later stage this concept was further refined following the recognition that the dose–response relationship was proportionate to body size (more specifically surface area) and a factor of 10 was used arbitrarily to convert the finding in, for example, the rat for the greater size of a man. It was also recognised that there were occasionally substantial quantitative differences in the metabolic pathways of man and rat, and a further arbitrary factor of 10 was added. Thus the permissible limit of a material in the human diet was calculated as the no-effect level in the experimental animal (or the most sensitive species if several species were used) divided by 100. Occasionally this factor is varied according to the expert judgement of a regulatory committee, but 100 is the figure commonly used. The resultant figure is often referred to as the 'acceptable daily intake' expressed as a dose per unit body weight.

There have been a number of consequences for toxicology since this concept was introduced. First, manufacturers, faced with the costs of toxicological analyses, have settled for the quickest route to having their products accepted—namely to determine the no-effect level—and have not considered other aspects of potential toxicity. This has reduced toxicological investigation to a 'check-list' operation with very little scientific input. The consequence has been the very slow development of toxicology as a science and its virtual relegation to high-grade technology.

Secondly, the technology itself has flourished so that there has been a tremendous development of techniques to detect minor variations from normal. This has led, in part, to confusion as to the significance of some observations, but for the most part, and as a consequence of the lack of scientific underpinning, many such effects are regarded as abnormal. One other consequence arising from the greater ability to measure biological functions is a marked extension of the list of studies now required to characterise potential toxicity, a list that is still increasing.

Thirdly, there have been even greater advances in the techniques of analytical chemistry. It is now possible to measure changes in biological chemistry at many orders of magnitude of concentration below former limits. This has had two direct consequences—greater perplexity in the biological interpretation of hitherto undetected effects (such as minor changes in serum chemistry) and a realisation that observed biological effects attributed to a given tissue concentration are now known to occur at much lesser concentrations because the sensitivity of analyses is greater.

The overall consequences of these developments have been a marked increase of the extent, range and analytical integrity of the studies required to ensure absence of toxicity, with the associated increases in cost, manpower deployment, time and numbers of experimental animals. Other developments have taken place that add to the problems of cost. The increasing complexity of the experiments involved has required much more attention to statistical analysis. This has, in general, led to an increase in animal numbers in an attempt to determine the statistical validity of the minor biological changes now identifiable. Although the latest thinking in statistical analyses recognises that economy is possible on the basis of multifactorial analyses, these have not yet been incorporated into regulatory requirements.

Finally, there has been the inception of 'good laboratory practice' and the impositions this makes on administrative and documentary efforts required in any given set of experiments.

FUTURE DEVELOPMENTS

The developments of toxicity testing as so far described have resulted in a number of effects that have influenced and will further influence the practice of experimental toxicology.

First, there is the public perception of the numbers of animals used in toxicity studies. Although there has always been uneasy acceptance of the need to use animals in experiments designed to safeguard human health and safety, there has also been a vociferous minority that objected strongly to such usage. Coincidental with the anniversary of the Act of Parliament 1874 that controls animal experiments in the United Kingdom there was a change in public attitudes that led to a questioning of some of the practices involved. As so often happens, this was rarely expressed in scientific or even rational terms, but there can be no denial of the genuine emotional reaction experienced by many. That this was (and is) sometimes expressed in violence is distressing, but the underlying anxiety seems real. This anxiety now has a political aspect in that several Members of Parliament have been successfully lobbied and the revised Act has some provisions that acknowledge the anti-experiment presence. The political involvement will ensure continued activity in this field, with the possibility of continued influence on food safety experiments.

Secondly, the escalation of toxicological requirements with the attendant costs has resulted in a severe reduction of research and development of food chemicals. Further, the research required to keep certain compounds in the range is not being undertaken, so the number of 'approved' additives is declining. This, together with the activities of some journalists who see career opportunities in undermining public confidence in the quality of the food supply, will result in the greater use of fewer additives—a situation that may be counterproductive in terms of safety. On the other hand, such a trend may well accelerate the development and widespread acceptance of non-chemical methods of achieving additive functions such as refrigeration, irradiation, vacuum packing etc.

Thirdly, there is a growing trend among some scientists to question the validity of the conventional toxicological approach in the prediction of human hazard. The recognition of food intolerance and allergies has highlighted the unavailability of animal models for these conditions. The recent obsession with the concept of the unbalanced diet as a source of human illness, particularly degenerative illness, has also pointed up the deficiencies in animal models. Regrettably, the development of epidemiology has not reached the stage where causes of morbidity can be attributed even for single factor effects, much less the multifactorial problems that underlie many nutritional diseases. Even for single chemicals, the records of exposure render much interpretation of dubious significance.

The future of food toxicology will devolve upon several important developments.

(1) *In vitro* techniques will serve two purposes, first to reduce further the use of experimental animals and second to move toxicological analyses much more towards the assessment of the biochemical effects that underlie toxic manifestations. This, of necessity, means a move away from the blanket search for any conceivable biological effect towards more targeted assessments related to known human disease. An example of this type of analysis is the development of *in vitro* methods to detect the induction of abnormal DNA (with all that that entails) for the detection of potential carcinogens. It may be envisaged that, as the underlying biochemical basis of human disease becomes better elucidated, so *in vitro* models to detect such biochemical events will be devised. This might extend, for example in the case of potential carcinogens, to the detection of specific oncogenes formed by the interaction of a food chemical and a sensitive *in vitro* model.

It may be envisaged that other disease processes will lend themselves to an analysis of possible chemical involvement by similar techniques. If, for example, atherosclerosis is dependent on the development of deficiency in lipoprotein receptors, *in vitro* methods could be devised for measuring this effect—in this case probably not through the action of a chemical agent but through a combination of excess fatty acid and ageing.

It is to be expected that the development of such models will increasingly employ human tissues. Such developments will be hindered by the wide genetic variability of man, and may well require much greater development of the concepts of human tissue typing. On the other hand, the development and availability of a wide range of human tissues available for culture may allow the selection of cells with the requisite sensitivity. Given that many intracellular activities are the result of genetically determined control mediated by RNA, it is not impossible that many of the degenerative diseases are the result of abnormal gene expression. Methods will certainly become available to assess this, though whether the abnormal expression can be chemically induced (vis-à-vis oncogenes) remains to be established.

Developments of this nature will have two important effects. First there will be a reduction of animal experiments. This will bring benefits to beleaguered scientists and vote-hungry politicians but will have the consequence that there will be fewer toxicological assays in whole-body systems. If reasonable predictions of biological effects are to be achieved there will need to be much more attention paid to the mechanisms of effects, for in the absence of observable whole-animal results the prediction of toxicity requires the identification of principal mechanisms.

The second effect therefore will be the increased use of *in vitro* systems to identify and measure cellular mechanisms of toxicity—a development that is, in any case, long overdue.

(2) Notwithstanding an increased usage of *in vitro* techniques that are deployed with greater scientific objectivity, it will be some time before such systems are sufficiently available or sufficiently comprehensive to obviate whole-animal studies. Given, however, the difficulty of using experimental animals to predict human effects, and given the wide genetic variability of human beings, it seems likely that much more work will have to be done on human volunteers. This is likely to be even more the case if food chemical toxicology moves much more into the realm of nutritional toxicology—that is the toxic effects (disease producing) of dietary components. Despite the anxieties generated by what may be regarded as human experimentation, this seems not to bother many so-called 'food activists' who think nothing

of advocating outlandish and often bizarre diets with no thought of the possibly traumatic effects. There should therefore be no impediment to the properly controlled and ethically approved human studies to evaluate certain nutritional hypotheses. It is certainly important that such issues are addressed as a matter of some urgency if the requisite guidelines are to be in place in good time.

(3) Despite the onslaught of politically motivated attacks on the food industry, the advance of food technology is unlikely to be abated. This, coupled with the development of biotechnology, will result in a range of new foodstuffs, or familiar items produced by new techniques. It is to be expected that these will lead to much ponderous deliberation by the various regulatory mechanisms concerned with safety. It is unlikely that conventional toxicological techniques will be appropriate to solve such problems but the developments described in (1) and (2) above will. It will be more satisfactory if the nutritional performance of new foods is taken as the main assessment. This of necessity will involve animal growth studies, and there are few toxic materials that sustain normal growth when incorporated into the diet at the levels of nutritional components. (Carcinogenic hormones are an obvious exception.) Such studies coupled with *in vitro* experiments and eventually studies in human volunteers would ensure adequate safety and adequate nutritional performance without the financial and temporal handicaps of routine toxicity tests.

CONCLUSION

In essence, the future of food toxicology is in the field of nutritional toxicology and particularly in relating diet to degenerative diseases. The conventional approach to toxicity testing based upon large-scale animal experimentation has not only impeded the development of toxicology as a science but has priced itself out of the market as far as food chemicals are concerned. The development of new techniques directed more specifically at human effects and related initially to known human disease promises to bring closer together the studies of toxic mechanisms and the biochemical basis of human disease, both centred on intracellular aberrations. These changes will be accelerated by public and political attitudes to animal experimentation and dietary safety.

INDEX

449